# PHILOSOPHICAL FOUNDATIONS OF HEALTH EDUCATION

## JILL M. BLACK

## STEVE R. FURNEY

## HELEN M. GRAF

## ANN E. NOLTE

### EDITORS

### FOREWORD BY VALERIE A. UBBES

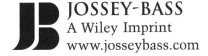

JOSSEY-BASS
A Wiley Imprint
www.josseybass.com

Published by Jossey-Bass
A Wiley Imprint
989 Market Street, San Francisco, CA 94103–1741—www.josseybass.com

*Library of Congress Cataloging-in-Publication Data*

Philosophical foundations of health education / Jill M. Black . . . [et al.], editors ; foreword by Valerie A. Ubbes.
    p.   cm.
Includes bibliographical references and index.
ISBN-978-0-470-43678-3 (pbk.)
  1. Health education.   I. Black, Jill M., 1959-
RA440.P485 2010
613—dc22

2009027722

Printed in the United States of America
FIRST EDITION
PB Printing        10  9  8  7  6  5  4  3  2  1

# CONTENTS

# PART 2
## DEVELOPING A PHILOSOPHY OF HEALTH EDUCATION 45

# PART 3
## COGNITIVE APPROACHES IN HEALTH EDUCATION 91

# FIGURES, TABLES, AND EXHIBITS

## FIGURES

## TABLES

## EXHIBITS

Dedicated posthumously to the following members of the
American Association for Health Education and
leaders in the profession:

William Carlyon
Peter Cortese
William H. Creswell Jr.
William M. Kane
Robert D. Russell
Elena M. Sliepcevich

And in particular to Ann Nolte whose love of history and
philosophy provided the impetus and motivation
for this book.

# FOREWORD

Of the many human activities that derive pleasure, our caring choice of words in human communication can culminate in tactful thoughts and actions. Tact refers to a sense of touch [L. tactus, to touch] and also includes a delicate perception of saying and doing the right thing without offending. Tact also implies skill in dealing with persons or challenging situations with a poised composure and adroit diplomacy. Historically and today as dignitaries travel from place to place to represent a national or domestic perspective, ambassadors interact responsibly with personal and social graces favorable for each situation. Usually an ambassador carries a written document to establish the objective goals and expectations for the exchange. Gifts and concrete objects are also shared to transition and bridge a conversation toward the hopeful outcome of the main message. In musical communication, a segue is used to imply how a tone or melody moves without a break into the next section or piece, much like this preface does for this book.

With the compilation of this book, it seems reasonable to reflect on the historical action of our professional ambassadors who have transitioned health education from the twentieth to the twenty-first century. An integration of their personal and professional philosophies is found in this first-time collection of published works.

Each one of us shares our personal and professional stories when we interact in real time at professional conferences, meetings, and symposia. Are we not all ambassadors of our own storied lives as we share our tales of who we are and what we do? In doctoral seminars with professor emeritus Dr. Mary K. Beyrer, I learned that "people make history" and thus people ultimately become the subject of our profession. This text brings together the messengers and their messages in order to educate for health in individual, community, and global contexts. We are fortunate to have this collection of philosophical works that have been written by respected professionals from their place and time in history. As these ambassadors profess the importance of health education for a community of learners both now and beyond, the editors of this book "re-present" both past and current thinking since 1953.

As professionals come together to share their ideas in spoken and written narratives, we continue to synthesize and refine our messages for health education. With diplomacy, we can all learn to leave a space in history to honor our subjective stories and more objective theories while negotiating and interrogating ideas for our collective futures. This book affords us a scholarly discourse for engaging philosophical ideas across time from four major perspectives. For the first time, we will be able to compare and contrast a body of published works in a more in-depth way. By making these papers available in one place, the editors of this volume help to open new pathways to our storytelling and theoretical musing.

As we investigate the crossroad between story and theory in our professional community, may we honor and respect the sophisticated thinking of our ambassadors [L. ambactus, helpers] who have brought into view different vistas for health education while bearing their gifts for philosophical discourse.

Valerie A. Ubbes, PhD, CHES
Miami University

# INTRODUCTION

Philosophy has been defined as (1) a love and pursuit of wisdom by intellectual means and moral self-discipline, (2) an investigation of the nature, causes, or principles of reality, knowledge, or values, based on logical reasoning rather than empirical methods, (3) a system of thought based on or involving critical inquiry, or according to William James, "philosophy is the unusually stubborn attempt to think clearly." Thinking critically about different philosophical beliefs and perspectives involves intellectual strategies to probe the basic nature of a problem or a situation. This means that the reader will need to make observations, assumptions, and comparisons and contrasts to try to uncover the relationships between the parts and the whole (Sloane, MacHale, & DiSpezio, 2002). Philosophy provides a foundation for all academic disciplines. It seeks to shed light on questions such as Who am I? What is real? What and how do I learn or teach? How should people live? What is it to be healthy? It deals with issues and problems that cannot be addressed adequately by appealing to experience and scientific study alone. Philosophical inquiry requires that we question our assumptions, our beliefs, and our reasons for believing them.

Over the past thirty years, health educators have been calling for a professional philosophy for the health education profession (Oberteuffer, 1977; Landwer, 1981; Balog, 1982; Rash, 1985; Timmreck, Cole, James, & Butterworth, 1987, 1988; Shirreffs, 1988; AAHE, 1992; Welle, Russell, & Kittleson, 1995; Coalition of National Health Education Organizations, 1999; AAHE, 2005 [see Appendix B]; Gambescia, 2007). Welle and her colleagues (1995) stated that "health educators perform a multiplicity of roles in a variety of settings, a single philosophy does not seem possible or even particularly desirable. Rather, what the health education profession needs is a clear delineation of the major existing philosophies and an analysis of the current trends in health education philosophies."

In his 2007 SOPHE presidential address, Stephen Gambescia asked, "Do we have a philosophy of health education?" He suggests that we should think critically about three major questions: (1) How do I know what I know (epistemology)? (2) What should I do; how shall I behave (ethics [see Appendix D] and morality)? And (3) How do I interact with others; and what is my relationship to them (governance)? He goes on to emphasize the importance that we, as a profession, should "discover our own philosophy of health education" (Gambescia, 2007).

This publication offers just such an opportunity. The readings are organized into parts for your critical review: personal philosophies of selected health educators (Part 1), commentaries on philosophical perspectives in health education (Part 2), and discussions of a range of philosophical issues that are relevant to the practice of health education (Parts 3 to 6). These last four parts are organized around four philosophical perspectives found repeatedly in the health education literature and identified by Welle and her colleagues (1995), including cognitive approaches (Part 3), behavior change (Part 4), freeing/functioning (Part 5), and social change (Part 6). (For a brief comparison of these perspectives, see Appendix A, Philosophy of Health Education Grid.)

We encourage you to read each selection carefully, analyze the points raised, and consider the values identified and discussed by each of the authors. The essay beginning each part includes an overview of the articles and highlights their challenges to the reader.

After reading each selection, consider the following questions.

1. Summarize the key points of the article.

   Discuss the key ideas from the article with a classmate. (What?)

2. Compare the concepts discussed in the selection to your philosophical beliefs.

   What are the relationships, if any, between what you believe about practicing health education and what the author states about health education? (So What?)

3. What are the implications? (Now What?)

   How does this material inform your practice of health education?

4. Relationships

   What themes emerged as you read this material?

5. Applications

   How can you utilize this material?

## REFERENCES

AAHE Board of Directors. (1992). A point of view for health education. *Journal of Health Education, 23*(1), 4–6.

American Association of Health Education. (2005). Philosophy of health education: A position statement of the American Association of Health Education (AAHE). Retrieved from http://www.aahperd.org/aahe/pdf_files/pos_pap/Philosophy.pdf.

American Association of Health Education. (2008). Health literacy: A position statement of the American Association of Health Education (AAHE). Retrieved from http://www.aahperd.org/aahe/pdf_files/pos_pap/HealthLiteracy.pdf.

Balog, J. (1982). Conceptual questions in health education and philosophical inquiry. *Health Education, 13*(2), 201–204.

Coalition of National Health Education Organizations. (1999). Code of ethics for the health education profession. Retrieved from http://www.cnheo.org/code2.pdf.

Gambescia, S. F. (2007). Discovering a philosophy of health education. *Health Education & Behavior, 34*(5), 718–722.

Landwer, G. E. (1981). Where do you want to go? *Journal of School Health, 51*(8), 529–531.

Oberteuffer, D. (1977). Concepts and Conviction. Washington, DC: AAPHERD Publications.

Rash, J. K. (1985). Philosophical bases for health education. *Health Education, 16*(2), 48–49.

Shirreffs, J. H. (1988). The nature and meaning of health education. In L. Rubinson & W. F. Alles (Eds.), Health education: Foundations for the future (pp. 35–62). Prospect Heights, IL: Waveland Press.

Sloane, P., MacHale, D., & DiSpezio, M. (2002). The ultimate lateral and critical thinking puzzle book. New York: Sterling.

Timmreck, T. C., Cole, G. E., James, G., & Butterworth, D. D. (1987). The health education and health promotion movement: A theoretical jungle. *Health Education, 18*(5), 24–28.

Timmreck, T. C., Cole, G. E., James, G., & Butterworth, D. D. (1988). Health education and health promotion: A look at the jungle of supportive fields, philosophies and theoretical foundations. *Health Education, 18*(6), 23–28.

Welle, H. M., Russell, R. D., & Kittleson, M. J. (1995). Philosophical trends in health education: Implications for the 21st century. *Journal of Health Education, 26*(6), 326–332.

# THE EDITORS

**Jill M. Black**, PhD, CHES, FAAHE is a Fellow of the American Association for Health Education, a former member of the AAHE Board of Directors, and current chair of the AAHE History and Philosophy Committee. She is an associate professor of Health Education at Cleveland State University, where she is the coordinator of Cleveland State's Community Health Education Graduate Program. She holds a BA in Mass Communications, a BS in Health, Physical Education, and Recreation, and a master's degree in Health Promotion from the University of Oklahoma. She received her PhD in Community Health Education from Southern Illinois University at Carbondale. She has published more than 30 articles and presented more than 60 professional presentations at local, state, regional, and national meetings. Her specific areas of specialization include the history and philosophy of health education, professional preparation of health educators, program planning and evaluation, health promotion and wellness, foundations and methods of community health, aging and gerontology issues, stress management, and other related issues.

**Steven R. Furney,** EdD is a professor at Texas State University in San Marcos. where he has been on the faculty since 1980. He serves as the director of health education and teaches in the areas of health education and health promotion. His teaching has been recognized with the Texas State University Presidential Award for Excellence in Teaching, the Texas AAHPERD College Health Educator of the Year Award, the Southern District AAHPERD College/University Health Educator of the Year Award, and the National AAHE College Health Educator of the Year Award. Dr. Furney has filled many professional leadership roles at the state, district, and national levels. In Texas, he served as president for the 75th anniversary diamond jubilee celebration year in 1998. In Southern District AAHPERD, he was president in 2001. He has served the Alliance as a member of the AAHE Board of Directors from 2003 to 2006 and through work on various committees including the AAHPERD Strategic Planning Committee and the AAHE Scholarship, Fellows, Nominations, Ethics and History and Philosophy Committees. The professional bodies for which he has served have recognized him with the AAHPERD Honor Award, the AAHE Professional Service Award, the AAHE Health Education Professional of the Year Award for Administration, the AAHE Fellow, the Southern District AAHPERD Health Professional of the Year for Administration, the Southern District Honor Award, the Texas AAHPERD David K. Brace Award, the Texas AAHPERD Honor Award, and the Texas AAHPERD Scholar Award.

**Helen M. Graf,** PhD, is an associate professor at Georgia Southern University in Statesboro. She serves as the program director for all undergraduate programs in the

Department of Health and Kinesiology. She holds a BS and M S in Food and Nutrition Science and a PhD in Community Health from Southern Illinois University at Carbondale. Her dissertation was titled *An Exploration of Philosophical Trends and Preferences in Health Education.* In 2003, Helen was awarded the Georgia Southern University's Excellence in Service Award. Currently, Dr. Graf has 62 publications including peer-reviewed articles, book chapters, books, and conference proceedings (among others); 16 grants totaling $470,000.00; and 93 national and international presentations. Dr. Graf has served as vice chair of National Commission of Health Education Credentialing (NCHEC), Inc; executive editor for the NCHEC Bulletin, steering committee member for the Competency Update Project, and member of the History and Philosophy Committee of AAHPERD. Dr. Graf's research interests lie in professional preparation, stress in young adults, research methodology, and statistics. She holds certifications in coaching and officiating with USATF and serves as the local high school cross country coach.

**Ann E. Nolte**, PhD, CHES, FAAHE, was a Distinguished Professor, Illinois State University. She was also a Fellow of the American Association for Health Education, a Distinguished Fellow of the Society for Public Health Education, and a Fellow of the American School Health Association. Her career in health education spanned more than 40 years and included teaching positions from high school to university settings and numerous achievements, honors, and awards. Dr. Nolte's research interests were numerous. She officially retired from Illinois State University in 1990, but remained very active in her profession. She is most appreciated for her extensive work on the philosophical foundations and historical perspectives of health education, a movement she both chronicled and shaped for modern higher education. Dr. Nolte served as president of the American Association for Health Education, 1980 through 1982, and was named the AAHE Scholar in 1983. Her scholar address was titled, "In Relationship: Freedom and Health." Dr. Nolte was a founding member of the AAHE History and Philosophy Committee and served the AAHE as historian from 1974 until her death in 2009.

# PHILOSOPHICAL FOUNDATIONS OF HEALTH EDUCATION

# PART

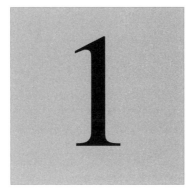

# PHILOSOPHICAL PERSPECTIVES IN HEALTH EDUCATION

*Thinking philosophically involves many analytical skills, such as critical inquiry, reasoning, and logic. When these skills are applied to a body of knowledge, such as health education, it reveals the values, ethics, and dynamics of life as applied to an individual functioning within an environment and culture. Basically, it is the what, how, when, where, and why of health education to which the health educator must respond as he or she practices as a professional. Examining the philosophical beliefs of key leaders, both past and present can inform our understanding of the development of the profession and aid us in the development of our own personal and professional philosophy (Black, 2006).*

*These readings explore different ways of thinking about health and education. Each author addresses different aspects of health and education. Extrapolating the substance of these articles will reveal a wide range of different values and beliefs. Examining these beliefs and determining which ones are meaningful for you and your future as a health educator is the beginning of a foundation for your professional life. Maintaining this foundation in essence is the application of your philosophy and the continual reexamination of your beliefs in light of advancements in basic science and behavioral sciences.*

## ARTICLES

The articles in this section provide a sampling of different ways of thinking about health and education. Bensley (1993) provides a personalized view of health education and discusses both his personal and professional philosophical perspective. Rash (1985) and Wilgoose (1985) focus more on the foundations of health education. In "Three Essential Questions in Defining a Personal Philosophy," Pigg (1993) provides a general discussion on philosophy, ethics, morals and religion and discusses his personal view of the implications for health education. Carroll (1993) provides a bit of health education history as a platform to discuss what he calls "guiding principles of health and health education." These four principles are personal empowerment, life affirmation, interconnectedness, and an admission of some of the limitations of health education. Thomas (1984) closes this section with a philosophical overview of holistic health and an analysis of the writings of three health education philosophers, Jesse F. Williams, Howard Hoyman, and Delbert Oberteuffer, and their views that related to holistic health. These six articles provide a sampling of both personal and professional philosophies of selected health educators and identify some of the key issues that readers might face when beginning to develop their own personal and professional philosophy of health education.

## CHALLENGE TO THE READER

A philosophy may fluctuate over time. This is a normal process and represents the growing and developing life of the professional. The continuing examination and validation of one's beliefs (philosophy) is a healthy process for a professional health educator.

# 1

# THIS I BELIEVE: A PHILOSOPHY OF HEALTH EDUCATION

## LOREN B. BENSLEY JR.

During my undergraduate years, I was given an assignment by a professor to write my philosophy of education. When asked to participate in this monograph series on philosophies of health education, I turned to the assignment that I had done thirty-six years ago. Being a collector of trivia, I knew exactly where to find the assignment. When I read my philosophy, I was amazed at how simple yet clear I stated my beliefs and mission in education. My philosophy reflected that of an inexperienced, naive young man who valued and believed that by choosing to be a teacher, one would have the opportunity to make a difference in others' lives. As a teacher of health, I believed that I could change attitudes of young people so they might resist the temptations which would result in poor decision making. As I continued to read the assignment given to me thirty-six years ago, I realized that I still believed in the optimism that I had as a student preparing to be a teacher of health education. Reading my philosophy created a feeling of pride and satisfaction that the mission I had set forth to accomplish has been, to a certain extent, achieved. I am pleased that over the years I haven't become a pessimist or one who has become discouraged with the educational system with its many flaws. It is interesting, while at the same time gratifying, that the values and beliefs of my present philosophy of health education are nothing but an exaggeration of what I believed as an undergraduate about to enter the profession of education. If there has been any change in these beliefs, it has been a stronger commitment based on my professional and life experiences. What is set forth in the statement that you are about to read is not a new philosophy of health education but one that has existed for a long time and has been resurrected to share with others what I stand for, what I believe in, and what I strive to accomplish.

In developing a personal philosophy of health education, it is necessary to first understand what *philosophy* means. Philosophy can be defined as a state of mind based on your values and beliefs. This in turn is based on a variety of factors which include culture, religion, education, morals, environment, experiences, and family. It is also determined by people who have influenced you, how you feel about yourself and others, your spirit, your optimism or pessimism, your independence, and your family. It is a synthesis of all learning that makes you who you are and what you believe. In other words, a philosophy reflects your values and beliefs which determine your mission and purpose for being, or basic theory, or viewpoint based on logical reasoning.

My personal philosophy of health education includes all of what I am, what I value, and what I believe and stand for in relation to health and education. In other words, in order for me to establish my philosophy of education it was necessary to identify the multitude of factors that have formulated what I believe in, which in turn, has given me direction in establishing my credo or my mission. According to Shirreffs (1976) "all philosophizing begins with the person becoming aware of his/her existence which precedes the establishment of essence in that individual." This being the case, self-examination of our existence will help us discover our essence, or our being. Put another way, the reason for our existence reflects our values and beliefs that influence the direction of our professional being or mission.

What then are my values and beliefs, and how have they influenced the development of my philosophy of health education? Those things that I value have evolved from a multitude of life experiences. Values which have shaped my philosophy of health education are justice and equality, self-esteem, education and learning, kindness and forgiveness, a higher spirit, helping others, family unity, goodness and morals, freedom and autonomy, self-improvement and self-discipline. Undoubtedly there are other values that I hold in high regard, but lack of space limits an extensive list. Each of these values give me a foundation for my existence and can be identified in my philosophical approach to health education.

My philosophy of health education also has been greatly influenced by other values such as the literature of the profession, conferences I attended, involvement in professional associations, and most importantly colleagues. Their teachings, writings, and personalities reflect my existence as a health educator. In addition, my philosophy of health education has been influenced by the philosophies of many whom I respect and consider dear colleagues. A personal philosophy includes more than identified values. It also must include what people believe in, or in another perspective, what they stand for. In other words, it is all a health educator represents or communicates through their lifestyle, their teaching or professional involvement and commitment.

I believe health education offers an individual an invitation to be and become—to reaffirm the self and become committed to the development of individual potential through decision making and action (Shirreffs, 1976). I am committed to the philosophy of existentialism as an approach to health education. Shirreffs (1976) states that "the existential health educator sees his/her function as one of awakening learners to their own capacities and of providing opportunities for them to be responsible for their own learning opportunities and/or ignorance. The existential health educator provides opportunities in which each student can 'be' and 'become' in an atmosphere of freedom coupled with responsibilities. He/she helps students to understand that each individual is ultimately responsible for what he/she becomes. We cannot force individuals to behave in ways conducive to attaining and maintaining wellness, but we can offer knowledge and promote awareness to individuals regarding responsibilities for health-related behavior."

I believe the ultimate goal of health education is to provide learning experiences from which one can develop skills and knowledge to make informed decisions which will maintain or better their health, or the health of others. It is important that the health educator provide these experiences without being a dictator of moral behavior. On the other hand, it is my belief that too often health educators are neutral and end up sitting on the fence regarding critical issues. There are times when a health educator should take sides, especially when they stand for certain principles, values, and standards that he or she believes can make a difference in the health of individuals or communities. When this occurs, information must be communicated in a way that gives guidance to those making health decisions. This is especially true with young people who are confused regarding their own morals and values as they relate to their health.

I believe that health education must be more than dissemination of information. The existentialists believe that the health educator's interaction centers around the clients in assisting them in personal learning quests (Youngs, 1992). Health educators must provide the opportunity for individuals to act intelligently on their decisions. All too often health education exists in a vacuum. In other words opportunities to implement that which is learned are nonexistent. Environments must be established to serve as a vehicle to put into action choices to improve lifestyles. One without the other is incomplete.

I'm also a strong believer that health educators must provide a role model for their constituency. The statement that "I can't hear what you're saying because of what I see" has no place in health education. Those of us who are health educators must strive to maintain a level of wellness within our own limitations and indulge in personal lifestyles which foster good health.

I believe the study of behavioral psychology is a must in order to understand the nature of those we educate. The future of health education will go beyond presenting facts. All too often health education falls short of its objective and goals. This is because we have failed to consider the variables that contribute to unhealthy behavior such as poor self-esteem, lack of internal locus of control, poor social skills, and so forth that lead to undesirable behaviors. Furthermore, we have not examined the factors that contribute to the aforementioned variables such as one's spirit and purpose and meaning of life. As health educators, we must work within this element of human existence. We must cease addressing the behaviors that cause ill health and focus on the reasons for the behavior.

We also must become knowledgeable regarding resiliency which people have in overcoming adversities. The potential for prevention lies in understanding the reasons why some people are not damaged by deprivation (Rutter and others, 1979). The resiliency model described by Richardson and others (1990) has great promise and must be a part of the practice of health education.

Much has been written and practiced, especially by Asians, regarding the connection between the mind and body. The concept of psychoneuroimmunology is an example of the improvement of one's health status as a result of positive thinking. This was demonstrated by Cousins (1979) in introducing the mind-body connection to Western medicine in his book *Anatomy of an Illness*. I believe the future success of health education will depend on how well we adapt the science of human behavior to mental, physical, social, and spiritual wellness.

In conclusion, I am content to reaffirm a simplified philosophy that I held over three decades ago. It is refreshing to realize that after thirty-four years in the profession my original philosophy has not changed but has been strengthened and reinforced by new educational theories, medical advancements, and most importantly, new developments in human behavior. This confirms what I have always believed, that I am no smarter that I was as an entry-level professional: however, I know I am much wiser as a result of my experiences and professional friendships with colleagues who have taught me by example and challenged my beliefs. Of special importance in the development of my thinking and beliefs have been my students who have diligently listened to me profess. It is through them that I've grown and learned to appreciate the reexamination of what I believe to be the truth. My students serve as my inspiration and love for teaching and the profession. Our future is in their hands. Their beliefs and values, their philosophies will shape the profession for decades to come.

## REFERENCES

Cousins, N. (1979). *Anatomy of an illness*. New York: Bantam Books.

Richardson, G. E., Neiger, B., Jensen, S., & Kumpfer, K. (1990). The resiliency model. *Health Education, 21*(6), 33–39.

Rutter. M., Maughan, B., Mortimore, P., & Ouston, J., with Smith, A. (1979). *Fifteen thousand hours: Secondary schools and their effects on children*. Cambridge, MA: Harvard University Press.

Shirreffs, J. (1976). A philosophical approach to health education. *The Eta Sigma Gamman*, Spring, 21–23.

Youngs, B. (1992). *The six vital ingredients of self-esteem*. Rolling Hills Estates, CA: Jalmar Press.

# CHAPTER

## 2

# PHILOSOPHICAL BASES
# FOR HEALTH EDUCATION

## J. KEOGH RASH

The profession of health education is relatively young and as yet has not clearly defined its purposes and goals. Since a clarification of basic beliefs is essential to the definition of goals and purposes, it is time to examine our beliefs and define our purposes and set some goals for the profession. What do we believe about health?

The World Health Organization has defined *health* as "complete physical, mental, and social well-being, and not merely freedom from disease or infirmity." The Joint Committee on Health Problems in Education of the National Education Association and the American Medical Association in an early report (1941) emphasized the "physical, mental, social, and moral" aspects of health.

The comparatively recent development of the psychosomatic emphasis in medical science supported by the emphasis on a satisfactory spiritual philosophy seems to justify a broad interpretation of health. In light of this interpretation, *health* is here defined as "physical, emotional, spiritual, and social well-being."

## FOURFOLD SYMMETRY

To illustrate the fourfold nature of health, we may think of life as represented by a sphere, with segments consisting of the four aspects of health—physical, emotional, spiritual, and social. Only as long as the parts of the sphere remain in balance and symmetry is maintained may the ball be thrown or rolled accurately.

In this age of speed, it is not difficult to realize the importance of symmetry if the ball is to roll along life's highway with any degree of stability. The driver of a speeding automobile soon realizes the importance of a balanced wheel. The presence of a boot in an automobile tire may not be noticed at low speeds, but as speed is increased the extra weight of the boot is multiplied by centrifugal force, creating an intolerable, hazardous condition.

This is not unlike the health picture for an individual. Failure to maintain symmetry through neglect of any aspect of health results in an unbalanced individual. Such an individual may get along very well under ordinary circumstances, but in times of catastrophe or under the pressure of the present stresses of life, he runs a great risk of cracking up and will certainly do so if the stress becomes great enough.

Symmetry in the sphere of health as maintained or achieved by proper attention to the fourfold development is increasingly vital as the pace of life continues to accelerate. Failure to give attention to conservation of any aspect of health places the individual in jeopardy. Each individual must give proper attention to being a well-rounded individual.

It is important that we recognize the interrelatedness of the four aspects of health. As recognized in the development of psychosomatic medicine, no single aspect of life exists independently of the others. Physical, emotional, social, and spiritual well-being are so interrelated and interdependent as at times to be indistinguishable. In health, many factors appear in more than one aspect. Above all, health is not and cannot be static or compartmentalized.

## THE CROWN OF HEALTH

Health would seem to be the most important single aspect of life. In terms of monetary or property value, fame, influence, or prestige, it is impossible to place a value on health. There is an old Egyptian saying which illustrates the importance and common feeling about health: "Health is a crown upon the well man's head but no one can see it but a sick man." Nothing in life is so taken for granted when possessed, or so sorely missed when gone, as is health.

This fact suggests an important consideration in health education, a philosophical basis. If health is so commonly the concern of the sick only, it may be that we are failing to emphasize those aspects of health which are challenging to well persons. Furthermore, we are certainly failing to take advantage of teachable moments. For example, few hospitals and almost no physicians have a health educator on their staff to assist the patient or his family in the solution of health problems or in living within known limitations.

## HEALTH EDUCATION

The American Association of School Administrators has suggested that "the goal of intelligent self-direction of health behavior by every person in our society is an ideal toward which to strive." In other words, the health-educated individual will be able to intelligently direct his own behavior concerning physical, emotional, spiritual, and social problems. Health behavior, in this instance, includes such things as personal hygiene, selection and purchase of health supplies, medical services, acceptable attitudes in social relationships, and a satisfactory and stabilizing spiritual experience. This does not imply meeting all of one's needs by himself. Indeed, this would not be intelligent direction if one were to try.

Within the school program there are two broad classifications of health education, direct and indirect. Indirect health education (incidental or concomitant learnings) accrues from one's everyday experiences; this is the kind of education represented by getting accustomed to clean surroundings and feeling uncomfortable when they are not clean. Direct health education is health instruction—the process of providing opportunities for learning experiences which will favorably influence knowledge, attitudes, and practices resulting in intelligent self-direction of health behavior.

Health instruction may be thought of as the process, health education as the result. Health instruction may be provided effectively in health education courses (the concentrated health course) or in units or lessons in other (usually related) courses. In the latter, the method employed may be either through direct teaching or through correlation, that is, showing the relationship of the health problem to the subject being studied.

Isn't every teacher a health teacher? We might also justifiably ask, isn't every teacher an English teacher, a mathematics teacher, or a history teacher? The answer is both yes and no: *yes*, to the extent that every teacher should make use of opportunities to strengthen the learnings in these areas, to correct errors, and to insist on proper usage, but *no* in the sense that it is not possible for everyone to be responsible for everything. We have not as yet been able to provide enough teachers thoroughly grounded in all aspects of knowledge to ensure the successful conduct of a completely integrated program of education. If, or perhaps when, we are able to staff our schools with teachers each of whom is a composite grammarian-mathematician-scientist-historian-sociologist-health educator, at approximately the master's degree level in each area, we might assume that we have a staff capable of conducting the completely integrated program, thus making everyone a health teacher.

In the meantime, except for the lower elementary grades, we would do well to direct our efforts toward providing direct health instruction plus coordination of the efforts of all who are working in areas related to health education. At the same time, all school personnel must see their relationships to health.

Health is not an end in itself; it is a means to the end of a fuller, richer, more enjoyable life which will make possible a higher service to mankind. Furthermore, it is a safe assumption that health will not be conserved by making it the primary objective of life. Important as it is, it loses its proper place in our perspective of life and remains like the will-o'-the-wisp, always just outside one's grasp when it becomes the primary objective.

## CONSERVATION OF HEALTH

The nature of health is such that efforts of health education should be directed toward conserving health. With some notable exceptions, one's quality of health is seldom better than that with which one is endowed at birth. Like a spool of thread of unknown length it may be unwound at varying speeds. Too frequently the thread is broken and life ends without playing out the maximum potential. Disease, stress, deprivation, dissipation, unhygienic living, overwork, loss of sleep, and other seemingly minor factors take their toll and unwind the spool at an accelerated rate.

Medical science may at times need to be called on to assist nature in restoring the healthful condition of the organism. Health education can be of assistance to medical science through the development of intelligent self-direction of health behavior, thus conserving health and rendering less likely the need for restoring health. It is important that health education be distinguished from the practice of medicine. We should understand that one of the most important contributions of health education is to promote intelligent recognition of the need for medical attention and proper selection and use of health services.

Just as health education can result from other educational experiences, so are there concomitants resulting from health instruction. In terms of the objectives of education, health instruction will be recognized as making direct and significant contribution to the objectives of health, citizenship, worthy home membership, and ethical character. It may also contribute, but perhaps less directly, to the objectives of vocation, worthy use of leisure time, and command of fundamental processes.

Health instruction provides countless opportunities for the liberal or cultural education. However, we must not lose the proper perspective for health education. *Its aim is intelligent self-direction of health behavior.* To the extent it is able to realize this aim, it may be said to be successful and justifiable as an integral part of the educational program.

Originally printed in the *Journal of Health, Physical Education, Recreation*, January 1960.

# CHAPTER

3

# THREE ESSENTIAL QUESTIONS IN DEFINING A PERSONAL PHILOSOPHY

### R. MORGAN PIGG JR.

Early on Christmas morning, 1959, my dad and I got into the car and began an important journey in my understanding of life. Heavy snow had fallen on Christmas Eve. Dad drove slowly for hours through the Tennessee hills until we stopped outside a sharecropper's shack near the Alabama state line. A large man emerged from the shack and labored through the fresh snow toward our car. A little boy not more than four followed several feet behind in his footsteps.

Dad opened the trunk, took out a new tricycle, and gave it to the man. The little boy watched from a distance. The men shook hands. Neither said much. As we drove away I watched out the back window as the little boy plowed through the snow on his new tricycle. Even at age twelve, I knew something special had happened. That Christmas morning remains a defining moment in my life.

## PHILOSOPHY DEFINED

Philosophy involves the intellectual pursuit of wisdom and knowledge. It represents one of four terms related to defining human behavior. *Philosophy* involves a process to identify, classify, and explain knowledge. *Ethics* defines acceptable and unacceptable behavior within the norms of a particular group. *Morality* sets standards for right and wrong in human behavior. *Religion*, or spiritualism, addresses good and evil behavior, often in terms of eternal consequences.

Thus, philosophy describes human existence without necessarily judging it. Judgment comes in the form of ethics (acceptable//unacceptable), morality (right/wrong), or religion (good/evil). The four terms should not be confused since they represent related but distinct concepts. Therefore, avoid considering the concepts collectively as in "philosophy and ethics."

Ancient philosophers loved knowledge and devoted their lives to the search for meaning in human existence. Defining three central components—reality, truth, and value—formed the basis for that search. Over time three traditional schools of philosophical thought emerged: idealism, realism, and pragmatism. Contemporary schools of thought include existentialism, naturalism, humanism, theism, and eclecticism. While the schools differ in detail, all approach reality, truth, and value by addressing considerations such as the relationship of human beings to nature, the relationship between individuals and society, the relationship between mind and body, sources and consequences of human behavior, the absolute or relative nature of values, the meaning of the physical world, the role of science in defining human existence, and the nature and involvement of God in human existence.

## THREE ESSENTIAL QUESTIONS

While studying philosophy as an academic subject can prove interesting, the process may provide students with limited help in forming a personal philosophy. Formal courses often focus on the history of philosophy, rather than developing methods of philosophical thought among the students. They study the writings of past philosophers, or what others have written about those philosophers. They spend time talking about philosophy, rather than developing their own abilities as philosophical thinkers. Consequently, they gain knowledge but fundamental questions go unanswered. They leave the course better appreciating Plato or Idealism, but lacking confidence in their own explanation of human existence. Unfortunately, the abstract nature of the experience can discourage students from further contemplation.

Philosophy need not be an abstract process. You and I still face the same fundamental question as did Plato or other great philosophers: "What is the origin, nature, and purpose of human existence?" Or, treating the matter as three essential questions: Where did I come from? Why am I here? and What happens to me after I die? To be viable, any philosophy must provide satisfactory answers to these questions.

Given the knowledge available today, we have at least as good a chance, or perhaps a better chance, to successfully answer the questions as did the ancient philosophers. Answers to question one (Where did I come from?) fall into three categories: creation, evolution, and fate. Options one and two both require faith since neither can be proven with complete satisfaction, especially to an unreceptive listener. If creation, then by whom? If evolution, then from what and to what? Fate merely accepts, without explanation. Answers to questions two and three (Why am I here? Where am I going?) derive from the answer to question one since, logically, the explanation of origin will influence one's views of current and future events.

## IMPLICATIONS FOR HEALTH EDUCATION

What role does philosophy play in Health Education? Think of philosophy as the solid foundation upon which we build the house of professional practice. We need both to be successful.

Professional preparation programs in Health Education have improved dramatically the past several years, particularly in developing student knowledge and skills. Our major students display impressive ability in areas such as conceptualizing the discipline, planning and evaluating interventions to document effectiveness, applying computer technology to instruction, and acknowledging the importance of cultural diversity.

Yet, much of the improvement centers on the "how" rather than the "why" of Health Education. We provide a strong defense for the process of Health Education, but prove less effective in presenting a fundamental rationale for its existence. For example, we can confirm the effectiveness of smoking-cessation strategies, but we falter in providing a convincing rationale for assisting the individual smoker. Beyond offering general comments about reducing medical care costs or contributing to self-actualization, we often fail to show why that one smoker is worth the effort. Discussions of health as a right, for example, are premature without first confirming the inherent worth of the person for whom we advocate that right.

Accepting individuals as unique and valuable, regardless of their circumstances, provides a foundation for dealing positively and professionally with our students, patients, and clients. The concepts of anonymity, confidentiality, informed consent, and voluntary participation in research are particularly important in this regard. Likewise, personal philosophy allows us to confidently address important topics more specific to the field such as defining the concept of optimal health, examining the relationship between free will and determinism, or explaining why one smoker is important. Philosophy won't always give specific answers, but it provides a context for answering questions and making decisions.

Professors frequently ask students to speak or write about their professional philosophy of Health Education, often with no link to personal philosophy. Consequently, these experiences sometime remind us of efforts to define *patriotism* or *family*. As a young professional, I found the dichotomy disconcerting since in my own thinking the two philosophies invariably merged. Today, students still struggle to reconcile that dichotomy. Once we understand that personal philosophy begets professional philosophy, then we understand the application of philosophy to professional practice.

Using the three essential questions posed previously as a guide, students can develop a foundation upon which to derive a personal philosophy. For example, let me share with you briefly the essence of the personal philosophy that gives direction to my professional practice. I believe Creation provides the most reasonable explanation for human existence (Where did I come from?). Deity endows each human being with a life force, or soul, making every human being inherently unique arid valuable. Human beings exist to serve Deity, and we render that service in part by helping other human beings in our common journey toward an eternal existence (Why am I here?). Through successful service, we serve Deity for eternity in the afterlife (Where am I going?). I also believe in ultimate justice, where good eventually triumphs.

A clear philosophy of the purpose for human existence can significantly influence our approach to personal and professional relationships. For example, a professor labors against an impossible deadline to complete a critical project when a student knocks, sticks her head in the door, and asks, "Do you have a minute?" In this situation, you know two things. First, you don't have a minute, and second, even if you do, the matter will take more than a minute. What do you do? Time management tells us to lock the door, pull the shade, and turn off the light, but a philosophy that views the individual with respect and value says to help now, or at least make certain the need isn't urgent or life-threatening.

Some would question the preceding example, suggesting we should take time for ourselves. While we all need time for ourselves, Americans have elevated self-care to an art form. Since helping others usually requires sacrifice, a clear philosophy confirms the purpose and importance of serving. While anyone can render acts of service, those who work from a sense of right and duty (or love) often serve with contentment and conviction for a lifetime. In this sense, service represents as much an attitude as an act. Even on "bad days," a philosophy grounded in service sustains us in helping our students, patients, and clients—especially when they don't deserve it or appreciate it. Conversely, service without substance eventually fades, leaving the individual frustrated and disillusioned.

## CONCLUSION

I'm reminded again of that time with my dad on a snowy Christmas Day in 1959. Dad was not a politician or social activist. He just believed in people. He respected them, accepted them, and related to them as individuals regardless of their circumstances. He particularly loved children. That year, dad worked at a furniture store. The sharecropper had bought the tricycle as a Christmas present for his son, but he had no car and the snowstorm prevented his picking it up on Christmas Eve. Dad knew that without the tricycle, the little boy would have no Christmas. He saw a need, and he met it. That act was especially significant in 1959. The little boy was Black.

Dad died on October 6, 1992, at age 80 following a ten-year struggle with countless health problems. The experience jaded my view of modern medicine, but Dad didn't complain. Rather, he accepted the situation and endeared himself to the countless medical workers who filled his life. His passing left a small hole in the universe, not so much for his worldly accomplishments, but for the quality of his character. He successfully answered life's three essential questions. I often pose this question to my students: "If we could master all the knowledge of a great university, yet not provide a reasonable explanation for the reality of human existence, what have we learned?"

What kind of hole will you and I leave in the universe? If we can face that proposition with confidence, then we understand life, and we are ready to apply our philosophy to the professional practice of Health Education in any setting under any circumstances.

## SELECTED READINGS

David, R. (1990). The fate of the soul and the fate of the social order: The waning spirit of American youth. *Journal of School Health, 60*(5), 205–207.

Gunderson, S., & Kreuter, M. W. (1982). Is anyone there. Does anyone care. *(Journal of) Health Education, 13*(2), 3–5.

Hicks, D. A. (1982). Eta Sigma Gammans—Teach, research, serve. *The Eta Sigma Gamman, 14*(2), 3–5.

Hoyman, H. S. (1966). The spiritual dimension of man's health in today's world. *Journal of School Health, 36*(2), 52–63.

Keene, C. H. (1938). For what ends shall we live. *Journal of School Health, 8*(8), 232–234.

Kreuter, M. W. (1979). A case for philosophy. *Journal of School Health, 29*(2), 115–116.

Leight, R. L. (1984). Three pragmatic philosophers. *The Educational Forum*, Winter, 191–206.

Nolte, A. E. (1984). In relationship—Freedom and love. *(Journal of) Health Education, 15*(5), 3–5.

Oberteuffer, D. K. (1953). Philosophy and principles of the school health program. *Journal of School Health, 23*(4), 103–109.

O'Connor, K. T. (1988). For want of a mentor. *Nursing Outlook, 36*(1), 38–39.

Philosophy, ethics and futurism in health education (special feature). (1980). *(Journal of) Health Education, 11*(2), 1–25.

Philosophical direction for health education (special feature). (1978). *(Journal of) Health Education, 9*(1), 1–36.

Pigg, R. M. (1987). The successful servant. *The Eta Sigma Gamman, 19*(2), 20–21.

Pinch, W, J. (1986). Quality of life as a philosophical position. *Health Values, 10*(6), 3–7.

Rash, J. K. (1970). The image of the health educator. *Journal of School Health, 40*(10), 538.

Salk, J. (1972). What do we mean by *health? Journal of School Health, 42*(10), 582–584.

# CHAPTER

## 4

# HEALTH EDUCATION
# AS A BASIC

## CARL E. WILLGOOSE

There is an enlightening expression from Sanskrit that indicates that a day "well lived" is what determines all tomorrows. The concept is not new, for optimum health and human functioning have always depended upon the intricacies of one's way of life. Thus the late Rene Dubos writes enthusiastically of the celebrated life—a life of direction and adaptation, excitement and dynamism in action, human awareness, and fully spirited men and women who acknowledge their fragilities and sensitivities and appreciate beyond a doubt the complex relationship between *being able* and *well-being*.

Unfortunately, society has not always defined *well-being* in terms of human vitality and productivity. Historically it has been disease-oriented and discussed in terms of infectious organisms, degenerative conditions, and defective organs. In recent years disease has been more broadly considered as a total organism's lack of ease—disease with numerous behavioral overtones of a psychosomatic nature and relating to such significant health items as chronic fatigue, obesity, hypertension, industrial backache, and physical fitness. It is this shortcoming in functional ability to perform that has been a worldwide major deterrent to the reduction in human misery and to the advance of civilization.

*Note:* This article is intended to be read for its philosophical perspective. Originally published in 1985, it may contain factual material or examples that are dated.

## HEALTH ADVANCEMENT IN A COMPLEX SOCIETY

The whole of an individual's capacity for expression is involved in the health spectrum. It is multidimensional—anthropological, biological, psychological, economic, and even political. The truth of the old English adage is once again appropriate: "Where indeed is illness bred, in the heart or in the head, or in the body politic." Thus all human relationships between a community and its environment are somehow health related. There are no set boundaries. Social unrest, inadequate sanitation, and urban dehumanization are as significant in terms of well-being as a bleeding ulcer, a coronary thrombosis, or advanced paranoia.

Several decades ago Aldous Huxley worried about man blowing himself to smithereens, and he warned that science and scientific know-how are not sufficient for prudent individuals' survival. On numerous occasions Norman Cousins has presented essentially the same view as he calls for a concept of health that embraces the way we live.

It is clearer than ever before, that despite the many exciting biomedical advances, it is necessary to *prevent* illness.

There is today general agreement on the basic need to educate people at all ages about healthful living, for as the President's Committee on Health Education demonstrated, it is no longer possible to stem the tide of human illness and despair with improved medical and surgical techniques, more hospitals and social workers, and more sophisticated health care centers. The committee's message signaled a significant change—a call for prevention. There is evidence that this can be accomplished with an adventurous, broad-spectrum approach to all human illness and health from the more popular topics of malnutrition, drug dependency, cancer, and aging to those issues shrouded in ignorance, superstition, and indifference.

Referring again to Dubos, one is impressed with the observation that human beings can never adapt biologically to the diseases of civilization, but through "creative adaptation" they can shape their lives. Constant attention to the aspects of daily lifestyle, individually and collectively, has revealed that significant educational impact can be made on a person's overall physical and mental capacity. In cardiorespiratory epidemiology alone, studies have invariably incriminated certain components of lifestyle such as sedentary living and obesity as major risk factors. Moreover, as much as 50 percent of mortality from the ten leading causes of death in the United States can be traced to lifestyle.

## THE PUBLIC HEALTH REVOLUTION

To revolutionize is to break with the past—to change the face of an operation. Over the last several decades this is precisely what has occurred in health activities of the public, particularly in the educational dimension. This prevention effort has been spurred on by an alarmed concern for such national health issues as the rising cost of health care, the changing patterns of illness and causes of death in America, the urgency of health problems of youth, the amazing gullibility of the consumer, and "value illness" as a primary concern in contemporary health education.

Health education risk reduction programs are becoming effective because of improved coordination among health departments, schools of public health, medical colleges, local hospitals, and various private sector professional and voluntary health organizations. In a recent study by the Center for Health Promotion and Education, Centers for Disease Control, it was shown that health professionals were interested in a wide number of health topics but were primarily interested in risk reduction, stress management, nutrition, and exercise—topics they believed to be most susceptible to a comprehensive educational approach. Clearly, a cooperative education for health works. It can be measured by a variety of successful outcomes:

**Stroke Mortality:** Over a twelve-year period there has been a 42 percent decrease.

**Heart Disease Mortality:** Over a twelve-year period there has been a 24 percent decrease. Heart attacks are still the nation's number one killer.

**Alcohol:** There is a fundamental change in attitudes about alcohol consumption. Both discussion and action continue relative to raising the drinking age to 21, banning happy hours, stiffening drunk-driving penalties, making people who serve alcohol liable for the actions of guests, and prohibiting drinking while driving. There is evidence that people are starting to use alcohol in a more responsible fashion, and the National Institute on Drug Abuse reported a decline in regular drinking among high school seniors in the previous year.

**Youth Death Rates:** Unheralded in the popular press is the drop in the death rate for adolescents and young adults, 15- to 24-year-olds—due chiefly to the decline in automobile accidents and suicides.

**Drugs:** Teenagers are increasingly aware of drug-related health risks, more opposed to legalizing drug use, and less likely to cave in to peer pressure than in the past according to the findings from the alcohol and drug abuse program of the Department of Health and Human Services. Marijuana usage among the young has gone down, but drug use by American youth is highest in the Western world.

**Smoking:** Fewer people are smoking than ever. The teenage decline began in 1977 with a major effort by the National Interagency Council on Smoking and Health. Smoking is still responsible for about one-third of all coronary disease and all cancer deaths—and it is almost universally acquired during childhood and early adolescence.

**Child Restraints:** Almost half the states have adopted child restraint laws, resulting in a remarkable reduction of child injuries from automobile accidents.

**Seat Belts:** Mandatory seat belt laws have come about because of an informed public that has called for change.

**Exercise:** Thousands of people have adopted an exercise program to, among other things, strengthen the heart, regulate metabolic functions, control blood sugar, combat anxiety or depression, bolster immune defense, and strengthen bone and muscle. The exercise boom continues.

**Infant Mortality Rates:** In three years the rate has dropped from 13 per 1,000 live births to 11.

**Industrial Health/Wellness Programs:** Employee health promotion programs are helping to decrease individual and company health care costs. Financial costs relative to alcoholism and employee premature deaths are down, and absenteeism has been markedly reduced.

**Aging:** Older people are responding to the need for better nutrition and physical activity and are realizing more and more that their health is not at the mercy of their genes. Result: they are living longer. By the year 2000 there will be nearly 59 million Americans aged 50 to 74, a tremendous increase over present numbers.

**Stress Adaptation:** Through relaxation techniques and other healthful practices individuals are being helped to adapt to worry, anxiety, apprehension, fear, hate, jealousy, and anger.

**Sexuality:** The educational impact of sexual understanding in terms of health and happiness is substantial. Teenage pregnancies and out-of-wedlock births frequently relate to toxemia, prolonged labor, low birth weight, and mental retardation. Sexually transmitted diseases strike the 15-to-19-year-old group very hard. Gonorrhea and genital herpes rates are not dropping very much.

**Weight Control:** Great numbers of individuals and groups are giving attention to overweight and obesity. In the Tecumseh, Michigan, study—an epidemiological investigation of an entire community—there was found a strong relationship between the lack of activity and fatness as it contributed to high serum cholesterol levels and poor heart rate response to moderate exercise.

**Environment:** An informed public is making progress in cleaning up and creating a healthful environment. However, Congress is currently faced with the need to reauthorize virtually all the nation's landmark environmental laws, including the Clean Air Act, Safe Drinking Water Act, Toxic Substances Control Act, and the Superfund hazardous waste clean-up program.

**Health Maintenance Organizations (HMOs):** Unlike conventional insurance, the HMO offers total health coverage. It provides all services, a realistic way to budget for health care, and family health education programs that are frequently quite elaborate.

The sine qua non of a revolution—the health of the citizen or anything else—is the visible change in human values, beliefs, judgments, and commitments. The most stupendous of man's inventions, said Joseph Krutch, was not the wheel, or the lever, but the values by which he has lived. Although health values are not always articulately expressed, they are appearing more and more in the day-to-day attitudes of people of all ages and all convictions. Indeed, an increasing number of people are testing inherited health values against new and fresh circumstances. Moreover, they are asking questions. What are the potentialities of a fully able human being? What connection do we see between the fully able citizen and the development of the society itself?

## HEALTH EDUCATION IN THE SCHOOLS

As a result of the recent studies and reports pertaining to shortcomings in educational practices and curriculum in the nation's schools, there has been a very noticeable cry to meet the needs of thousands of children completing school who cannot read properly, write a check, and construct an appropriate sentence. The goal is to get the schools "back-to-basics."

What is basic? Is not health education a *basic* need? Doesn't back-to-basics really mean a return to fundamentals, to longstanding, long understood, and long supported educational goals? Is it not true that every set of educational goals, from ages past to the present, has had the health objective heading the list? From Herbert Spencer (*What Knowledge Is of Most Worth?*) and Horace Mann to the enlightened pronouncements of the American Academy of Pediatrics, American Medical Association, and American Public Health Association, the support for formal health education has been clearly stated.

There is today a need to point out at every opportunity that health education, in both schools and community organizations, is indeed a basic—an essential educational concern no less important than the fundamental processes of calculating and communicating. Moreover, the effort to seek a comprehensive and coordinated school and community health education should not be lost in the all too often emotional school board battles over curriculum and style, but should be directed toward reviewing reportable evidence of studies and new programs that can be implemented locally. To do otherwise is to permit health education to slip by default to a "frill" level course one can take or leave, and miss the opportunity to treat the health and wellness dimension as one of the longstanding basics in education.

It is the combined effort of school and community forces on the school population that is coordinated by school personnel in terms of health services, healthful school environment, and health education. It is health education that is the organization of learning experiences that ultimately influence health attitudes and practices. It is an applied science that relates research findings to the lives of people by narrowing the gap between what is known and what is practiced. It is both a process and a program concerned with human values and behavior that are openly and subtly associated with such items as ecology and environmental well-being, nutrition and growth, mental health, mood-modifying substances, safe living, consumer health, sexuality, and the comprehensive treatment of major health problems of youth and adults. Health education was recently defined by the National Center for Health Education as "the process of assisting individuals, acting separately and collectively, to make informed decisions about matters affecting their personal health and that of others." The long-range goal of health education, therefore, is to prepare persons with the wherewithal to work toward their life objectives because they possess

1. optimum organic health and the vitality to meet emergencies,

2. mental well-being to meet the stresses of modern life,

3. adaptability to and social awareness of the requirements of group living,

4. attitudes and values leading to optimum health behavior, and

5. moral and ethical qualities contributing to life in a democratic society.

## EXHIBIT 4.1 Five National Health Goals

### Healthy Infants

*Goal:* To continue to improve infant health and, by 1990, to reduce infant mortality by at least 35 percent, to fewer than nine deaths per 1,000 live births.

### Healthy Children

*Goal:* To improve child health, foster optimal childhood development and, by 1990, to reduce deaths among children ages 1 to 14 by at least 20 percent, to fewer than 34 per 100,000.

### Healthy Adolescents and Young Adults

*Goal:* To improve the health and health habits of adolescents and young adults and, by 1990, to reduce deaths among people ages 15 to 24 by at least 20 percent, to fewer than 93 per 100,000.

### Healthy Adults

*Goal:* To improve the health of adults and, by 1990, to reduce deaths among people ages 25 to 64 by at least 25 percent, to fewer than 400 per 100,000.

### Healthy Older Adults

*Goal:* To improve the health of and quality of life for older adults and, by 1990, to reduce the average annual number of days of restricted activity due to acute and chronic conditions by 20 percent, to fewer than 30 days per year for people aged 65 and older.

Source: Bureau of Health Education, U.S. Public Health Service, *The Surgeon General's Report on Health Promotion and Disease Prevention*

**FIGURE 4.1**    **Comprehensive School Health Education**

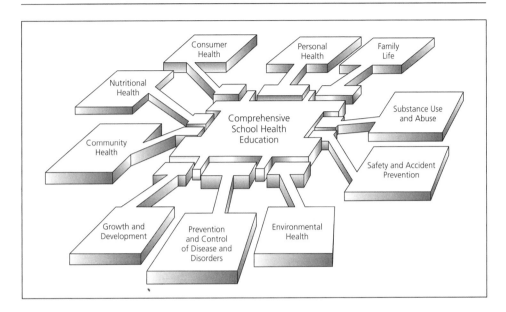

## A COMPREHENSIVE PROGRAM

Obviously, the health education effort will always be a multidisciplinary endeavor, for it is a study of what Whitehead long ago described as "life in all of its manifestations." This might seem to indicate that the health dimension in a school could be nicely handled by dividing it up among science, physical education, and social studies personnel. After all, science teachers examine the human body, physical educators deal directly with the benefits of exercise and physical fitness, and social studies frequently involves a study of community factors essential to well-being.

However, research over the years has demonstrated that health education is poorly handled in isolated and single-topic fashion. It requires direct attention in the classroom with full subject matter status. This is chiefly because the topic of health and wellness is both subtle and dramatic, both obvious and hidden, and means many things to many people, which requires an in-depth treatment.

In order to assure an orderly and progressive consideration for the various major health topics, it has proven effective to call for a comprehensive school health program that avoids "bandwagon" approaches, crash programs, and piecemeal efforts focused on one or two topics that may be enjoying popularity at a particular time. It is a program in which health learning strategies are planned at every grade level and in which there is a concern for student goals, course content, resources, evaluation procedures, and the managerial function of health education coordinators. It is this shift from the fragmented health teaching ventures to proper scope and sequential programs that has had the support of the American Academy of Pediatrics since 1973 and more recently the American Public Health Association and the Association for the Advancement of Health Education (AAHPERD). Recent efforts by the National Congress of Parents and Teachers and the Center for Health Promotion and Education, Centers for Disease Control in Atlanta to publicize demonstration projects have been instrumental in gaining support for school health education as well as appropriately prepared health teachers.

Especially significant in recent years is the manner in which national professional school health education organizations have worked together to promote comprehensive programs and develop definitive statements describing concepts and processes of instruction. (See Helpful Sources for specific guidelines.) These organizations have been influential in bringing about a considerable number of health curriculum changes toward the more balanced programs, and by doing so have provided thousands of students with the chance to appreciate the multitude of delicate particulars of the healthful lifestyles. Failing to seek such a balanced curriculum is to miss what Nobel laureate Jacques Monod considers vital—recognition of distinction between objective knowledge and the realm of values.

Ultimately, the determination of which is a major health topic and which is a minor one will have to be made by curriculum developers locally. There are roughly twelve to fourteen health areas that are worthy of graduated programming for student exploration and reflection, from the early grades through secondary school. A number of state curriculum guides spell out these major health areas rather well, that is, New York, Oregon, Pennsylvania, Massachusetts, and Alabama. A suggested listing of major topics follows.

*Elementary Grades* (P—Primary, I—Intermediate)

1. Personal cleanliness and appearance (P, I)

2. Physical activity, sleep, rest, and relaxation (P, I)

3. Nutrition and growth (P, I)

4. Dental health (P, I)

5. Body structure and operation (P, I)

6. Prevention and control of disease (P, I)

7. Safety and first aid (P, I)

8. Mental health (P, I)

9. Sex and family living education (P, I)

10. Environmental health (P, I)

11. Tobacco, alcohol, and drugs (I)

12. Consumer health (I)

*Secondary Grades 7 to 12*
*Area I: Physical Health*

1. Physical activity, sleep, rest, and relaxation

2. Nutrition and growth

3. Dental health

4. Body structure and operation (including special senses and skin care)

5. Prevention and control of disease

*Area II: Mental Health*

6. Mental health (including death education)

7. Alcohol and drugs

8. Smoking education

9. Sex and family living education

*Area III: Environmental and Consumer Health*

10. Environmental health

11. Consumer health

12. World health

13. Health careers

*Area IV: Safety Education*

14. Safety education

## SCHOOL AND COMMUNITY HEALTH PLANNING

There are numerous official and voluntary health organizations in the country today that are anxious to be of assistance in the school health program. These groups can be especially valuable at a time when the school is in the process of revising a course of study or preparing new curriculum materials. Agencies having to do with child health, vital statistics, nutrition, accident prevention, fire protection, consumer health, drug abuse, alcoholism, cancer, heart conditions, mental health, air and water pollution, respiratory disorders, and the other diseases of mankind all have a real interest in assisting school health coordinators and teachers to be more effective. Using the expertise of all community groups and seeking to achieve balance in the contributions from all sources is to anticipate a state of harmony, so well-defined by the early Greeks as "an orchestration of many powers."

The act of collaboration affords ordinary people a voice in the schools and reduces feelings of powerlessness resulting from frequently unresponsive bureaucracies, and it discovers community perceptions of local health problems and their bearing on students and families. The nationwide effort to promote the community-based drug programs certainly supports the practice of school-community planning to meet a local health situation. Other examples of school-community collaboration are plentiful. In Louisiana the Comprehensive Health Education Guide was developed with the express help of multicultural groups so that it would be completely useful when implemented. In Pennsylvania, the Pennsylvania Health Curriculum Progression Chart was prepared from outcome statements at the state level and reflects the different geographical regions and ethnic and cultural differences within the state.

Finally, it should be acknowledged that people have to struggle together to reach common goals. Conrad knew this well when he wrote that "man is born; he struggles; he dies."—a pretty short life history. The key word here is *struggles*. Life is a struggle—a struggle to generate the capacity to perform well and to achieve a certain happiness.

## RECOMMENDATIONS

School administrators, policy makers, and school board personnel will find it appropriate to

1. Review existing school health education practices and consider the need to revise and update programs in the light of student lifestyles and current national and local health problems.

2. Establish a working committee consisting of both school personnel and community members who have a strong interest in health and health-related happenings within the community and will function to favorably influence school health education.

## HELPFUL SOURCES

*A healthy child: The key to the basics*. (1984). Kent, OH: American School Health Association (P.O. Box 708, Kent, OH 44240).

Bruess, C. E., & Laing. S. J. (1983). Promotion of health education programs. *Health Education, 14*(2): 26–30.

*Comprehensive school health education* (Report by the National Professional School Health Education Organization). (1984). *Health Education, 15*(6), 4–8.

*Health education curriculum progression*. (1980). New York: National Center for Health Education (30 E. 29th St., New York, NY 10016).

*Health education: Guidelines for planning health education programs, K–12*. (1983). Kent, OH: American School Health Association (P.O. Box 708, Kent, OH 44240).

Livingood, W. C. (1984). The school health curriculum project: Its theory, practice and measurement experience as a health education curriculum. *Health Education, 15*(2), 9–13.

*National School Health Service program, special report number 1.* (1985). Princeton, NJ: The Robert Wood Johnson Foundation (P.O. Box 2316, Princeton, NJ 08540).

Noak, M. (1982). *State policy support for school health education.* Denver: Education Commission of the States.

U.S. Department of Health and Human Services. (1980). *Objectives for the nation.* Washington, DC: U.S. Government Printing Office.

Willgoose, Carl E. (1982). *Health teaching in secondary schools* (3rd ed.). Philadelphia: Saunders.

Originally printed by the Association for the Advancement of Health Education, October 1985.

# 5

# SOME GUIDING PRINCIPLES ON HEALTH AND HEALTH EDUCATION: A PHILOSOPHICAL STATEMENT

### CHARLES R. CARROLL

Everything I ever needed to know about Health Education, or so I thought, I first learned at The Ohio State University. It was my good fortune to have enrolled in a teacher education course that emphasized the potential role of any secondary teacher to influence favorably the health-related knowledge, attitudes, and behaviors of students. This was a somewhat revolutionary concept for me—that the school could be a positive force in improving health status! Little did I realize at that time, when I was preparing to be a science educator, that thirty-five years later, I would have the opportunity to reflect on my "professional roots" that took hold quite by accident during a "golden age of health education" at Ohio State.

In so many ways, I owe my career to these energetic professionals: Drs. Mary Beyrer, Wesley Cushman, Robert Kaplan, Ann Nolte, Delbert Oberteuffer, Elena

Sliepcevich, and Marian Solleder. They inspired me, challenged me, and encouraged me for more than three decades. Although I am not really a collective clone of my former professors and associates, my philosophy, theories, and methodologies of health education are derived from the aforementioned individuals who remain as the number one force that still influences me the most today in my professional endeavors.

Over time, in different teaching environments, and under differing circumstances, my concepts of health education and even health itself have changed somewhat. Perhaps the term *evolved* would more appropriately describe my altered perceptions of these basic concepts. And yet, these newer constructs do not deviate too far from my earlier, original beliefs and understandings of what I am, what I try to do, and why I do or do not do certain things in my role as a health educator at Ball State University.

For instance, health itself has been defined by the World Health Organization as a state of complete physical, mental, and social well-being, not merely the absence of disease or infirmity. Though useful, this definition of health is not absolute, because health itself means different things to different people. Some "healthologists" describe health as a multidimensional condition including not only physical, but mental, social, and even spiritual aspects, thus recognizing the holistic, unified view of each person. Others view health as a commodity, a state or condition of the human individual to be used in the pursuit of personal or social goals. Here, health is viewed as a means to some end, rather than as an end in itself.

While all of these definitions have merit, I have come to view health in terms of "here-and-now" well-being as well as past and future well-being (Carroll & Miller, 1991). As such, I now emphasize the changing nature of health and one's potential role in improving health status and in the prevention of disease. Accordingly, I define health as a process of continuous change throughout one's life cycle.

From the very beginning of human life until death, the human organism is confronted with numerous forces that influence growth, development, maturity, well-being, and eventual decline. These dynamic, interacting hereditary and environmental forces may be either favorable or unfavorable, yet they determine the level of well-being that any one person experiences at any one time (Hoyman, 1965). Moreover, these interacting forces are continuous and bring about accommodations or adaptations within one's total self. Consequently, health may be perceived as an ever-changing process involving various interactions and adaptive responses. In essence, health is the ability to function both effectively and happily and as long as possible in a particular environment (Dubos, 1965). Now, this operational definition of health isn't too far removed from Oberteuffer and Beyrer's (1966) original, yet more succinct offering in which they defined health as "the condition of the organism which measures the degree to which its aggregate powers are able to function."

Having formulated a broad definition of health, I should now like to focus on some of my adventures and struggles in the process of health education—the attempt to help people apply what is known about health to their own lives. Initially, I would have described my undertakings as process-oriented, that is, helping students make informed decisions about personal and social health concerns and motivating them to do so. It wasn't long, however, until I inherited or was asked to develop a number of topic-specific health courses. Overnight, I had become a subject matter specialist in human sexuality, substance abuse, consumer health, and more recently, thanatology. Despite my tendency to overwhelm some students with subject matter, I still try to function as an "educational bridge" between fact and fancy, between concept and misconception, and between research and its application (Beyrer, 1985).

While I serve as a catalyst in decision making and clarification of ethical issues, I sometimes feel as if I am mainly a consultant on health-related matters. In fact, some of my best class sessions are spent in answering or commenting on a myriad of students' questions, not unlike Larry King's *Open Phone America* or Rush Limbaugh's *Open Line Friday*. On such occasions, I make pertinent applications, indicate connections between topics and between personal behaviors and potential consequences of actions, analyze facts and theories, and build concepts.

One of my colleagues, Dr. Wayne A. Payne of Ball State University, believes that some health educators assume the role of "secular minister." I think such a label often describes my major function in the classroom. It certainly beats the criticism of my harshest detractors who describe me as a benevolent "social engineer." In a sense, I nurture hope and resolve guilt. I disturb and shake people out of complacency; I raise consciousness and express outrage; I display concern and then raise more questions in genuine puzzlement. I have even cautioned students that those under the influence of alcohol and other drugs may engage in high-risk sexual behavior that could, in turn, result in death, especially if the HIV virus is transmitted and the infected person develops the Acquired Immune Deficiency Syndrome. In other words, sex "under the influence" can be deadly! Amen!

And now I should like to share with you four of the guiding principles that have helped me tremendously as I try to influence favorably the health-related knowledge, attitudes, and behaviors of college students during the last decade of the twentieth century.

## EMPOWERMENT

Recently, I have become intrigued with the concept of personal empowerment in relation to health education. In my attempt to become more skill-oriented in my teaching objectives and to become more of an enabler for my students, I have begun to emphasize behaviors that can enhance health and to deemphasize factual trivia that serve mainly as convenient bases for test questions. Although this skill focus is not a new goal of health education, the concept of empowerment is revitalizing, more consciousness-raising, and much more socially focused than the traditional educational approaches that stress individualism and actions that may eventually trickle down to preordained behavior change and lifestyle program (Fahlberg, Poulin, Girdano, & Dusek, 1991).

Although ideally developed for community health advocacy, as noted by Miner and Ward (1992), I can see the potential of empowerment as another means of "interpersonal" health education. As I view the concept, empowerment is an ongoing process of liberation, and maybe even one of democratization. It restores people's capacity to act with others to improve the quality of life. As people experience and engage in the empowerment process, they have the potential to grow and change.

Sometimes, empowerment levels the so-called playing field between patients and physicians or other caregivers. Smart patients are now encouraged to communicate with their doctors so they, the consuming patients, can get better treatment or decide to select other health care providers. Indeed, the whole field of patients' rights, including "informed consent," seems to be based on the social empowerment model which may eventually lead to a newly structured health care delivery system that views physicians more as health care consultants and less as miracle workers.

In my estimate, empowerment is also a potential remedy for the number-one problem that is often cited as interfering with mutually satisfying and rewarding relationships, and the number-one problem that is frequently at the very core of broken relationships, separations, and divorces. As you might have guessed, the problem is "poor communications"—a failure to speak up, to express needs, to resolve conflict, to say no without hurting one's partner, to demonstrate care and appreciation, and to share. These empowering communication skills are not meant to develop power over one another. They are intended to facilitate interactions between partners in an ongoing process of active listening and expression, a consciousness-raising challenge in promoting healthy sexuality. Perhaps the term *enablement* more accurately describes this function, but I like to think about ways I can empower my students to jointly resolve sexual harassment, driving under the influence of alcohol, and joining with others in a memorial society to arrange simple, dignified, and economical funeralization or body disposition after death.

## LIFE-AFFIRMATION

When I inherited the death-and-dying course at Ball State University nearly twenty years ago, I adopted an operational principle that is best described as "life-affirmation" in relation to the various topics of thanatology. I chose not to dwell on mortality. Rather, I have deliberately tried to emphasize the positive, life-enhancing aspects of death-related topics.

Through a variety of learning opportunities, I try to explain grief as a normal and desirable response to bereavement. In studying the meaning of death, I emphasize the importance of appreciating others while they are still here and while we still have time to share our thoughts and affection. In a study of the autopsy, I clarify how the dead can help the living via "gifting," and how a postmortem exam can establish an assessment of clinical medical practice as well as reveal genetic defects that could possibly affect the children of the deceased. And most importantly, in studying various psychological reactions often displayed by dying individuals, I propose ways of relating to the dying and helping the dying to live as fully as possible—often through inclusive activities and the promotion of decision making.

## INTERCONNECTEDNESS

Regardless of subject matter or course title, I try to demonstrate the many interconnections that exist between and among the topics that are generally considered within the health science curriculum. In a study of alcohol and other drug problems, I emphasize the potential effects of drug use on college performance and dropout rates as well as the influence of advertising on the mind-set of many Americans who believe firmly that one cannot have fun at a party without consuming alcoholic beverages. When the course deals with human sexuality, I also discuss the expenses of childbirthing, the selection of a marriage counselor or sex therapist, and the portrayal of sex roles in movies and television programs. Whenever the topic is weight control, cancer, cardiovascular health, or even mental health, there is always a need to evaluate news reports, radio and/or television guests, and newly released books that claim some novel remedy or recommended regimen. We must have some basic criteria by which to assess the latest cure or approach to health maintenance, especially when dealing with "alternative medicine." And when the topic is AIDS, I will focus not only on transmission of the HIV virus and specific prevention techniques, but also on the impact of this modern epidemic on the current health care system and on the psychological responses of the person with AIDS.

First introduced to the ideas of interconnectedness and conceptualization by analyzing the School Health Education Study, or SHES ("Health Education," 1969), I still try to demonstrate the linkages between many topical areas and prove that all health education is really consumer health education. The original SHES study also made me more conscious of the comprehensive nature of the health curriculum and of the continuing need for establishing behavioralized teaching objectives to guide my classroom activities.

## ADMISSION OF HEALTH EDUCATION LIMITATIONS

It didn't take long for me to realize that health education does not have all the answers to personal or social health problems. Sometimes we recommend certain modes of action or lifestyling changes that are quite impossible for our target audience to adopt, due to unavailability of resources or lack of accessibility to those resources. Increasingly, I even question my right to intrude on the privacy of others so they will more likely accept predetermined reforms of their health behaviors. As a health educator, I willingly admit that I do not have all the answers to promoting health and preventing disease. But that will not stop me from asking probing questions that disturb people out of their complacency.

There is yet another aspect of health education's limitation that I have begun to realize: the very best health education experience may not result in changed health-related behavior if there is a lack of environmental supports, such as health-promoting legislative initiatives and governmental policies, engineering technology, and regulation of mass media advertising and business practices. With regard to alcohol abuse,

I have become more aware of the epidemiology of alcohol problems as I learned that many local governments allow three or more liquor stores in the same city block. And in spite of disclaimers from advertisers, it has become apparent to me that malt liquors are more heavily targeted to specific ethnic minorities, especially in inner cities. I am alarmed at the fact that many campus newspapers derive more than one-third of their revenues from alcoholic beverage ads. Alcohol abuse prevention remains a major challenge to health education.

Health education must now join with other environmental programs in an ongoing effort to promote health and prevent disease. Health education alone cannot do the job!

## REFERENCES

Beyrer, M. (1985). A health education collage: Future focus. *Health Education, 16*(April/May), 92–93.

Carroll, C., & Miller, D. (1991). *Health: The science of human adaptation* (pp. 4–5). Dubuque, IA: Wm. C. Brown.

Dubos, R. (1965). *Man adapting* (p. 263). New Haven, CT: Yale University Press.

Fahlberg, L., Poulin, A., Girdano, D., & Dusek, D. (1991). Empowerment as an emerging approach in health education. *Journal of Health Education, 22*(May/June), 185–192.

Health education: A conceptual approach to curriculum design. (1969). *The School Health Education Study* (Elena Sliepcevich, director). St. Paul, MN: 3M Educational Press.

Hoyman, H. (1965). An ecological view of health and health education. *Journal of School Health, 35*(March), 112–115.

Miner, K., & Ward, S. (1992). Ecological health promotion: The promise of empowerment education. *Journal of Health Education, 23*(November/December): 429–432.

Oberteuffer, D., & Beyrer, M. (1966). *School health education* (4th. ed., p. 14). New York: Harper & Row.

# CHAPTER

6

# THE HOLISTIC PHILOSOPHY AND PERSPECTIVE OF SELECTED HEALTH EDUCATORS

### STEPHEN B. THOMAS

Emergence of the holistic health movement has provided health educators an opportunity to participate in the ideological struggle between philosophical viewpoints: the concept of health and primary prevention versus problem-oriented health care. Reflections upon the nature of the universe and the nature of humankind are also part of this philosophical debate.

The philosophy of holism was formulated by Jan C. Smuts (1870–1950), prime minister of South Africa (1919–1924; 1939–1948), in his only philosophical work, *Holism and Evolution* (1926). Holistic concepts are not new to health educators; yet the work of Smuts is obscure and not quoted in the professional literature of health education. This lack established the need for research into the comparative relationship between the holistic perspective of selected health educators and the philosophy of holism as expressed by Jan C. Smuts. It is hoped this research will contribute to a better understanding of the holistic world view and the concepts of wholeness within health education.

From review of related health education literature and examination of Smuts' work *Holism and Evolution*, five categories were identified that served as the framework for the comparative analysis. The categories were (1) the nature of the universe, (2) the nature of man, (3) the relation of mind to body, (4) the view of human personality, and (5) the view of cause and effect.

Criteria for the selection of writings of health educators were established. The published articles and research of Jesse F. Williams (1886–1966), Delbert Oberteuffer (1901–1981), and Howard Hoyman (1902–1993) were identified as having a holistic perspective and were examined within one or more of the five categories.

Juxtaposition and comparison were used to determine the consensus, consistency, and overall significance between Smuts' philosophy of holism and the holistic perspective of Williams, Oberteuffer, and Hoyman.

## THE NATURE OF THE UNIVERSE

Smuts held the position that our view of reality and the nature of the universe was in the process of fundamental change: a change which would, in the end, affect every sphere of human thought and conduct. He believed that the 1859 publication of Darwin's *Origin of Species* stood out boldly as the inauguration of this change. The Judeo-Christian tradition of American education is based upon the premise that God created the universe, the world, and humankind. Yet it was within this context that Williams and Hoyman published articles that affirmed the theory of evolution as the operative principle in the universe and human nature.

Smuts considered that the viewpoint of creative evolution provided the best explanation of the whole-making tendency in the universe. According to Smuts, holism was the creative principle evolution of new forms. He identified five fundamental phases of progressive holistic synthesis in the universe: (1) physical mixture, (2) chemical compounds, (3) organisms, (4) minds, and (5) personality. These phases were arranged in a hierarchy and conceived by Smuts as stepping stones where lower phases served as the basis for the higher ones. From this perspective, mere physical mixture evolved into chemical compounds, that served as the basis for organisms which evolved minds, finally culminating in the emergence of human personality. Smuts (1926) considered that the transition from matter (chemical compound) to life (organism) occurred by way of a mutation, a quantum leap forward between Kingdoms. He writes that in the transition

> between the chemical compound and the cell, we have found . . . only a mutation— the greatest mutation of all undoubtedly in the whole range of science, but essentially nothing more than a mutation. (p. 57)

This served as the premise from which Smuts advocated that matter, life, mind, and personality were linked through the evolutionary whole-making tendency of the universe. This aspect of Smuts' holistic perspective of the universe is similar to

Williams' (1942), who also viewed the universe from an evolutionary premise. Williams identified a hierarchy of evolutionary phases based upon the observations of anthropology. These phases are (1) primordial mud, (2) flat worm, (3) quadrupeds, (4) apes, (5) man.

Williams' phases of evolution roughly correspond to Smuts' phases. He presented his phases of evolution based upon his observation of Homo sapiens' ancestral heritage. Williams did not elaborate on the details or transitions from one phase to another. Williams' phases are specific and can be categorized under Smuts' phases but not vice versa. For example, Williams' phase flat worm is encompassed by Smuts' phase organism, but not all organisms are flat worms.

The difference between Smuts' and Williams' perspective on the universe is in detail of explanation. Fundamentally, they agree on the premise that the universe has evolved through progressive phases, culminating in the evolution of human beings.

Hoyman's (1974) perspective on the nature of the universe is consistent with Smuts' holistic view that the universe has evolved. Hoyman's perspective, based on his ecological model, incorporates the influence of the environment and the reciprocal relationship between living things as fundamental aspects to the nature of the universe. Smuts (1926) supported the science of ecology and recognized that "the environment has a silent, assimilative, transformative influence of a very profound and enduring character on all organic life" (p. 218). The science of ecology was young at the time when Smuts published his work in 1926. In this regard, Hoyman's ecologic model is an expansion upon Smuts' perspective. Smuts' holistic perspective and Hoyman's ecologic model are complementary to one another regarding the evolutionary nature of the universe. In addition, from Hoyman's perspective, the universe is dynamic, not static. He considered that we live in a universe in which the earth and humans are still evolving. Smuts reached this same conclusion after rejecting the mechanistic interpretations of the laws of conservation and least action and the creation and metaphysical explanations of the universe. These views were based on a static universe, an unfolding of what was implicitly given. Smuts' holistic perspective considered that creative evolution included the mind. This view is supported by Hoyman, who also considered that the evolving universe included the "noösphere (sphere of mind)."

There is consensus between Smuts and Hoyman about the nature of the universe. They both acknowledged the role of ecology as a science to understand the effect of environment on organic life. Both Smuts and Hoyman viewed the universe as dynamic and still evolving; in this view, they included the sphere of mind. The difference between Smuts' and Hoyman's perspective on the universe is in what each chose to emphasize. Smuts' holistic perspective focuses on the holistic principle in the universe responsible for the progressive evolution of matter, life, mind, and personality. Hoyman's ecological model focuses upon human beings and their relationship to other life forms, the environment, and the potential for an ecological crisis resulting from failure to adapt to the environment.

## THE NATURE OF HUMANKIND

The holistic concept of a human being as an integrated whole, intimately and synergistically related to the environment, represents a reorientation of thought from a mechanistic to an organic view of human nature.

There is consensus between Smuts and Oberteuffer (1953) regarding a human being's integrated, indivisible nature. Both considered a human as a whole, greater than the sum of his or her parts. Oberteuffer's viewpoint was based on his belief that a human is "a being indivisible and whole, and who retains his integrated character . . . in the face of an adverse environment." Smuts' holistic viewpoint was based upon his theory that Homo sapiens represented the highest evolutionary integration of organic body and psychic mind. According to Smuts, a human is essentially a unique whole, the fullest expression of holism which nature has yet realized (1926, p. 152).

There is consistency between Smuts and Oberteuffer in their rejection of mechanistic and atomistic explanations of Homo sapiens' nature. Smuts rejected the mechanistic view that a human's essential processes could be explained in physiochemical terms. Smuts held that the mechanistic explanation of human nature "is only by way of analogy from lower forms of experience and not because man's spiritual structure is in any way of a mechanistic type" (1926, p. 152). According to Smuts, a human being "is a spiritual holistic being not a mechanistic type" (p. 152). Oberteuffer rejected the atomistic view that a human's essence could be functionally segmented. According to Oberteuffer (1965), the atomist "pulled man apart. They separated him into mind, body and spirit." Oberteuffer(1953) held that to study the segmented parts would throw little understanding on the whole of human nature because "the whole is something different from and greater than the parts." According to Oberteuffer, man is essentially a unified integrated whole organism.

There is consensus between Smuts and Hoyman about human nature. According to Smuts (1926), in essence a human being is a "spiritual holistic being . . . with sui generis categories of the mental and ethical orders" (p. 152). Smuts' perspective is based upon the progressive, creative evolution of human kind. He believed that Homo sapiens is the highest expression of holism that nature has realized. According to Hoyman (1972a), a human is in essence a self-determined, autonomous, self-actualizing moral agent whose "self-conscious awareness brings in a sui generis quality to his behavior compared to other life forms." Both Smuts and Hoyman indicate that moral, ethical, and spiritual dimensions are at the essence of human nature.

There is consistency between Smuts and Hoyman in their rejection of teleological vitalist explanations of human nature. According to Smuts, vitalists conceived of an outside "force" which distinguishes living from non-living bodies. He considers the vitalistic view "an assimilation of the concept of life to ideas . . . which . . . should be obsolete" (1926, p. 161). Hoyman (1974) rejected the viewpoint of reductionism which viewed a human as "nothing but" a robot or machine or animal, etc. He also rejected the view of environmental determinism and the vitalist concept of purposeful design. According to Hoyman, "man...has no rigidly predetermined teleological existence or essence."

## THE RELATION OF MIND TO BODY

Conceptualizations of the relation between mind and body fill the voluminous works of philosophy and no less science. In his address to the mind-body problem, Smuts presents holism not as a new fact but as a new framework within which to view the facts. His philosophy integrates body and mind within the forward whole-making tendency of creative evolution. Williams and Oberteuffer made clear their holistic perspective that mind and body were integrated elements within the totality of the individual.

There is consensus between Smuts and Williams about the relation of mind to body. Smuts considered that the evolutionary phase of organism and mind became integrated in the human being. According to Smuts, the integration of organic and psychic elements was synthetic and that "disembodied mind and disminded body are impossible concepts, as either has meaning and function only in relation to the other" (p. 261).

Williams (1943) advocated the view that mind and body were integrated elements within the unified whole of the human organism. His perspective was based on the scientific premise of human organismic unity. According to Williams, "[The] body is always and inevitably dependent upon what we call mind . . . [and] mind can only lead what is available."

Both Smuts and Williams rejected the dualistic viewpoint which separated mind from body and considered them independent entities. Williams warned physical educators against the "back-to-the body" idea and the concept of physical fitness as an entity. According to Williams (1942), when physical educators believe in mind/body dualism, "we tie our hands behind our backs and stand mute and dumb before all that science says about organismic unity." He advocated that physical education could never go back to education of the body because the dualistic implications were contrary to the scientific facts about the human being considered as a whole. Williams (1943) held the view that physical educators and health educators must accept mind and body as unified within the whole of the human organism or "erect a mystical concept of body, separated and distinct from mind." Williams' perspective is consistent with Smuts' holistic view that mind and body are not independent reals but instead are integrated within the whole person. Smuts and Williams supported the pagan concept of the body and opposed the Socratic and early Christian viewpoint. According to Smuts (1926), the pagan view considered the body clean, wholesome, and the embodiment of pleasure. He believed this was a natural and proper view (p. 265). Williams (1935) writes that "we need to revive, even at the risk of being called pagans, the delights and integrations of . . . the whole individual." According to Smuts, the historic error was the philosophical separation of mind from body which began during the fall of Roman civilization and the introduction of Oriental superstitions. He believed that the perversion of the body as evil had its influence upon "the spirit of Christianity . . . and instead of the body being regarded as 'the temple of the Holy Spirit,' it came to be looked upon as a fitter tabernacle for the devil." According to

Williams, the Socratic view of the body as a "prison from which the disciplined mind should escape" was the concept developed by the early Christians which "became to them such a conviction that release from the flesh was the only way for happiness."

Smuts believed that science rehabilitated the body and established the premise for its integration with mind within the whole person. He considered that holism was the antithesis of dualism (1926, p. 266).

There is consensus between Smuts and Oberteuffer regarding mind/body relations. Oberteuffer (1938) writes that his perspective rests on the premise expounded by Aldous Huxley who stated "mind and body form a single organic whole. What happens in the mind affects the body and what happens in the body affects the mind." Oberteuffer (1945) considered that his view of an integrated mind and body was in harmony with John Dewey, who stated: "It is the *whole* child we are educating—not just memory centers." According to Oberteuffer (1953), "mind and body disappear as recognizable realities and in their stead comes the acknowledgment…[of] a whole being." His viewpoint is similar to Smuts' holistic concept that in essence there is no relationship between mind and body because "all such action is synthetic and holistic . . . and no explanation which ignores the whole…can be considered satisfactory" (p. 272).

There is consistency between Smuts' and Oberteuffer's rejection of dualistic philosophies. Smuts rejected the philosophies of vitalism and mechanism because their inherent dualism resulted in life and mind as nullities. Oberteuffer rejected the early Puritanic philosophy inherent in schools and colleges begun originally to train the mind. According to Oberteuffer (1945),

> the early form of American education was cut in the form of devotion to a dualistic intellectualism in which mind was an entity unrelated to the remainder of the organism.

Smuts considered that the philosophy of holism resolved the mind/body problem. He believed

> the real explanation [was] that Mind and Body are elements within the whole of Personality . . . . [T]he most important factor of all in the situation . . . is holistic Personality itself. (p. 262)

The perspectives of Williams and Oberteuffer do not contradict Smuts' holistic resolution of the mind/body problem. There is fundamental consensus and consistency among the views presented.

## THE VIEW OF HUMAN PERSONALITY

Smuts contends that within the history of creative evolution the human personality emerged as the last of the five fundamental phases of holistic synthesis in nature. It was the fastest whole of evolution based upon the prior structures of matter (physical mixture and chemical compounds), life (organisms) and mind (conscious and unconscious central control).

There is consensus between Smuts and Oberteuffer that the human personality is integrated and requires self-expression and self-realization for normal adjustment. Oberteuffer (1945) considered that the very nature of health education and physical education provided "the opportunity for normal personality adjustment and integration through and by the satisfactions arising out of self-expression."

Smuts considered personality the evolutionary outgrowth of the integrated mind and body of the individual. According to Smuts,

*[p]ersonality . . . is a new whole…the highest and completest of all wholes . . . a creative synthesis of . . . organic and psychical wholes . . . higher than any of its predecessors. (p. 263)*

He advocated the concept that "personality is fundamentally an organ of self-realization" and through self-expression it is able to achieve the objective of wholeness: "The object of a whole is more wholeness…more of its creative self, more self-realization" (p. 290).

There is consensus between Smuts and Hoyman about self-actualization (self-realization) and the evolutionary basis of the unique human personality. Hoyman (1971) considers a human being a unified, self-regulating, self-actualizing organism. According to Hoyman (1972a), "human personality and character are also evolutionary and ecologic emergents." Smuts considers that the evolution of personality is a unique phenomenon in the world and each human individual has a unique personality. Hoyman considers that "personality refers to the unique features that distinguish one person from another." According to Smuts, the personality achieves self-realization through harmony with the personal character. He states further:

*when through its own weakness the character is degraded and a course of conduct embarked on which constitutes a denial of that fundamental tendency and aspiration towards wholeness, the . . . personality…is often strong enough to rescue the individual and . . . convert him to . . . moral wholeness. (p. 300)*

Smuts' view of personal character is similar to Hoyman's (1972a), who writes that "*character* refers to the person judged in terms of ethical standards of right and wrong." Both Smuts and Hoyman agree that human personality is not static but still evolving. Hoyman (1972b) writes that personality is in a dynamic process of growth and maturation within the individual from "cradle to grave." Smuts (1926) considers that personality is in a constant state of evolution towards wholeness which requires "the elimination of disharmonious elements from the personality" (p. 291). There is a basic difference between Smuts' and Hoyman's views of the heredity source of personality. According to Hoyman (1974),

*the basic sources of personality are heredity and environment . . . . [H]owever as [a] . . . child . . . interacts with environment factors, a unique individual emerges whose . . . self-structure becomes a third force in shaping . . . further personality development and behavior.*

According to Smuts, personality is not inherited. He believes that the individual inherits a body and mental structure slightly different from parents and ancestors. But above this organic and psychic inheritance, there is an individual personality which makes a unique and different blend of the organic and psychic composition. Smuts (1926) writes:

> What we inherit is not a ready-made affair but a wide possibility and potency of molding ourselves in our lives . . . . What above all is inherited is freedom. (p. 247)

Smuts and Hoyman differ in the status given personality within the individual. Hoyman considers the "self" as the integrating core of personality. He writes: "The self is . . . not a separate agent or entity; and it involves both self-awareness and death awareness." According to Smuts, personality is the integrating core of mind and body. He considered personality the highest achievement of holistic synthesis in nature. Smuts (1926) viewed personality "as a whole which in its unique synthetic processes continuously performs . . . the creative transmutation of the lower into the higher in the holistic series" (p. 304). Smuts considered the evolutionary emergents of personality to be the absolute values of truth, beauty, and goodness, and the holistic ideals of self-realization, creativeness, freedom, and wholeness. Smuts' holistic perspective encompasses Hoyman's (1970) view that "spiritual and ethical values are central to human personality development and mental health."

Smuts and Hoyman complement each other in criticizing the view of psychology and education regarding personality. Hoyman (1972b) considered his viewpoint consistent with Arnold Toynbee, who "stressed depersonalization and the destruction of human personality as the most critical problem of our time." From this premise, Hoyman criticized the personality development approach used by health educators. He considered it too sporadic, superficial, and naïve to be of much justice to personality. Smuts criticized the analytic method of psychology, which generalized and averaged personality. According to Smuts (1926), psychology "deals with the human mind, not in its individual uniqueness . . . . the individual differences are . . . considered negligible" (p. 278). From this premise, Smuts advocated the establishment of a separate discipline for the study of personality. He suggests the name Personology for this new science of personality, whose domain would be psychology and all sciences which deal with the human mind and body. The method of Personology would be biographical, with the goal to study

> human personalities as living wholes and unities in successive phases of their development . . . . [s]ynthetically, rather than analytically in the manner of psychology. (p. 262)

Smuts' holistic perspective encompasses and complements the views of personality expressed by Hoyman and Oberteuffer.

## THE VIEW OF CAUSE AND EFFECT

Smuts' perspective on cause-and-effect was a continuation of his synthetic holistic philosophy and rejection of dualistic concepts. He considered that the mechanistic and vitalistic viewpoints isolated cause-and-effect as sharply defined entities in which

*everything between this cause and this effect was blotted out, and two sharp . . . situations of cause-and-effect were made to confront each other in every case of causation like two opposing forces. (p. 16)*

He criticized science and philosophy of the nineteenth century which applied the rigid categories of physics to the hazy phenomena of life and mind. From this premise, Smuts rejected the lineal stimulus-response (S-R) model of causation. He considered the (S-R) model mechanistic and narrow. Hoyman also rejected the (S-R) model of causation. According to Hoyman (1974), the lineal (S-R) model was too simplistic and limited to the individual's input-output behavior, without consideration for the intervening variables within the individual considered as a whole organism-personality.

Smuts' holistic model of causation is similar to Hoyman's model of ecological web of causation. Smuts used the analogy of magnetic fields of force to explain his concept:

*everything has its field, like itself, only more attenuated . . . . It is in these fields only that things really happen. It is the intermingling of fields which is creative or causal in nature as well as in life. (p. 18)*

From this premise, he advocated the holistic model of stimulus-organism-response (S-O-R). Smuts considered that the organism completely absorbs the stimulus and transforms it into itself, so that the response or behavior is a result of the total organism rather than the passive effect of the stimulus. Hoyman advocated the concept of an ecological web of multiple interacting variables as the basis of causation. According to Hoyman (1971), "the causal webs of human health, disease, aging, longevity, and death are all interlinked dynamic processes in the organism-personality and are far more complex than appear on the surface." Hoyman's view that causation takes place in the dynamic, ecological web of multiple variables is similar to Smuts' holistic view that causation occur within the intermingling fields of force. Both agree that models of causation must take into account multiple intervening variables. Both Smuts and Hoyman are consistent in their rejection of the single factor, lineal causation paradigm.

## RECOMMENDATIONS AND CONCLUSIONS

Smuts' philosophy of holism is a well-established world view that provides a sound basis for the development of health education theory and practice.

The holistic perspective of Williams, Oberteuffer, and Hoyman continues to be fundamental to basic concepts within the historical tradition of health education as it was evolved into a separate discipline from physical education. These perspectives should be integrated with Smuts' philosophy of holism.

The holistic perspective will help health educators accomplish the goals of facilitating health as a positive condition of the individual as a whole. The philosophical tenets of holism are conducive to health education curricula based upon the conceptual approach, for example, the School Health Education Study, 1967. Holism can be synthesized into a philosophical framework from which the spiritual dimension of health can be developed without contradicting the science of evolution.

In addition, we should research and develop Smuts' science of Personology and the method of biography as one means to determine the principles of health as a dynamic condition of the individual considered as a whole organism-personality (synthetically versus analytically). Holistic research designs for health education may be derived from the work of the general systems theorists, such as Ludwig von Bertalanffy; the studies of existential, humanistic psychologists; and those psychotherapists who advocate a holistic view of humankind—for example, Perls' Gestalt therapy, Assagioli's psychosynthesis, and Tournier's "whole person" therapy.

Within the historical and philosophical context of holism, we can develop a set of principles to guide our attitudes towards health, our teaching methods, and our understanding of the relationships between mind and body, teacher and student, human and environment, health educator and the health care delivery system.

The holistic worldview serves as the rational premise necessary to produce health education professionals devoted to the understanding and furtherance of health as a positive goal.

## REFERENCES

Hoyman, H. (1970). An editorial: Health and a living faith. *Journal of School Health, 40*(6), 279–280.

Hoyman, H. (1971). Human ecology and health education II. *Journal of School Health, 41*(10), 538–547.

Hoyman, H. (1972a). Health ethics and relevant issues. *Journal of School Health, 42*(8), 516–525.

Hoyman, H. (1972b). New frontiers in health education. *Journal of School Health, 43*(7), 423–430.

Hoyman, H. (1974). Models of human nature and their impact on health education. *Journal of School Health, 44*(7), 374–381.

Oberteuffer, D. (1938). Re-evaluation of the professional curriculum. *Journal of Health and Physical Education, 9*(8), 469–522.

Oberteuffer, D. (1945). Some contributions of physical education to an educated life. *Journal of Health and Physical Education, 16*(1), 3–57.

Oberteuffer, D. (1953). Philosophy and principles of the school health program. *Journal of School Health, 23*(4), 103–109.

Oberteuffer, D. (1965). A challenge to the profession. *Journal of Health and Physical Education, 26*(1), 3–12.

Smuts, J. C. (1926). *Holism and evolution.* New York: Macmillan.

Williams, J. F. (1935). Today's challenge to health and physical education. *Journal of Health and Physical Education, 6*(8), 10–63.

Williams, J. F. (1942). Persons in a plan. *Journal of Health and Physical Education, 13*(6), 349–365.

Williams, J. F. (1943). Physiological implications of fitness in women's athletics. *Journal of Health and Physical Education, 14*(9), 469–509.

# PART

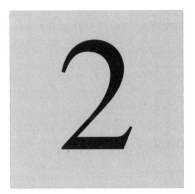

# DEVELOPING A PHILOSOPHY OF HEALTH EDUCATION

*Philosophy, as defined in the Oxford Dictionary of Current English (2006), is the study of the fundamental nature of knowledge, reality, and existence. It is an attitude (a way of thinking or feeling about someone or something) that guides a person's behavior. The study of philosophy aids individuals in the quest of understanding the world around and within as a whole entity.*

*Thus, if we are going to develop a philosophy of Health Education, we must consider some of the following issues: (1) human functioning—physically, mentally, emotionally, socially, culturally, or environmentally; (2) goals of humankind—the desirable future and the physical, social, emotional, cultural, or societal factors influencing it; (3) communication skills among varied populations—ages, parameters of life structure, and value systems.*

*Education and philosophy are fundamentally inseparable. Educational philosophy's unique emphasis is to examine the basic assumptions underlying particular areas of human knowledge. Philosophy within an educational context attempts to explain the ends and means of education in order to give guidelines to action. Philosophy helps to address the purpose, parameters, and content of the discipline.*

*The health educator must answer the question, What are the appropriate ways and means of health education in order to receive guidance for educational action? The answer lies in the philosophical approach one chooses and its corresponding underpinnings of beliefs about the purpose of health education, the role of the learner, role of the teacher, educational methodologies and content material.*

*Philosophical discourse in health education has been robust. A constant challenge to the health education profession is to clarify its philosophy in order to give the field clear direction and rationale. Health education philosophy helps to determine action and is the basis for a systematic development of goals and a foundation for values. A philosophy will provide you with direction for your continuing education, how you will function with other professionals, and how you will work with your designated population.*

## ARTICLES

The articles in this section present different personal views of philosophy and can provide you with ideas to consider for your evolving professional philosophy. Smith (2006) provides an historical overview of the development of key concepts in health education and emphasizes the need for health education students and practitioners to develop a personal philosophy of health education and to reflect on how that informs the development of their professional philosophy. Clark (1994) and Timmreck, Cole, James, & Butterworth (1988) suggest issues and challenges that they believe will influence the philosophical development of health education into and through the twenty-first century. They also call for a new way of thinking about these materials. Based on an examination of the health education literature, Welle, Russell, & Kittleson (1995), have identified five philosophical approaches that explore or demonstrate prevailing philosophical beliefs in health education. These perspectives have been incorporated in the organizational structure of this book.

## CHALLENGE TO THE READER

These four articles provide a bridge between concepts that influence the development of a personal philosophy and how these ideas can guide the continued development of professional philosophies as they are currently categorized in health education. Health educators will need to think critically about all of these issues and to continue to explore and develop emerging concepts.

# CHAPTER

## 7

# CONNECTING A PERSONAL PHILOSOPHY OF HEALTH TO THE PRACTICE OF HEALTH EDUCATION

**BECKY J. SMITH**

The World Health Organization (1946) defines *health* as "a state of complete, physical, mental, and social well-being and not merely the absence of disease or infirmity." Many health education and promotion professionals are familiar with this definition and accept it as their own. However, there are many definitions of health and it is useful to examine why they contain subtle differences and what those differences mean to health education professionals. Such an examination must build upon an understanding of the fundamental components central to the meaning of health. These components have been identified by individuals directly related to the field of health or health education and by scholars interested in the human condition.

In the past century, a number of scholars wrote about the nature and qualities of man to gain insight toward the meaning of health. Such scholars examined the entity and expression of health, thus providing health educators with a foundation for philosophical debate. Charles Darwin was one of the first renowned scientists to acknowledge the need for studying the human organism in relation to its environment. Not only was he concerned with the complete essence of man, but he also was interested in the overall environment, including natural and manmade elements (Muller, 1973). Jesse F. Williams, an early leader in the field of health and physical education during the 1920s, developed a perspective of health as "the quality of life that renders the individual fit to live most and serve best" and "a condition of the whole organism expressing its functions" (1935, pp. 10, 12). He felt that the development of health was contingent upon participation in quality experiences or activities by the whole organism. Through a compendium of articles spanning several decades, health education professionals such as Delbert Oberteuffer (1931), Mabel Rugen (1940), Howard Hoyman (1965; 1966), Robert Russell (1975), Russell & Hoffman (1981), Ann Nolte (1976), Richard Eberst (1984), and Jerrold Greenberg (1985) reinforced the holistic concept of health as the basis for sound health education.

One of the challenges inherent to implementation of a holistic approach to health and health education is language. The compartmentalization of language begins as we strive to define and discuss the various dimensions of human functioning which include, but are not limited to, physical, mental, spiritual, emotional, and social components (Eberst, 1984). As soon as different dimensions are identified and labeled, scientists begin to create measures to determine how well each of the dimensions is functioning. Biologists and kinesiologists develop measures for the physical dimension; psychologists, psychiatrists, and neurologists attempt to measure the mental dimension; and an even broader spectrum of professionals engage in describing and attempting to measure the social and spiritual dimensions of human functioning. In light of these measurements, health educators must question the potential and limitations of each dimension. Furthermore, health educators must continually challenge the definition of holistic health. For example, are individuals afflicted with paralysis considered "healthy" in accordance with the holistic model of health? Similarly, are individuals plagued by mental disabilities incapable of experiencing holistic health? These are the questions health educators must explore and resolve at a personal level before they can practice at an optimal level of effectiveness. There is no right or wrong answer to these questions, but each practitioner must have an answer that is consistent with his or her personal philosophy.

To illuminate the holistic concept of health, J. Keogh Rash stated, "Above all health is not and cannot be static or compartmentalized" (1960, p. 34). Rash's statement presents a challenge for health educators striving to act on behalf of their philosophical beliefs.

In past and current centuries, health educators have identified and developed various strategies to reflect their philosophical tenets. For example, a select group of health educators has focused on changing the unhealthy habits of individuals through behavior modification techniques (Green, Kreuter, Deeds, & Partridge, 1980; Greenberg. 2004; Hochbaum, 1981). Behavior change methods have ranged from reward and punishment to aversion therapy (Simons-Morton, Greene & Gottlieb, 1995). Other health educators have stressed the importance of changing individuals' attitudes about lifestyle factors that clearly have a great potential influence on health (such as smoking, nutrition, lack of exercise, and so on) (Ajzen & Fishbein, 1980). Another group of health educators has expanded the primary focus of health education to include the acquisition of credible information and the attainment of skills to utilize that information in support of healthy decision-making (that is, health literacy) (Joint Committee on National Health Education Standards, 1995). The logic behind the latter approach is that individuals can make future health-related decisions from the standpoint of having knowledge and skills (Bensley, 1993). All of these approaches have met with some success in helping people lead healthier lives, and yet, they also have fallen short in providing health educators with a consistent framework for understanding best practices in health education.

Where does all of this information leave the health education profession and, more importantly, the individual health educator? Essentially, this information leaves each health educator with a need for personal research and analysis about the human potential for health. Such research will help health educators identify, analyze, critique, and internalize the value of health-related concepts. When a health educator identifies and organizes concepts deemed as valuable in relation to health outcomes, he or she can begin to form a philosophical framework for functioning comfortably and effectively.

My personal journey through this exploration led me further and further into explorations of human potential and mind-body relationships within the science and social science disciplines. Such disciplines provide the basic knowledge health educators strive to apply in practice. My research transpired into a dissertation that examined the philosophical components of six renowned and highly relevant contemporary scholars including Rene Dubos, microbiologist, environmentalist, educator, and author; Erich Fromm, psychologist, educator, humanist, and author; Abraham Maslow, psychologist, educator, humanist, and author; Ashley Montagu, professor of anatomy and physical anthropology, educator, and author; Paul Tillich, philosopher, theologian, and author; and Paul Tournier, psychologist, physician, and author (Smith, 1976). My intent for this philosophical analysis was not to describe the scholars' contributions to my philosophy, but rather to develop an aggregate synopsis of their contributions to understanding the potential for health in mankind through their perspective of the qualities of man, human potential, and the expression of human qualities within individuals and society.

The philosophical components of these scholars reflected their perspectives regarding the expression of qualities inherent to man. The scholars' perceptions of man, human potential, and the expression of health within individuals and society, were explored. The selected scholars were chosen because of their unique and valuable professional contributions within and beyond their respective disciplines. Essentially, the scholars transcended the confines of their respective disciplines to study the holistic nature and well-being of man.

In essence, each scholar expressed belief that the development of human potential is equated with the evolutionary process of man's responses to environmental stimuli. The evolutionary process is partly a function of man's choice and partly a result of genetics and environmental influences.

Tillich and Tournier believed that part of the process also results directly from the grace of God. Each of the scholars emphatically stated that the development of our potential, within the limitations of our existence, is an essential need. If an individual does not reach his or her potential, then he or she will not achieve inner harmony and health. Development of human potential is infinitely significant to the development and maintenance of health.

Although the definitions of health developed by Dubos, Fromm, Maslow, Montagu, Tillich, and Tournier vary, they share strong commonalities. Their definitions support the concept that health is an expression of quality of life. When the positive quality of one or more life processes is hampered from external or internal sources, full development and actualization may falter and a greater potential for illness or disease may result.

Numerous barriers compromise the potential and expression of health. Perhaps the most paramount barrier perceived by the scholars is lack of opportunity for the development of full humanness. According to the scholars, not developing the capacity for full human functioning will be a source of distress, illness, and disease. As such, individuals must attempt to discover and embrace opportunities for developing their full human potential and expressing health and quality of life.

Studying these scholars helped me develop a personal understanding of how individuals express health and how the potential for health can manifest despite severe limitations in one or more dimension(s). I have come to believe that when external and internal elements that facilitate development of human potential are available, individuals are more likely to experience optimal health. This has helped me understand my role as a health educator responsible for assisting individuals, communities, and society. It also has led me to believe that nearly everyone expresses some level of health even when they are confronted with the most devastating circumstances. I prefer to look for that expression of health as a starting point for professional interaction, education, and enhancement of health rather than focus on existing debilitation.

## CONCLUSION

As stated earlier, each health education and promotion professional should study the dimensions of human functioning to develop a set of personal beliefs and subsequent framework for professional practice. The aforementioned framework represents a professional philosophy. The philosophy should provide a personal definition of health grounded in dimensions deemed important for addressing the complete essence of an individual. Once developed, the philosophy gives direction and provides a sense of professional comfort and expertise to the practitioner.

Health education professional preparation programs have a responsibility to provide a forum for the philosophical development of their students. Many students enter a graduate program with a professional philosophy that is functional for their needs. However, the majority of students (including those at the graduate level) have not consciously reflected on development of their personal philosophy of health and health education. The academic setting represents an ideal environment for the pursuit of philosophical development because it allows rich opportunities for collegial dialogue that expand and solidify individual thought. From both a programmatical and personal perspective, the development of philosophical frameworks is perhaps the most neglected professional endeavor in health education. However, it is never too late for an individual to invest time and effort in personally clarifying his or her philosophy. After all, the rewards are personally and professionally satisfying.

## REFERENCES

Ajzen, I., & Fishbein, M. (1980). *Understanding attitudes and predicting social behavior.* Englewood Cliffs, NJ: Prentice-Hall.

Bensley, L. B., Jr. (1993). This I believe: A philosophy of health education. Eta Sigma Gamma Monograph Series, *11*(1), 1–7.

Eberst, R. M. (1984). Defining health: A multidimensional model. *Journal of School Health, 54*(3), 6–11.

Green, L. W., Kreuter, M. W., Deeds, S. G., & Partridge, K. B. (1980). *Health education planning: A diagnostic approach.* Palo Alto, CA: Mayfield.

Greenberg, J. S. (1985). Health and wellness: A conceptual differentiation. *Journal of School Health, 55*(10), 403–406.

Greenberg, J. S. (2004). *Health education and health promotion: Learner-centered instructional strategies* (5th ed.). New York: McGraw-Hill.

Hochbaum, G. M. (1981). Behavior change as the goal of health education. *The Eta Sigma Gamman*, 3–6.

Hoyman, H. S. (1965). An ecologic view of health and health education. *Journal of School Health, 35*, 110–123.

Hoyman, H. S. (1966). The spiritual dimensions of man's health in today's world. *Journal of School Health, 36*(2), 52–63.

Joint Committee on National Health Education Standards. (1995). *National health education standards: Achieving health literacy.* Atlanta: American Cancer Society.

Muller, H. J. (1973). Reflections on re-reading Darwin. *Bulletin of the Atomic Scientists, 7*, 5–8.

Nolte, A. E. (1976). The relevance of Abraham Maslow's work to health education. *Health Education, 7*, 25–27.

Oberteuffer, D. (1931). Two problems in health education. *Journal of Health, Physical Education, and Recreation, 2*(2), 3–6, 46–47.

Oberteuffer, D. (1953). Philosophy and principles of the school health program. *Journal of School Health, 24*(4), 103–109.

Rash, J. K. (1960). Philosophical basis for health education. *Journal of Health, Physical Education, and Recreation, 1*, 34–35.

Rugen, M. E. (1940). Needed curriculum revision in the field of health education. *Journal of Health, Physical Education, and Recreation, 11*(9), 532–535.

Russell, R. D. (1975). *Health education: Project of joint committee on health promotion in education of the National Education Association and the American Medical Association.* Washington, DC: National Education Association.

Russell, R. D., & Hoffman, F. S. (1981). *Education in the 80s: Health education*. Washington, DC: National Education Association.

Simons-Morton, B. G., Greene, W. H., & Gottlieb, N. (1995). *Introduction to health education and health promotion* (2nd ed.). Prospect Heights, IL: Waveland Press.

Smith, B. J. (1976). *Selected writings and their relationship to an ontology of health: An analytical study.* Unpublished doctoral dissertation, University of Illinois, Urbana.

Williams, J. F. (1935). Today's challenge to health and physical education. *Journal of Health, Physical Education, and Recreation, 8*, 10–12.

World Health Organization. (1946). *WHO definition of health*. Retrieved from http://www.who.int/about/definition/en/print.html.

# CHAPTER

## 8

# HEALTH EDUCATORS AND THE FUTURE: LEAD, FOLLOW, OR GET OUT OF THE WAY

**NOREEN M. CLARK**

$B$ecause I live in Michigan, a reader might think that I stole the title of this article from Lee Iacocca (who used it in a car commercial) or that he stole the phrase from me. In fact, we both stole it from someone else.

Since this is an article about health education, the future, and leadership, I thought this was a good title. The point I want to make is that it is crucial that we provide invigorated leadership in health education as the twenty-first century draws near. If we don't shape the direction of events in health education, others less able will. The forces of change are moving quickly, and if we don't guide them, we'll have no choice but to follow or be pushed out of the way.

I am focusing this discussion in response to three questions:

1. What is the context for change between now [1994] and 2050—the trends that will reshape America in the next sixty years?

*Note:* This article is intended to be read for its pholosophical perspective. Originally published in 1994, it may contain factual material or examples that are dated.

2.  What kind of health education is needed as we move into the next century?

3.  What do health educators need to do to meet the future with confidence?

## FIVE THEMES THAT DRIVE CHANGE

This is a time of unprecedented change in the world. At least five things have been identified as central themes that drive change (Cox & Hoover, 1992). I'm going to suggest that in this moment, the practice of health education, and we as health educators, are confronted by all five—and because we are—as we move toward the new century we will fundamentally change the way we do business.

1.  Whether or not we recognize it, changes in society will cause *changes in our essential mission as health educators.* Our future task will not be to teach people facts—to focus on their cholesterol number—the mission will be to help them become more analytical thinkers, to be more able to deal with an uncertain and complex environment. We will become people's health enablers, helping them to manage new and confusing information and to make decisions in turbulent situations.

2.  Our *identity and image is changing.* In my professional lifetime, health behavior has moved from obscurity to the forefront of American culture. Health is "chic" and more and more Americans are meditating, eating right, and exercising. By association, we've been carried along on this wave to prominence, and we have the potential for increasing credibility with a large audience that will become even larger.

3.  Our *relationship to key stakeholders in the arena of health is changing.* The medical care establishment is slowly but surely experiencing an erosion of power. The public is rethinking its health goals—slowly but inevitably shifting from notions of longevity coupled with high tech medicine to notions of quality of life. We have the potential for newer and stronger partnerships with the people and communities who have always been the heath education constituents. Medicine by necessity will become partners with us. Collaboration and partnership have new, more powerful meaning for health education.

4.  There are *changes afoot in the way we work.* We are in the midst of a shift back to community-based health education interventions after more than a decade of focus on individual behavior. We have a renewed sense of urgency for helping to empower communities to find appropriate solutions to their health problems. At the same time we have an amazing array of technology at our disposal. We can reach people in new and powerful ways. I recently went to Washington, DC where, at the offices of the Red Cross, a television hookup connected me to AIDS educators around the country, and together we explored ways to improve community education for AIDS. Computers, fax, and television are changing the way

we work. Technology will be central to health education of the future but the emphasis will be technology for people, not *in spite of* people. User-friendly, people-focused technology *is* the future.

5. Finally, we are undergoing a massive *change in culture* in our society. We are literally looking different as a nation and the conventional majority values and norms are being challenged as we become a more diverse, more ethnic, more interesting culture. Health educators have long prided themselves with working across cultures and being sensitive to individual differences. The cultural changes that are in the works, however, are of a greater magnitude than any of us have experienced previously.

I want to look a bit closer at all these themes of change—the forces propelling us into the twenty-first century. We can begin with the last, the demographic changes we are undergoing which will transform us into a new culture. Let me provide a few statistics as a backdrop for discussing the trends I see occurring.

## MINORITIES, AGING, NEW TYPES OF FAMILIES, AND ACTIVISM

Two numbers almost tell it all:

1. By the year 2000, 35 percent of school age children will be what we conventionally have termed minority: African American, Latino, and Asian;

2. By the year 2000, one-fifth of the population will be over the age of 65.

These statistics deserve elaboration (see Gerber et al., 1989; Naisbitt & Aburdine, 1991; Miller, 1991). In 1985, 14.9 percent of all school children in America were Black—by 2000 this figure will be 16 percent. In 1985, 9.6 percent of school age children were Latino, by 2000 the number will be 16 percent. Fertility and immigration patterns indicate that Latinos and Asian Americans are the fastest growing minority groups in the country. By the year 2000, over 10 million people in the United States will be of Asian descent, and in California they will be the number-two minority group, exceeded only by Latinos.

The White non-Latino population is growing more slowly and is expected to have decreased from 73 percent in 1985 to 66 percent by the year 2000. In some areas the change is particularly vivid. In New York City, by 2005, 35 percent of the population will be Latino. Whites and Blacks will represent 25 percent each. By 2025 over 40 percent of New York City residents will be Latino, and figures for California will be similar. From these data it is clear that we are rapidly becoming a society where minorities are the majority.

In the late 1980s, 30 million Americans were over 65, and that is 12 percent of the population; by the year 2000 this group will be 20 percent. By 2025, people over 65 will outnumber teenagers two to one, and by 2030 one in every four people will be 65 years or older. By 2000, just around the corner, there will be five million Americans of 100 years or more. Willard Scott and the *Today Show* will not be able to wish them all happy birthday every morning. The over-85 set is a fast growing group. Two-thirds of it is female.

This unprecedented shift in age distribution has been called the "age wave" or the "graying of America." Whatever term you prefer, America literally is getting older. A trend tied to the age wave is the fact that we are outgrowing the youth culture.

Around 2010, when the baby boomers reach their 65th birthdays, we *really* will feel the shift to maturity. The boomers have been likened by demographers to a pig in a python. They are a great bulge moving through time and society. When they become senior citizens, their tastes, interest, concerns, and experiences will dominate America.

A few more interesting statistics: In 1988, 80 percent of white children lived with both parents, 50 percent of Black children lived with both parents, and 78 percent of Latino children did. There has been a fairly consistent decline in the number of children living with both parents that is expected to continue into the future.

The number of female-headed households is increasing. By the year 2000, 48 percent of Black households will be headed by females. Childbirths to unmarried women are increasing. This is the case only with Whites and Latinos, not with Black women.

There also are more single people than ever in the United States who are living alone. One quarter of all U.S. households are single adult households. Among other things, this statistic means that more and more Americans are delaying marriage.

By the year 2000, the under-age-five population will have declined to 16.9 million and is expected to stay below 17 million for the next sixty years.

Gay men and lesbians are a more and more vocal segment of our population. Figures generally used suggest that this group constitutes between 10 and 15 percent of Americans. Parenthetically, these individuals earn more household income, are more educated, and are more employed than the average American.

These data suggest that there is a fundamental change in the nature of American households—most of us need to rethink our concept of family. Families of the future will be smaller, nontraditional, and will operate with a new set of norms. Ties of friendship will become as thick as blood as different arrangements of people come together to help each other with childcare and eldercare. Older people functioning as families so they can attend to their mutual needs, cohabiting couples, single parents, gay and lesbian couples with children, all will demand new laws, new policies, new procedures, and new health education in recognition of these new types of family.

The demographic shifts we are experiencing are contributing to changing forces of influence in the country, and greater activism. Women are an ever-increasing power within society. We have made great strides over the years, but political events related to women's rights and sexual harassment in the recent past have seemed to galvanize women even more to exert their influence alongside men.

Most of the working women in this country are not the career-driven supermoms we see in the media. Most women are working less for the fulfillment of a career than because it now takes two incomes to meet the household budget without a setback in the standard of living. The wage gap persists (women earn about 66 percent of what men earn). This fact will continue to motivate women to push forward their agendas.

Obviously, minorities and women will exert even greater influence in all aspects of American life in the coming decades: in the media, in school, work, and music and art. Given the history of racism and discrimination in the United States, minority groups that have grown in numbers are organizing for parallel growth in political influence.

This means more and more citizens will be learning to be activists—to make their demands heard and influence felt. It also means there is potential for culture clash as different groups exert their wills.

In addition, older adults now and increasingly in the future will be organized and constitute a formidable political influence. Currently, the American Association of Retired Persons has a membership in excess of 30 million. Some writers have speculated about "age wars" in the future as we struggle to support the older generations—to meet their needs and demands—while at the same time serving their grandchildren and great grandchildren (Dychtwald, 1990).

As the years pass and the flower children of the 60s and baby boomers of the 70s reach maturity, there will be even more activism among the elderly, as these are groups for whom speaking out has been a tradition and fitness and good health a preoccupation.

Finally, one thing we all have in common is the environment. Public awareness—and in some cases wrath—is increasing daily about risks to the planet, not to mention ourselves.

There is a real feeling afoot, especially among the young, that society has been greedy and unthinking when it comes to the ecology. Americans lag behind Europeans in the way they have organized socially and politically around environmental issues. We will see more and more environmental activism in this country, and it will cross age, economic, regional, cultural, and partisan lines.

## NEW THINKING FOR A NEW FUTURE

This is a dynamic context in which all of us have to do the work of health education: activism, changing sources of influence, clashes across cultures and generations, competing values about what's right, and good, and necessary, extreme cynicism about politics and political leadership, and we can, of course, throw in a worrisome economy. All these accompany the dramatic demographic changes we're seeing.

Quite frankly, the turbulence of the current time depresses some people and scares others. It is hard to maintain a sense of security and confidence when the old way of doing business does not solve new problems. Why is it we have such trouble dealing with change and why do we see it as so disruptive?

Two writers, Ornstein and Ehrlich (1989), have speculated that the mismatch between what the society needs and what we actually do is a function of old minds confronting a new world.

I won't go into great detail about then-theories, but one or two ideas are instructive. They suggest that since the beginning of human time, we have had to condense the enormous amounts of information available in the environment into manageable dimensions. We've had to develop a kind of mental shorthand. They call this creating caricatures of reality. Because we can't deal with all the stimuli in any given experience, we tend to retain the elements of reality that are most proximate and simple to understand. We haven't developed long-term memories or much tolerance for complexity. We tend to trivialize things and make them local. The media, of course, has made the whole world our neighborhood, and events in the far corners of the globe are experienced as if they were next door. We quail at the news of terrorist attacks thousands of miles away, highly unlikely to occur to any of us—they become a kind of public obsession and dominate the news—while we ignore much more salient occurrences such as slow but significant increases over time in the number of homeless Americans, or the gradual thinning of the ozone layer—tragedies that really are occurring in our own backyards.

We respond to the immediate and simplified caricature of a menacing terrorist and overlook the dull statistics that indicate over time the development of fundamental societal problems. Our learned response is to notice and personalize discrepancies, emergencies, scarcity, anything we are told is "news." We have to develop a new way of thinking to live up to the challenges of the future. We have to give up being short-term thinkers and develop the long view, to analyze situations rather than personalize them. We have to look far enough back in time to understand our development as a society and to see the trends that are evolving that help or threaten our quality of life. We have to plan for long-term solutions as opposed to expecting the sitcom 30-minute resolution for serious societal problems.

For those of us in public health and education, this means we have to help people to give up the search for instant cures and for preventive panaceas. We have to stop behaving as if organized medical care is responsible for longevity and enhancing health status. We all know that the changes in death rates and levels of health we have seen over the past decades have been a result of better sanitation, better nutrition, changed behavior, and better environmental conditions, and not new developments in medical technology. The general public, however, doesn't get this. They ignore or fail to see that improvements come from gradual non-newsworthy changes in behavior and the social and physical environment. We have to help people forego the hype. Hype has become the hallmark of modern life, and we consistently confuse important issues with unimportant ones.

We have to help people to understand and rectify the human predilection for using simple caricatures. We have to help them to take the long view, analyze statistics, understand different cultures, think probabilistically. This is an especially important role for those of us working with children.

## THE LOOK OF THE NEW HEALTH EDUCATION

What will health education look like when it is created by health educators whose thinking has caught up with the new world we are living in? Health education will be empowering. Let me suggest some key words that will characterize it: values, process, cost effectiveness, quality of life, integration, and multi-level.

## Values

Many of the problems we are confronting as a society are a matter of values. The pro-choice movement is a matter of values. Operation Rescue is a matter of values. Economic growth versus protection of the ecology—values. Money for the military versus money for health programs—values. Alas, scientific advances only complicate the question of values.

There are no formulae for doing what's right. Being right requires careful thought, humility, and hard work.

As a society we have to get agreements on what is important, what we value. It's not a matter of your values being better than mine. It's a matter of creating a society where both our values can co-exist. I was reading an article (Simon, 1992) about the woman who is the head of the American Librarians Association. She said, "Three areas that seem to be the focus of a great deal of censorship are sex education, satanism and witchcraft, and health education." Health education is going to have to go to the ground for some values—for example, the right to know. We can't possibly do our work if we can't address the issues. I'm sure you're aware that we are the only developed country that runs obscure ads on television about AIDS—the basic message is "learn about AIDS"—great, from whom? In other countries, in Europe at least, people are given the facts, and the what's needed to protect oneself is clearly presented. In this country, TV can show murder and mayhem but not condoms.

Health education of the future will place more emphasis on values clarification—in helping people to be courageous, to find out what they really value, to make informed choices.

In helping people to get clear about their values, we also have to account for culture and the different way values are played out in different cultures. We have to focus on the things that make people feel valued and respected. A lot has been said about being politically correct. But, political correctness can risk trivializing an important principle. What we have to focus on is not creating so many new politically correct labels that we're afraid to talk to each other—but on creating dignity and respect for all. A colleague of mine has put it very well. He says, "[W]e (health educators) have to begin with developing an awareness and knowledge of culture which implies a non-judgmental acceptance of the worth of all ethnic groups—a willingness to see people as much as human beings as members of a particular group. . . . [T]he final stage is to be able to perform a specific task while taking culture into account such that the outcome is better than it would have been had the role of the client's culture not been considered" (Neighbors, 1992). This is the kind of value that empowering health education reflects. And health education has to re-dedicate itself to finding processes that reach individuals who embrace different values.

## Process

The core of health education practice in the future will be helping people learn how to learn. The rapid production of information—the technological explosions occurring monthly mean that facts get outdated before they're disseminated. What's effective practice one week is ineffective the next. Life is not as simple as following a formula for risk reduction or anything else. Health education in the new century will help people learn how to use data, how to be analytical, how to make judgments, how to tailor their own solutions to their own needs, in short, to learn how to learn.

## Cost

There will be, however, no give on the issue of cost. Health education interventions will need to prove themselves as not only affordable, but generating cost savings. We will confront a three-way paradox if there is such a thing: reach large audiences with programs that are at the same time relevant to cultural differences and cost effective. The need for solid demonstration research will be as great or greater than it has always been. The need for efficient practice will not lessen.

## Quality of Life

The measure of successful health education in the future will be whether or not people judge the quality of their lives to be better because of it. There will be a major paradigm shift where health and medical care will be deemed effective if people feel they are functioning optimally and are happy. Knowledge tests, attitude scales, objective tests of health status, and measures of health care utilization will only be relevant as they relate to individual and community views about the quality of life. To define quality, we'll work even more closely with our clients to understand how they want their lives to be and how they perceive health education as useful to them.

## Integration and Multi-level Services and Education

We need to perfect our mechanisms for designing and delivering multi-level approaches to priority health problems, approaches that make health education optimum. We have to develop approaches that adequately address the complexity of the health problems we face. With apologies to Simons-Morton and colleagues (1988), I will try to summarize their observations on how we can have major impact on health problems by addressing several strata of a problem at once. They suggest that our health education has to work on at least three levels: governmental, organizational, and individual. We have to consciously target "key" government and community leaders, organizational decision makers, individuals at risk. We need governments that are operating on the basis of healthful policies, regulations, and programs. We need organizations that enact healthful policies, maintain healthful facilities, implement healthful programs. We need individuals who are healthful in their behavior, and in the physical and psychological aspects of their life. All these levels must be involved to engender improved health status in the society.

We already have experience with multi-component, multi-level programs. Smoking cessation is a good example. Our efforts in the United States have included information campaigns, smoking restrictions, health provider counseling, incentives such as reduced insurance premiums, smoking cessation clinics, and school health education.

Another area is one I'm familiar with, asthma education. The National Institutes of Health is undertaking a national asthma education program which is producing media campaigns and informative materials; a major professional education effort is underway, as is patient education provided by hospitals. There are efforts to change school system policies prohibiting asthma medicine-taking at school; there are family education programs being made available by voluntary organizations; there is involvement of major professional associations such as the Thoracic Society and the School Nurse Association; there is a push for changes in reimbursement policies to cover asthma self-management education.

These multi-faceted programs targeted at several levels of influence will be the norm in the future. Our efforts have to become larger, to have wider impact (Cofield, 1992; U.S. Department of Health and Human Services, 1990), to be delivered through partnership and collaboration with all the relevant organizations and groups. We will see these integrated, multi-level efforts in school health also (Behrman, 1992). There is growing recognition of the need to integrate education, health, and social services within our school system. We're moving beyond the notion that one system—schools—can address all the needs of kids, to the idea of partnerships of systems in which the school will be the fulcrum. Despite the current controversies about schools as the place for delivering health services and effective sex education, schools in the future will be key in collaborations to serve kids health and social service needs. The gap between school and community services will by economic and moral necessity close. The lines between school and community, and school work and real life, will disappear.

## LEADERSHIP FOR HEALTH EDUCATION

These observations bring us inevitably to the question of leadership. The failure of leadership in the United States is a big topic of conversation. At least one pundit has noted that leadership has been confused with parroting out-of-context findings of public opinion polls. Political leaders listen to the pollsters, determine the direction of the latest survey, adopt those opinions for the moment, and purport to be leading the parade. This isn't leadership—it's the exact opposite.

In health education, we have to create leadership and shape the flow of change (Beckhard & Pritchard, 1992), change that is responsive and sensitive to the people we serve. How do we do this? We have to start with ourselves personally. We have to exercise leadership and help to develop it in others. What is leadership anyway? One expert in the field of business put it this way: "[A]n effective leader is the person who has a long and well-integrated memory, constantly open to new input" (Hine, 1991). A leader shows the way, guides, causes progress, creates a path, influences, begins.

Here is one writer's version (Cox & Hoover, 1992) of the ten commandments of leadership. I think they describe how a health educator becomes personally powerful:

1. cultivate a high standard of personal ethics;

2. maintain a high level of energy (don't get worn out by the petty issues, but trust your own judgment on these and see the big picture);

3. know what your working priorities are so you can remain stable under pressure;

4. have courage (isn't it the Marines who say, "do what you fear or fear will be in charge");

5. have commitment and dedication (no one ever worked himself to death on a job he loved);

6. go with the urge to create because innovators own the future;

7. have a goal;

8. maintain enthusiasm (this is mostly important because it's contagious);

9. stay level-headed, which means see things as they really are, not as you wish they were;

10. help others to grow—an open exchange of ideas leads to synergy and synergy means change.

As health education leaders, what should we do to meet the future with confidence? A 1992 paper by ASTDPHE president Brick Lancaster presented some ideas. In it he stated that a fundamental task for health education is to close the gap between practice and research. In brief, he recommended that we create many kinds of opportunities for researchers and practitioners to talk to each other and influence each others' work. He recommended that practitioners give up their anti-intellectual ways and utilize findings from health education research more often and more effectively. He recommended that researchers forego their "we're too sophisticated for you" attitude and develop research that is more based on realities as they exist in the communities we're supposed to be serving. He gave examples of ways in which practitioners and researchers have forged collaborations and both groups have benefited. He also suggested that we create a national health education agenda perhaps by establishing a public and private partnership of academic, government, voluntary, and private organizations. This is a great idea, and I would recommend a technology subcommittee. Why not establish advanced technology groups: collaborations between researchers and practitioners that emphasize how people can use technology to learn. We need a group to (1) identify promising technology; (2) rethink existing paradigms for education and explore how various forms of technology could transform the way things are done now; (3) share the vision broadly in the field of health education; (4) anticipate consequences of use of technology and find ways to reduce any potentially negative effects; and (5) transfer and disseminate health education technology that proves effective.

What are other things we must do? Tool up and keep up. Most of us take part in conferences and continuing education. These are ways of keeping up. What is it that we're not doing? Getting out into the community that we want to reach to find out what is really going on there? Learning to use a computer or a new program? Reading the most recent issue of a health education journal? Getting some innovative health education started in your organization, even though you think the cards are stacked against you? Creating a partnership with another organization even though there's been no collaboration in the past? Tool up, tool up, the twenty-first century is around the corner.

## SOME CONCLUDING OBSERVATIONS

Physicists say that electrons can move both forward and backward in time. Using this analogy one could say that the future is not out there in front of us but resides in this very moment—wasn't it Pogo who said we have met the future and it's us?

With this idea in mind, there are some tasks I think are especially important for every health education leader. We need to think through the topics that need to be added to our health education programs to keep them salient in the coming decade and create new ones to address new needs.

One can think of a range of topics: health practices sensitive to issues in minority or aging populations; integrating physical/mental/emotional aspects of health; environmental safety and health; family relationships; ethical decision making; cultural aspects of health issues; new approaches to forestalling health problems through risk reduction; self-management of chronic diseases, including HIV; dying (activist older adults will want to have as much say over the circumstances of their death as they've had over their life—people will quite literally want to learn how to die); genetic counseling and use of genetic information in decision making; the relationship of new medical procedures to quality of life—one could go on and on.

We also need to explore new channels for getting health education into the action. A number of channels will be on the forefront in the next thirty years: *activism*—we need to capitalize on all the power and energy that's out there for our health education agendas; the *workplace*—proposals for health insurance will only increase the need to get effective health education into the place of employment; *health care organizations*—there is more and more receptivity to the idea that health education makes a difference in the management of disease—this venue will remain an important setting for our programs; *peer education*—the huge number of older adults already functioning as peer educators is a hint of the power of peer education to come; *technology*—the possibilities are exciting.

Why do we need a sense of the future? To keep an eye on life and try to nudge incessant change toward a direction we recognize as progress. "No person can lead other people except by showing them a future. A leader is a merchant of hope." This speaks to my admonition to us all to lead health education into the new century.

And, related to the idea of following or getting out of the way, "even if you're on the right track, you'll get run over if you just sit there, 'cause the times they are a'changing."

## REFERENCES

Beckhard, R., & Pritchard, W. (1992). *Changing the essence: The art of creating and leading fundamental change in organizations*. San Francisco: Jossey Bass.

Behrman, R. (ed.). (1992, Spring). *The future of children*. Center for the Future of Children, David and Lucile Packard Foundation, 2(1).

Cofield, G. (1992, Feb.–Mar.). Can public health combat today's health problems? *NewsReport*, National Research Council, *42*(2), 22–24.

Cox, D., & Hoover, J. (1992). *Leadership when the heat's on*. New York: McGraw-Hill.

Dychtwald, K. (1990). *Age wave: How the newest important trend of our time will change your future*. New York: Bantam.

Gerber, J., Wolff, J., Kiores, W., & Brown, G. (1989). *Lifetrends: Your future for the next 30 years*. New York: Stonesong Press.

Hine, T. (1991). *Facing tomorrow: What the future has been, what the future can be*. New York: Knopf.

Lancaster, B. (1991). Closing the gap between research and practice: A commentary. *Health Education Quarterly, 19*(3).

Naisbitt, J., & Aburdine, P. (1991). *Megatrends 2000*. New York: Morrow.

Neighbors, W. (1992, Apr. 18). Some thoughts on the concept of cultural competence (personal communication).

Ornstein, R., & Ehrlich, P. (1989). *New world new mind*. New York: Simon & Schuster.

Miller, E. (1991). *Future vision: The 189 most important trends of the 1990s*. Dubuque, IA: Kendall/ Hunt.

Schroth, R., & Mui, C. (1991, Nov./Dec.). Focusing on the future: Advanced technology groups. *Indications, 8*(2).

Simon, J. (1992, Apr.). Far from meek and mousy, The American Library Association is a staunch upholder of the right. *Northwest Airlines*.

Simons-Morton, D. C., Simons-Morton, B. G., Parcel, G. S., & Bunker, J. F. (1988, Aug.). Influencing personal and environmental conditions for community health: A multi-level intervention model. *Family and Community Health*, 25–35.

U.S. Department of Health and Human Services, Public Health Service. (1990). Healthy people 2000: New objectives to promote health, prevent disease. *Prevention Report*.

This article is based on an address to the Association of State and Territorial Directors of Health Education and Centers for Disease Control, Kansas City, Missouri, May 20,1992. Originally printed in *Journal of Health Education*, May/June 1994.

# CHAPTER

## 9

# HEALTH EDUCATION AND HEALTH PROMOTION: A LOOK AT THE JUNGLE OF SUPPORTIVE FIELDS, PHILOSOPHIES AND THEORETICAL FOUNDATIONS

THOMAS C. TIMMRECK
GALEN E. COLE
GORDON JAMES
DIANE D. BUTTERWORTH

Historically, health education (instruction for hygiene) was founded on concerns such as the lack of physical fitness in school children or military inductees. Habits such as drug and alcohol use, viewed detrimental to society and especially children, were also a focus of many original health education activities. Health education, with its early ties to physical education and medicine, evolved to the point where health education was associated with physical education and mostly abandoned by medicine. When medicine lost its obsession with the "miracle drug" penicillin, and not being able to "cure" viral infections, it again recognized that education toward prevention "works" and that the mind is connected with the body, influencing disease and healing processes, and that behavior and lifestyle are associated with health status. Health education once again became more acceptable to medical science.

As chronic diseases continued to have a heavy impact on the nation's health status and as chronic diseases, coupled with an aging population, began using the health care dollar at a rate beyond all predictions, prevention, health education, and health promotion began to take on new meanings. With many disease states no longer caused by microorganisms, health education soon became a possible solution to many medical problems facing the nation, especially the preventable and behaviorally founded diseases and syndromes.

Health education and health promotion represent a behavioral science discipline, which offers a unique preventive perspective, knowledgeable enough in the medical sciences to effectively educate and divert groups of people from needing expensive clinical medicine. Thus health education and promotion have become more behavioral science than medical science with physical education and fitness being an important but minor focus of concern from the holistic perspective.

Health education for many years has promoted "health" from a holistic perspective. Now "holism," "lifestyle," and "wellness" are being embraced by many segments of the helping professions, medicine, and business. Because of the global concern for health and lifestyle, the fields of health psychology, behavioral medicine, medical/health anthropology, medical sociology, education, and human services, and others also claim a similar perspective, resulting in a jungle of theories, philosophies, and approaches. Health education, needing a clear identity, has tried to decide which aspects of these various disciplines to accept, embrace, adapt, or reject. It is obvious that many theories and approaches from these various disciplines are of great use and benefit to health education and health promotion. The dilemma faced by health education is to discern which or how much of the theory of related or supportive fields to accept and apply while avoiding becoming or duplicating that discipline. The result is a jungle of theory for health education to utilize from other supportive disciplines. However, the theory in a health education or health promotion context is not clearly delineated, nor is it organized in a manner that is clear. Consequently health education lacks direction and a well-organized theoretical base from which to develop the field. Health education research, certification, competency-based training, teaching and process development, planning, and evaluation are not done in an organized manner because there is no common basis of philosophy and theory upon which to rely (Timmreck, Cole, James, & Butterworth, 1987). Health education's uniqueness beyond related fields lies in its ability to marry the field of behavior science to medical science knowledge and in turn provide educational, counseling, and behavior change skills in a variety of settings that will have the greatest impact on preventing future illness, disability, and death.

## BEHAVIORAL SCIENCE CONTRIBUTION

When instruction for health was found to be less effective than desired, and with disease states related to lifestyle and behaviorally founded conditions, new developments in other fields that were applicable were quickly noticed. One area that was appropriate for health education to observe was the behavioral sciences. Behavioral science is a broad field encompassing all of psychology, anthropology, sociology/education, and the sub-areas of each and related fields—that part of knowledge and study that deals with the actions and interactions of all of mankind and on an individual, group, or community-wide basis. Certain aspects or segments of theory and application from the various behavioral science fields seemed to be natural for health education and health promotion.

In psychology the behavioralists introduced learning theory, behavior modification, then behavior therapy, opening the door for health education to embrace "behavioral change." These new ideas were incorporated into the already tangled health education processes, although changing a person's behavior after a crisis occurs (such as when a heart attack victim stops smoking) is considered tertiary prevention. Even though this is not primary prevention and is treating the problem after the fact, health education embraces these types of activities (Vojtecky, 1984).

Behavior change as an adaptation from behavior therapy assumes that education based on learning theory has the potential of influencing and changing behavior. In turn, education for health is considered a useful intervention that can be applied where attempts to change unhealthy behaviors are warranted. Proponents of this approach accept a pre-determined set of values which are assumed to contribute to the health status of the individual and health status in general (Simons & Padres, 1980; Parcel & Baranowski, 1981). Some proponents of the field (Ward, 1981) believe that health education should reflect more than a pupil's knowledge or lack of it, behavior change being one goal of prevention and health education.

Obviously there are major differences in various approaches to health education practice. Although proponents of the various approaches espouse health knowledge and see health education as having an important role in terms of informing specified individuals or groups in matters regarding health, a major difference exists between these groups regarding the issue of behavior change. The behavior change group accepts the challenge of attempting to rid society of undesirable health behavior by implementing educational and behavior-modifying interventions in an attempt to produce a healthier population. However, along with accepting this challenge, the behavior change camp also increases the risk of failure due to inherent complexities of the behavior change process.

All these approaches to health education and promotion are commendable and necessary. However, future trends resulting from current economic downturns will require more accountability from health educators to justify health promotion efforts and show that efforts are cost effective. The future health educator will have to "produce" in order to qualify for scarce monies regardless of the sector, public or private. Behavioral change approaches are most likely the area of health education to come under the scrutiny of cost effective performance appraisal, especially in hospitals and the worksite where accountability is measured in terms of productivity, funds produced, clientele seen, costs contained, and increased efficiency and effectiveness (Parlette, Glogow, & D'Onofrio, 1981). Behavior change in the form of behavior modification and behavioral therapy is also the tool of counseling psychology, clinical psychology, marriage and family counselors, social workers, psychiatrists, and psychiatric nurses, all of which are licensed clinical fields, thus putting health education in an uncomfortable position as being considered not a clinical area nor licensed to practice.

Educational psychology has been useful to health education in its understanding of processes that occur in the teaching side and learning end of health education activities or in health promotion programs involving individual or group instruction. Counseling approaches, techniques, and methodology which has roots in counseling, psychology, social work, marriage and family counseling have been looked to also for patient education and health counseling aspects of the broader health education field.

A long-standing approach to health education centers around cognitive development, another fundamental principle of psychology. As used in health education, cognitive development is directed toward making students more independent thinkers and learners. Viewed from a cognitive perspective, health education is directed at enhancing the intellectual domain as it relates to health. Students are taught concepts, learning techniques, and are shown how to assemble bits and pieces of knowledge to arrive at rational conclusions. Cognitive psychology added to the entanglement of the field attempts to increase awareness among learners concerning the position that health and lifestyle occupy in an individual's experiences and goals. However, it does not address behavior directly. Thus the recipient of health education is provided with an opportunity to address intellectually health related concerns deemed important to his or her well-being. Through cognitive awareness, the gap between lack of knowledge about health matters and new findings and learnings can be closed more than with only learned knowledge reinforced.

Health education long has been dependent on certain areas of the social sciences, mostly sociology, social psychology, anthropology, and marriage and family life. Community health education particularly has benefited from findings and theories of these fields. Community health education clearly deals with groups, systems of people, communities, and the various strata of the populations aligned, not by boundaries of city or counties, but by age, sex, race, income, minority status, disease commonalities, or culture.

## EDUCATION'S CONTRIBUTION

Teaching methods, processes, skills, approaches, techniques, and education theory always have been the mainstay and foundation for health education, especially school health instruction aspects. Due to the extensiveness and complexity of the contribution provided by education, only a brief mention is provided here, as a separate paper would be required to address this subject. Psychology and behavioral sciences provide a foundation for many aspects of education. Education in turn provides health education with much of its founding principles. Thus the lines which separate these two supportive fields are unclear. A clear delineation of how both of these have contributed to health education is also an entangled thicket. Yet almost all dynamics that occur in the health education process—that is, health instruction, community health education, patient education, health counseling, and various aspects of health promotion—rely on education theory and underlying educational psychology principles. Health education historically found that concepts, like activities from the bottom of the "cone of learning" and experiential learning, were much more effective than approaches used in "hard science" subjects which rely on a certain amount of role learning.

## BIOMEDICAL SCIENCE'S CONTRIBUTION

One of the first areas where preventive medicine and health education have been effective and moderately well received is in the area of communicable disease prevention. The marriage of disease prevention and health education was natural. The understanding of the cause, epidemiology, and communication of disease and how the transmission of disease can be prevented requires an understanding of the biological and medical sciences on the health educator's part. The health educator has to be able to communicate with professionals in the medical and health care community, all of whom rely on a biomedical educational foundation. Medical terminology and health care administration skills and knowledge are fundamental to successful community health education and health promotion (yet are missing from most curriculums). Credibility in all aspects of health education, from school health instruction to health counseling to management of community health education programs, relies on some competency in the biomedical sciences.

## MANAGEMENT'S AND MARKETING'S CONTRIBUTION

Community health education, wellness programs, and health promotion projects do not rely on a single person to have sole knowledge of health topics and health and medical content areas. Moreover, employers of persons expected to do health education activities outside the health instruction setting expect the health educator to have management and administration skills which minimally include accounting, budgeting, human relations/management, computer science, organization/program development, controlling, supervision, and coordinating. Having an extensive amount of knowledge and understanding about health topics and content areas does not get management of the program accomplished nor help show the boss, board of directors, or administrator that the health promotion program is cost effective. This area has been lacking in many health education programs, and today much resistance has been shown in acceptance of the need for administration training. The management need is ignored by the academic community in all of its tradition and pomposity, while graduating health educators face the real world and the job market without marketable administrative skills demanded by employers. Marketing of health education has been viewed as being akin to unethical practice in the field. If health education is to be effective in changing values and behaviors, it must embrace vigorously any field that will further the cause. The interfacing of marketing with health education is long overdue. If as much money and effort were put into health promotion through recognized marketing methods as has been put into promoting the use of tobacco and other disease promoting products, the picture of the health status of the country possibly would be different. The lack of use of the media and marketing is obvious by its absence in health education (except on a rare occasion or unique disease outbreak such as AIDS). Television can and should have a major impact on the quality of life of all persons and should be utilized to advantage. There is hardly a person of any age or educational level who does not know something about AIDS or hunger in Africa, primarily because of television news reporting, clearly demonstrating once again the impact that television can have in health education and health promotion activities.

Management's research on motivation has much to contribute to the field of health education and promotion, yet rarely is discussed. Health education is faced with motivating persons to activate a healthy lifestyle, to motivate people to change behavior, and motivate people to maintain positive health behavior already in practice. Motivation is an area from which health education could further develop and create a theoretical foundation (Timmreck, 1977; Timmreck & Randal, 1983).

Rarely considered in the jungle of health education and promotion theory and practice is management's expectation of outcome. That is, does the health educator/ promoter have a positive or negative productivity level in comparison with other professionals or workers? Are health educators and their programs a cost center (costing the organization) or a profit center (financially effective)? These are concerns of administration and management and are essential for future survival of all health education programs outside school health instruction (Parlette et al., 1981).

## FIELDS RELATED TO HEALTH EDUCATION

Health education has had only limited success in the field of patient education. Nursing has been successful in laying solid claim to the area. Nursing has the clinical training, and physicians who order patient education put much more trust in the nurse than the health educator, as the latter usually has little or no clinical training and thus limited credibility with most physicians.

Another infringement felt by health education has been the advent of several new related fields. Psychology has developed the field of health psychology. Behavioral health, a field less clearly attached to psychology, but clearly founded in the behavioral science aspects of health and medicine, is gaining prominence. The medical field has developed the area of behavioral medicine, combining education, counseling, and medicine. Further, how does the Association of Teachers of Preventive Medicine fit into the scheme of health education, or does health education fit into it? How do medical sociology and medical anthropology fit in with health education other than providing good training or supportive theory? Community psychology and social work also have been involved in health education and preventive-medicine-type activities. How do these fit in? (Doley, Meredith, & Ciminero, 1982; Bartlett & Windsor, 1985; Kane, 1974; McGuire, 1981; Millon, Green, & Maegher, 1982). These questions have an answer, yet need to be contemplated and the answers sought so that the identity of the health education field not be lost and a clear theoretical direction can be established.

## THEORETICAL PRESENTATION IN THE LITERATURE

One way the theoretical foundation of health education will be established is through the literary aspects of the professions. Without the cooperation and support of current periodicals, theory will not be advanced and the current status quo position will remain. Current major journals of the field need to examine more closely the types of articles they choose to publish. One of the purposes of professional societies' information vehicles (major journals, monographs, and special issues) is to advance the theoretical basis of the profession. It is known that theoretical-foundation-type articles may be refused for publication in favor of process or more attractive articles that in the opinions of the editors are more likely to be attractive to the readership. An analysis of publication activity of the two major journals (*Health Education* and *Health Education Quarterly*) for the last five years provides some insight through a comparison of the numbers of articles published in several categories, including the one entitled "theoretical" (see Table 9.1 and Table 9.2).

TABLE 9.1.  **Types of Articles Published in *Health Education*, 1981–1985**

| Content | Process | Research | Theory | History | Yr |
|---|---|---|---|---|---|
| 15 | 32 | 18 | 7 | 2 | 1985* |
| 13 | 27 | 19 | 5 | 2 | 1984 |
| 36 | 42 | 18 | 6 | 1 | 1983 |
| 33 | 33 | 9 | 8 | 3 | 1982 |
| 15 | 39 | 9 | 8 | 3 | 1981 |
| 112 | 173 | 73 | 34 | 11 | 5-year total |

*Excludes special centennial issue

**TABLE 9.2**   **Types of Articles Published in *Health Education Quarterly,*
1981–1985***

| Content | Process | Research | Theory | History | Yr |
|---------|---------|----------|--------|---------|-----|
| 2 | 4 | 7 | 3 | 0 | 1985 |
| 5 | 8 | 14 | 2 | 0 | 1984 |
| 2 | 3 | 6 | 3 | 0 | 1983 |
| 4 | 4 | 11 | 1 | 0 | 1982 |
| 6 | 11 | 3 | 4 | 0 | 1981 |
| 19 | 30 | 41 | 13 | 0 | 5-year total |

*Excludes special cancer issue

   Brief definitions of the headings/terms of the charts are necessary for clarification. A theoretical article, to an editor of a journal, likely would be one which presents learnings, information, or new findings, not a research article. However, in this article, the term *theoretical* means those articles which provide a philosophical and theoretical body of knowledge, one that provides substance and knowledge for the basis and foundation of the field of health education and health promotion. "Content" articles provide information other than research, a did-you-know article, new learnings in the content areas of health education that can utilize the process aspect of the field in order to deliver information. "Process" articles are the how-to-do-it articles which provide teaching and presentation ideas, techniques, skills, methods, roles, or program development ideas. "Research" articles are the ones that use a research design, use descriptive or inferential statistics in their presentations, and show that research actually was conducted. "History" articles advance an understanding of the beginnings of the profession by presenting what was done in the past (see Table 9.1 and Table 9.2).
   The journals of the profession should consider their current [1988] posture in accepting/rejecting theoretical articles (as per the definition above) in relation to the other types of articles, thereby fulfilling their responsibility to contribute more to advancing the theoretical basis of the profession. Another solution is to consider the approach the American Academy of Management has taken, that is to have two journals, one for the informational articles and another professional journal for research and primarily academic articles.

## WHY HEALTH EDUCATION THEORY?

Theory is essential to any profession. It provides direction and organizes knowledge into a pattern so that facts, information, data, observed activities, and learnings are interconnected in a manner which takes on meaning that would not exist in isolation. Thus interconnected learnings provide a basis, foundation, reason, and direction for process activities and research endeavors. Health education has struggled to find recognition as a separate discipline (Kreuter, 1979). The profession has focused on "process," taking learnings from other professions and fields and incorporating these into health education methods and health promotion activities. Process is as much a part of health education as theory ought to be. Unfortunately, process is picked as the major area of focus because it is more fun and exciting than theory. However, without a clear theoretical basis for the process, research and process methods become isolated and fragmented activities. Health education/health promotion, of all professions, is in a position to grasp and organize learning from the various fields it relies upon. Theory sheds light on similarities in knowledge and processes which appear dissimilar and disjointed, yet are heavily depended upon. Thus theory would be the machete which would cut through and organize the jungle currently experienced by the field (Organ & Hamner, 1982). When a diverse and fragmented body of knowledge exists, as in health education and health promotion, sound theory becomes useful as a means of summarizing diverse information into a body of knowledge. Theory allows a profession to gather and handle large amounts of information and empirical data having a limited number of propositions (Shaw, 1970). If health education were to be based theoretically, it would have quick and easy approaches to presenting what we have learned and believe about health education. This, in turn, would change the focus from so much attention paid to process aspects of health education to turning the jungle of fragmented information into useful data (Lipnickey, 1985; Lorig, 1985). In national conferences, professional publications, textbooks, and in the classroom, health education professionals cry out for more research. They plead "to be recognized as a profession." "We must justify and verify our credibility through research," is the cry. "The only way the medical profession and others will accept and recognize health education as a separate profession is to demonstrate our worth through hard research." With an element of truth in this cry, it is a mere echo in the classroom as the broader prayer rings empty, for the research is fragmented and provides little direction for the profession as a whole since it is not based on a solid organized theoretical health education foundation. For clarification, it is not to say that much of the research is not based in a recognized theoretical basis from another field, as it often is. A theoretical direction is the basis for any solid research project. If a clearer health education theoretical base became available, we would be prompted to do research which furthered the field instead of conducting research which is done out of personal or committee interest, an approach to be tolerated in a new and developing field (Oberteuffer, 1985).

If health education research could be done from a health education theoretical base, research would be prompted which would cut through the thicket of mimicking other fields and advance from a developing field to a more established one. This research approach would demonstrate a new direction and new perspective while not duplicating related professions. Instead of mimicking other respective support fields, a self-established theory for health education would allow the development of real and functional applications in and for the health education field. If a theoretical basis for health education research becomes available, health education researchers will explore new hypotheses about phenomenon and issues important to the advancement of health education and health promotion. Questions concerning the advancement of health education and health promotion, which otherwise would have been glossed over, would never be asked. As research is pondered, it would be able to cut through the jungle and develop a true health education research basis. If such accomplishments occurred, the profession would move beyond simplistic, superficial, obvious, and trivial research questions to more inquisitive, profound, and important hypotheses. Accepting pragmatic aspects of the current profession's theoretical status, it is wise to accept the research as it is done and utilize it to the best advantage of health education. Since the field is still in the developmental stage of theory development, it must use whatever approaches and sources that are appropriate. From the Role Delineation Project one can realize that many disciplines can and do use health education skills, methods, and approaches. Health education pulls together an amalgamation of skill development from many supportive fields so it can be applied to health education efforts.

Health education theory does not stop with mere analysis of findings and crunching of data, nor with ideas which originally gave birth to the research. It goes further by offering tentative inferences, profound observations, and predictions about how findings impact health education theory and relate to future implications.

Without a theoretical foundation for health education research, we get lost in its jungle since little direction is offered as to what to study, how to study it, or how to make inferences from it that contribute to the theoretical body of knowledge. If the health education researcher really wants to advance the field and have it recognized and accepted by the world and other professions, he or she must first operate in the conceptual world, using sound assumptions and logic, then arrive at effective yet pragmatic conclusions about the relationships of health education variables to the information and data it relies on. The informal theoretical state of health education needs organizing, summarizing, and guiding functions as a formal theory. The need for integrating a theoretical conceptual framework, a framework that links processes and activities is an essential tool for health education and health promotion and should not be discounted.

Health education and health promotion need to continue efforts toward further developing health education theory. Meanwhile, gathering and recognizing research appropriate for the use of health education also must be furthered.

A final belief that some professionals in the field hold is that health education lacks in a uniqueness that will allow the field to be divorced from the supportive disciplines. Our uniqueness, when it does occur, is in the application and process of theories and knowledge from other fields. As an eclectic discipline, we do represent an amalgamation of theories and practices from supportive fields. This fact is probably the main reason for lack of certification; with no real, unique clinical skills and a body of knowledge that is not our own, certification is probably not a real possibility. The task at hand is to separate the theories, concepts, skills, methods, approaches and knowledge from other fields and integrate them into one organized, usable, and recognizable discipline. If we rely on the philosophy and theories of other disciplines and have a mutual interdependency, we need not only to accept and recognize this phenomenon, but also to organize it so that sound theory and research results. Since health education is plagued by lack of uniqueness, the Role Delineation Project and interest in certification may not be realistic goals nor easily accomplished.

Because theory development in the health education discipline is still in its infancy, it must take on the full range of development, from proactive and retrospective exploration of supportive areas, to delineation of current activities, to planning future directions. In the field of health education we need to keep the doors open to a constant questioning and challenging of the discipline and not settle for the status quo. The religiosity flavor found in promoting the cause of well-being for a nation, quality of life for the community, and a healthy lifestyle for the individual cannot afford to be blinded by any resistance to self-criticism. Being self-critical can be the key to advancement of the profession. Only by questioning and a search for theory, activities, and research will learned growth and development occur. A close-minded religiosity-type approach to health education will deny the self-challenging and questioning that allows a healthy growth and direction. Since health education has the unique position of bringing together theory from "the supportive areas," only through critical self-questioning will it as a discipline develop enough to be able to formulate the philosophy, theory, skills, and learnings in a useful, organized, and practical manner.

## REFERENCES

Bartlett, E. E., & Windsor, R. A. (1985, Fall). Health education and medicine: Competition or Cooperation? *Health Education Quarterly, 12*(3), 219–229.

Doley, D. M., Meredith, R. L., & Ciminero, A. R. (Eds.). (1982). *Behavioral medicine*. New York: Plenum Press.

Kane, R. L. (Ed.). (1974). The behavioral sciences and preventive medicine. *Proceedings of the Conference of the John E. Fogarty International Center for Advanced Study in the Health Sciences and the Association of Teachers of Preventive Medicine*. Bethesda, MD: National Institutes of Health, Department of Health, Education, and Welfare.

Kreuter, M. W. (1979, February). A case for philosophy. *Journal of School Health*, p. 116.

Lipnickey, S. C. (1985, October–November). Health education to the third power (cubed). *Health Education, 16*(5), 47–49.

Lorig, K. (1985, Fall). Some notions about assumptions underlying health education. *Health Education Quarterly, 12*(3), 231–243.

McGuire, W. J. (1981, May–June). Behavioral medicine, public health and communication theories. *Health Education, 12*(3), 8.

Millon, T., Green, C., & Maegher, R. (1982). *Handbook of clinical health psychology*. New York: Plenum Press.

Oberteuffer, D. (1985, April–May). Two problems in health education. *Health Education, 16*, 50–53.

Organ, D. W., & Hamner, W. C. (1982). *Organizational behavior*. Plano, TX: Business Publications.

Parcel, G., & Baranowski, T. (1981, May–June). Social learning theory and health education. *Health Education, 12*(3), 14–18.

Parlette, N., Glogow, E., & D'Onofrio, C. (1981, Summer). Public health administration and health education training need more integration. *Health Education Quarterly, 8*(2), 123–146.

Shaw, M. E., & Costanzo, P. R. (1970). *Theories of social psychology*. New York: McGraw-Hill.

Simons, R. C., & Padres, H. (Eds.). (1980). *Understanding human behavior in health and illness*. Baltimore: Williams and Wilkins.

Timmreck, T. C. (1977). Motivation-hygiene theory adapted for education. *High School Journal, 61*, 105–110.

Timmreck, T. C. (1986). *Dictionary of health services management* (2nd ed.). Owings Mills, MD: National Health Publishing.

Timmreck, T. C., Cole, G. E., James, G., & Butterworth, D. D. (1987). The health education and health promotion movement: A theoretical jungle. *Health Education, 18*(5), 24–28.

Timmreck, T. C., & Randal, J. (1983). Motivation, management, and the supervisor nurse. *Supervisory Nurse, 12*, 28–31.

Vojtecky, M. A. (1984, Fall–Winter). An adaptation of Bigge's classification of learning theories to health education and an analysis of theory underlying recent health education programs. *Health Education Quarterly, 10*(3/4), 247–262.

Ward, W. B. (1981, May–June). Determining health education impact through proxy measures of behavior change. *Health Education, 12*(3), 19–23.

# CHAPTER

# 10

# PHILOSOPHICAL TRENDS IN HEALTH EDUCATION: IMPLICATIONS FOR THE TWENTY-FIRST CENTURY

HELEN M. WELLE

ROBERT D. RUSSELL

MARK J. KITTLESON

These are exciting times for the health education profession. Increasing demands are being placed upon the health education profession to assist in health promotion and disease prevention strategies (U.S. Department of Health and Human Services, 1991), and a strong self-directedness will assure successful participation for the profession. Yet health education has been accused of defining itself in a reactionary mode, alternating its mission and philosophy as the situation demands (Kreuter, 1979). Oberteuffer (1977) stated that a discipline without a philosophy lacks direction. Shirreffs (1988) articulated that a clearly delineated mission and philosophy of health education would determine participation in various national health efforts. Our profession is at a critical stage of self-evaluation, of which philosophical inquiry is a key element. Answers to the questions of what health education is (mission) and how one accomplishes this (philosophy) will determine the place of health education now and in the future.

Over the past twenty years there has been persistent, continuous outcry by the leaders in health education for the need to define a philosophy for the profession (Oberteuffer, 1977; Balog, 1982; Rash, 1985; Timmreck, Cole, James, & Butterworth, 1987, 1988). Some professionals have indicated that a clearly stated health education philosophy would help guide the profession in its activities (Landwer, 1981; AAHE Board of Directors, 1992). Yet as health educators perform a multiplicity of roles in a variety of settings, a single philosophy of health education does not seem possible or even particularly desirable. Rather, what the health education profession needs is a clear delineation of the major existing philosophies and an analysis of current trends in health education philosophies.

*Philosophical inquiry will be needed to move us to our rightful place as an instrument for improving the health of the nation and its people.*

*Shirreffs, 1988, p. 38*

## BACKGROUND

Numerous accounts of personal philosophies of health educators exist (Beyrer & Nolte, 1993). Yet very few health educators have attempted to decipher overall trends of health education philosophical options (Russell, 1976; Shirreffs, 1988; Kittleson & Ragon, 1993). Russell (1976) presented six philosophical positions represented on three continuums: *decision making* versus *specific behavior, behavior change* versus *behavior reinforcement*, and *functioning* versus *rule following*. Shirreffs (1988) contended that the health education profession has three major philosophies: *information-giving, behavior change*, and *social change*. Kittleson and Ragon (1993) concurred with these three and added a fourth: *decision making*.

Certain threads of congruency are noted within health education philosophical discussions. *Cognitive-based* philosophy is historically the most well-rooted (Shirreffs, 1988). This approach allows a large base of knowledge to be transferred relatively quickly and is viewed as a foundation upon which other philosophies can be built (Creswell & Newman, 1989; Kolbe, 1982). *Decision-making* philosophy became a prominent force in the mid-1970s as an alternative to *cognitive-based* philosophy (Dalis & Strasser, 1977). *Decision-making* philosophy is viewed as a systematic approach to education, designed to equip learners with certain skills which enable them to make self-satisfying decisions. Green, Kreuter, Deeds, and Partridge (1980) legitimized *behavior change* as an appropriate ways and means for health education. Examples of successful *behavior change* philosophy in all types of health education settings have inundated professional journals for the past fifteen years. In 1975, Russell defined *functioning* as a viable health education philosophy. This philosophy of health education is interested in how people function totally, despite some practices not generally correlated with health. Greenberg (1978) reiterated these beliefs, establishing a health education philosophy that he entitled *freeing*. Finally, the *social change* philosophy developed by Freudenberg and advocated by O'Rourke (1989) was identified as a persistent and pervasive philosophy in the discipline. *Social change* philosophy proposed to expand health education's purpose to include a political function and to recognize social variables that influence individual health. Thus, five dominant health education philosophies that encompassed most of the current philosophical trends for the profession are *cognitive-based, decision-making, behavior change, freeing/functioning*, and *social change*. Table 10.1 presents a brief description of these philosophies, as given to the participants in this study.

In order to expound and explore the theoretical bases of health education philosophies, a literature review was conducted on other educational disciplines that similarly operate from a variety of philosophical assumptions. Philosophically, the educational profession most closely aligned to health education was adult education. According to prominent adult educators, there exist five dominant adult education philosophies: liberal *(cognitive-based)*, behaviorist *(behavior change)*, progressive *(decision-making)*, humanistic *(freeing/functioning)*, and radical *(social change)* (Elias & Merriam, 1980). Health education philosophies are analogous to adult education philosophies, with variations observed in name (as noted in above italics) and historical evolution. In adult education, clarification of the theoretical bases of each philosophical paradigm included delineation of the following categories: purpose, methods, key words/concepts, role of teacher, role of learner, and historical evolution (Elias & Merriam, 1980). This groundwork was utilized by the researchers to help differentiate the health education philosophies.

*Every health educator has a philosophy of health education somewhere which is giving direction. For it to become more useful and fruitful, its possessors must work consciously with it.*

Nolte, 1976, p. 26

## METHODS

The study utilized a quasi-experimental descriptive approach. Data collection and analysis included quantitative and qualitative methodological triangulation (Patton, 1990). The purpose of the study was to ascertain if there is a single dominant philosophy ascribed to by health educators and to discover any variations in philosophical preferences between health education academicians and practitioners. The five categories of health education philosophies were (1) *cognitive-based*, (2) *decision-making*, (3) *behavior change*, (4) *freeing/functioning*, and (5) *social change*. In fall 1994, a survey was mailed to health educators randomly selected from the following two national lists: the 1992 Eta Sigma Gamma (ESG) National Directory of College and University Health Education Programs and Faculties and the 1992 Membership Directory of the Society for Public Health Educators (SOPHE). For the purpose of the study, subjects found on both lists were deleted from the SOPHE list prior to sample selection to ensure integrity of two groups of health educators: academicians and practitioners. Survey sampling technique for this study involved proportionate stratified random sampling. Twelve percent of members from both lists elicited sample sizes of 98 for ESG faculty and 107 for SOPHE members, for a total of 205 subjects.

## TABLE 10.1   The Five Health Education Philosophies

| Philosophy | Description |
| --- | --- |
| Cognitive-based | Content focused, emphasizes factual information and the expansion of the health knowledge base of the individual. |
| Decision-making | Designed to teach systematic problem-solving skills and decision-making processes that can be applied to health-related decisions. |
| Behavior Change | Emphasizes behavioral modification through such methods as self-monitoring, behavioral contracts, and goal setting. Program objectives are quantifiable and measurable. |
| Freeing/Functioning | Designed to help learners make self-directed and autonomous health decisions. Emphasizes concepts of freedom, individuality, and lifelong learning. |
| Social Change | Proposes education as a force for achieving social change. Health education is closely connected with emphasis on raising awareness for responsible social action. |

The Health Education Philosophy Inventory (HEPI) was developed to ascertain philosophical beliefs and preferences of health educators. (Requests for copies of HEPI can be sent to Dr. Helen Graf at Georgia Southern University.) Instrument items included five vignettes and their corresponding philosophical continuum, open-ended questions, a rank order exercise, and a demographics sheet (see the box for a sample vignette). Each vignette represented a different health education setting, topic, and two philosophies. The corresponding philosophical continuum gave the health educator an array of choices between two health education philosophies. Vignettes were fashioned so that respondents were forced, unknowingly, to make choices that reflected certain health education philosophies. Within these educational situations, health educators made "blind" choices for philosophical preferences in the "real world." Exhibit 10.1 is a sample of a vignette included in the inventory. Participants were asked to complete the rank order exercise last, so as not to influence choices made in the vignettes. The rank order exercise briefly described each philosophy (see Table 10.1) and requested participants to rank them. A score of one indicated a philosophy closest to beliefs, and a score of five indicated philosophy least like beliefs.

**EXHIBIT 10.1** **Sample Vignette from Health Education Philosophy Inventory**

**Setting: University/College**

Recent studies indicate that success in meeting Healthy People Objectives for the 1980s was mainly attributable to legislation which mandated certain health related behaviors, i.e., car seats for children, air bags in vehicles, raising legal drinking age, lowering restrictions for Medicaid eligibility, etc. You are teaching a college general education Healthful Living Course which typically defines health in terms of individual choices. This course adopts a holistic approach to health education by stressing the interconnectedness of all health dimensions and the development of full human potential. Would you restructure your course to spend time addressing more societal concerns of health? How would you divide the percentage of time dedicated to individual choices and societal health concerns?

| 100% Individual | 50%/50% | 100% Societal |
| Health Concerns (IHC) | IHC/SHC | Health Concerns (SHC) |

Place a mark (X) on the continuum where it would most accurately describe your beliefs/actions as a health educator in this setting.

Please describe the reason you chose your action:

_____

_____

_____

## VALIDITY AND RELIABILITY

HEPI was sent to a panel of five experts to determine consensual validity. Expert panel reviewers consisted of five nationally renowned health educators. The vignettes, continuum, and rank exercise were demonstrated to accurately reflect and measure preferences and beliefs of the five health education philosophies. Reliability for the content analysis was ascertained by determining inter-coder and intra-coder reliability (Krippendorf, 1980). Mean percentile agreement for inter-coder reliability was .93, while intra-coder reliability was .97. Reliability for this study was considered high.

## RESULTS

Total number of responses was 106, or 51.7 percent. Seven of the inventories were returned blank, thus reducing response number of usable forms to 99 or 48.3 percent. Practitioners' return rate ($n = 53$, 49.5 percent) was slightly higher than the return rate of academicians ($n = 46$, 46.9 percent). High response rate for a rather arduous and time-consuming mailed questionnaire indicated interest by the profession to engage in philosophical inquiry. Average time for completion of the inventory was twenty minutes.

Participants in the study represented a nationwide selection of health education practitioners and academicians. Table 10.2 depicts frequencies and percentages for demographic variables requested in the HEPI, overall and by group. Statistics revealed that the study was well-balanced and representative of the field. The majority of the participants were female ($n = 55$, 56.7 percent) and Caucasian ($n = 87$, 90.6 percent). All participants had a minimum of a bachelor's degree, with 45 percent with a master's degree and 54 percent with a doctorate. Primary health education setting included university/college ($n = 56$, 57.7 percent), followed by community ($n = 28$, 28.9 percent). The number of practitioners ($n = 34$, 64.2 percent) who were CUES was higher than the number of academicians ($n = 21$, 45.7 percent) who were CHES, though the combined rate averaged 57.3 percent. The mean age of participants was 47.5 years old, ranging from 21 to 72 years. Mean years of work experience in the health education profession was reported as 17.9. Data indicated that participants in the study were well-educated, experienced professionals.

Content analysis procedure divided participants' responses to the educational situations in the vignettes as supportive, eclectic, or alternative of the health education philosophy, as determined by markings on the continuum. In the HEPI, each philosophy was addressed twice within the series of vignettes. Thus, from a sample size of 99, support for each philosophy could reach as high as 198 if all respondents responded to all vignettes. Philosophical preference in educational settings, as depicted by the series of vignettes, was *behavior change* ($n = 74$, 39.78 percent), followed by *freeing/functioning* ($n = 69$, 35.75 percent) (see Table 10.3). Variations in philosophical preferences among health education practitioners and academicians were reported by means and standard deviations. ANOVAs (see Table 10.4) determined significant difference in *freeing/functioning* philosophy ($p < .05$). Academicians were more likely to make educational decisions based on the principles consistent with this philosophy. Significant differences were also discovered in *behavior change* and *social change* ($p < .10$). Practitioners preferred *social change*, while academicians demonstrated stronger agreement with *behavior change*.

Means were utilized to determine group ranking of philosophical beliefs as stated in the rank order exercise (see Table 10. 5). Preferred philosophies of health educators in this exercise were *decision-making* followed by *behavior change*. Spearman-rho correlation coefficient and independent *t*-tests discovered no significant differences in rank order of philosophical beliefs among health educators who were practitioners or academicians.

## FINDINGS AND DISCUSSIONS

Two potentially opposing philosophies, *behavior change* and *freeing/functioning*, vie for position of single, dominant preferred health education philosophy as determined by choices in educational settings. Significant differences ($f = 7.93$, $p < .05$) in

## TABLE 10.2 **Demographic Data for Overall Sample and by Group**

| Variable | Overall Frequency | % | Practitioners Frequency | % | Academicians Frequency | % |
|---|---|---|---|---|---|---|
| **Gender** | | | | | | |
| Male | 42 | 43.3 | 15 | 28.3 | 27 | 58.7 |
| Female | 55 | 56.7 | 38 | 71.7 | 17 | 39.9 |
| **Ethnic Background** | | | | | | |
| African American | 1 | 1.0 | 0 | 0.0 | 1 | 2.2 |
| Caucasian | 87 | 90.6 | 47 | 88.7 | 40 | 86.9 |
| Other | 8 | 8.3 | 6 | 11.3 | 2 | 4.3 |
| **Academic Degrees** | | | | | | |
| Bachelor's | 1 | 1.0 | 1 | 5.7 | 0 | 0.0 |
| Master's | 44 | 45.4 | 37 | 69.8 | 7 | 15.2 |
| Doctorate | 52 | 53.6 | 15 | 28.3 | 37 | 80.4 |
| **Health Education Setting** | | | | | | |
| Worksite | 3 | 3.1 | 3 | 5.7 | 0 | 0.0 |
| School | 1 | 1.0 | 1 | 1.9 | 0 | 0.0 |
| Community | 28 | 28.9 | 27 | 50.9 | 1 | 2.1 |
| Clinical | 4 | 4.1 | 4 | 7.5 | 0 | 0.0 |
| University | 56 | 57.7 | 13 | 24.5 | 43 | 93.5 |
| Other | 5 | 5.2 | 5 | 9.4 | 0 | 0.0 |
| **CHES Certified** | | | | | | |
| Yes | 55 | 57.3 | 34 | 64.2 | 21 | 45.7 |
| No | 41 | 42.7 | 19 | 35.8 | 22 | 47.8 |

*Note:* Less than 100% response in some categories was due to missing data from respondents.

TABLE 10.3 **Philosophical Preferences of Health Educators in Educational Situations**

| Philosophy | N | Frequency | Percentage |
|---|---|---|---|
| Behavior Change | 186 | 74 | 39.78 |
| Freeing/Functioning | 193 | 69 | 35.75 |
| Cognitive-Based | 188 | 56 | 29.79 |
| Decision-Making | 185 | 47 | 25.41 |
| Social Change | 193 | 40 | 20.73 |

Note: Less than 100% response in some categories is due to missing data from respondents.

TABLE 10.4 **Statistical Significance of Differences among Philosophical Preferences of Health Educators as Determined in Educational Situations**

| Source of Variation | df | One-way Analysis of Variance | | |
| | | Sums of Squares | F | Prob > F |
|---|---|---|---|---|
| Cognitive-Based | 1 | 3.71 | 0.38 | 0.5394 |
| Decision-Making | 1 | 16.77 | 1.13 | 0.2897 |
| Behavior Change | 1 | 30.00 | 2.94 | 0.0897** |
| Freeing/Functioning | 1 | 22.06 | 7.93 | 0.0059*[a] |
| Social Change | 1 | 29.24 | 3.11 | 0.0813** |

[a] Scheffe analysis indicated significant difference.
*$p < .05$
**$p < .10$

**TABLE 10.5**   Health Education Philosophical Preferences in Rank Order Reported Overall and by Group

| Ranking | Overall | Practitioners | Academicians |
|---------|---------|---------------|--------------|
| 1 | Decision-Making | Decision-Making | Decision-Making |
| 2 | Behavior Change | Behavior Change | Behavior Change |
| 3 | Social Change | Social Change | Freeing/Functioning |
| 4 | Freeing/Functioning | Freeing/Functioning | Social Change |
| 5 | Cognitive-Based | Cognitive-Based | Cognitive-Based |

Note: 1=philosophy closest to beliefs
      5=philosophy least like beliefs

educational choices were noted between academicians and practitioners, which represented health educators making very different choices given the same options. Practitioners tended to make educational decisions that favor *behavior change* or *social change*. This suggested that in the educational setting, practitioners were more aware of or more focused on change as something to work toward. Academicians' decisions reflected *freeing/functioning* educational principles, which promote learners' choice and self-directedness. These findings reflect well what one would anticipate the differences between the two types of health educators represented in this sample to be.

In stark contrast, analysis of the rank order exercise found that health educators professed identical philosophical beliefs. Both practitioners and academicians listed *decision-making* and *behavior change* philosophy as first and second preferences. These similarities are striking. The emergence of two distinct groups of health educators, namely, SOPHE and the Association for the Advancement of Health Education (AAHE), developed historically in different ways in different settings. Practitioners and academicians tend to perceive themselves as very different. This study suggested contrary evidence, that these two groups of health educators agree on important fundamental issues: the purpose of health education, role of teacher and learner, and educational methodologies.

*Decision-making* philosophy mirrors principles that health educators believe are of primary importance. *Decision-making* philosophy encompasses problem-solving, lifelong learning, pragmatic knowledge, and inductive methodologies (Elias & Merriam, 1980; Kittleson & Ragon, 1993). These philosophical beliefs were not

reflected in practice as depicted by choices made in response to the education scenarios depicted by the vignettes. For example, even though subjects stated that
*decision-making* was the philosophy closest to their beliefs in the rank order exercise, choices made in response to the vignettes reflected the philosophies of *behavior change* or *social change*. Very few written comments were given to justify
decision-making philosophy. This suggested that although health educators hold the
principles of *decision-making* as ideals, application of this philosophy in educational
settings did not result. Overall, the ability of learners to decide their own fate was
desired, yet it did not seem appropriate to any of the particular health education settings offered for judgment. This philosophical trend is pervasive and important for
health education. For example, the theme for the 1995 national convention of the
American Public Health Association (APHA) [was] Decision-Making in Public
Health: Priorities, Power, and Ethics. How health educators choose to put *decision-
making* principles into action will greatly affect the health education profession into
the next century.

Health educators, regardless of stated philosophical beliefs, often change philosophy according to health education setting: Philosophy is considered the foundation
that guides and gives directions in educational situations (Nolte, 1976). For the sample
population in this study, theoretical professional philosophy had little apparent impact
on educational decisions as offered in the vignettes. Many health educators are "action
people" rather than philosophers. They do what works, pragmatically, without much
philosophical forethought. Health education professionals also seem to let alternative
or external factors dictate educational decisions.

Health educators, even ones with strong philosophical beliefs, demonstrated great
adaptive ability. If health educators cannot bend/blend a little, they could do more
harm for the overall profession than good. An example of this might be sexuality education in the schools. If health educators are too rigid, they might alienate a group they
could potentially impact. On the other hand, are philosophical principles compromised
too much? The determining factor in this dilemma is that health educators need to recognize the philosophy of the agency and determine if it is too different from personal
philosophy. In a certain setting, can a health educator make the adaption and be
comfortable with it?

Health educators are comfortable in many settings adopting an eclectic approach
to directing learning. The importance of eclecticism in health education has been theo-
rized, yet never proven (Russell, 1975, 1976). Health educators who adopted this
approach demonstrated comfort in pulling bits and pieces of all/any philosophies to
justify their educational decisions. There are advantages and disadvantages in a profession that operates eclectically. Timmreck and his colleagues (1987, 1988) hypothesized that for health education to become a distinct profession, the adaptation of
eclecticism could hurt this development. This "lack of distinction" as a profession
clearly hampers participation in a number of contemporary issues. For example, health
education as a profession was largely ignored in the recent health care reform debate.
How can external organizations and institutions obtain input or help from a discipline

without knowing what it does? Conversely, the versatility of health education has allowed the profession inroads in many different settings or realms. Whether eclecticism is a strength or weakness is yet to be determined.

## SUMMARY AND IMPLICATIONS

An initial step has been taken to explore the philosophical trends and preferences of health education professionals. Philosophical inquiry, both individually and collectively, is of utmost importance to professional development. Several findings in this study are worth highlighting. Differences were anticipated and found in actions between health education practitioners and academicians. An unexpected similarity of stated philosophical beliefs among health educators was discovered. Philosophical preferences of health educators that work in other settings, that is, school, worksite, and clinical, need to be investigated. The researchers hope that this study will serve as a catalyst for future philosophical studies and to verify the findings of this study.

Health educators must remember that every single educational choice reflects a philosophical principle or belief. Educational choices carry important philosophical assumptions about the purpose of health education, the teacher, and also the learner. Thus, health educators should take the time necessary for individual philosophical inquiry, in order to be able to clearly articulate what principles guide them professionally. Setting seems to greatly affect educational purpose and goals. Different settings may produce a need for different philosophies. Every health educator should be aware of which elements of their individual philosophies they are willing to compromise for a particular setting, and which they are not. To assist one in making these decisions, health education professional preparation programs should include avenues of exploration into philosophical inquiry, at both the graduate and undergraduate levels in ways appropriate to maturity and experience.

These are exciting times for health education. The twenty-first century will be a test for the profession: a test of its versatility, adaptability, and responsiveness to the ever-changing demands of health education practice. Will more information and technology in the twenty-first century make for more human homogeneity or for a greater range of differences? Will culture become more democratic or autocratic, encouraging more freedom of thought and action or more specific behaviors and non-behaviors? Perhaps knowledge of philosophical alternatives and how these are applied will be the means of keeping the profession viable and relevant to a future about which there are many diverging speculations.

## REFERENCES

AAHE Board of Directors. (1992). A point of view for health education. *Journal of Health Education, 23*(1), 4–6.

Balog, J. (1982). Conceptual questions in health education and philosophical inquiry. *Journal of Health Education, 13*(2), 201–204.

Beyrer, M. K., & Nolte, A. E. (Eds.). (1993). Reflections: The philosophies of health educators of the 1990s. *The Eta Sigma Gamma Monograph Series, 11*(2).

Creswell, W. H., & Newman, I. M. (1989). *School health practice.* St. Louis, MO: Times Mirror/Mosby College.

Dalis, G. T., & Strasser, B. B. (1977). *Teaching strategies for values awareness and decision making in health education.* Thorofare, NJ: Charles B. Slack.

Elias, J. L., & Merriam, S. (1980). *Philosophical foundations of adult education.* Huntington, NY: Robert E. Krieger.

Green, L. W., Kreuter, M. W., Deeds, S. G., & Partridge, K. B. (1980). *Health education planning: A diagnostic approach.* Palo Alto, CA: Mayfield.

Greenberg, J. S. (1978). Health education as freeing. *Health Education, 9*(2), 20–21.

Kittleson, M. J., & Ragon, B. M. (1993). *Teaching strategies for the health educator.* Unpublished manuscript.

Kolbe, L.J.. (1982). What can we expect from school health education? *Journal of School Health, 52*(3), 145–150.

Kreuter, M. W. (1979). A case for philosophy. *Journal of School Health, 49*(2), 116.

Krippendorff, K. (1980). *Content analysis: An introduction to its methodology.* Beverly Hills, CA: Sage.

Landwer, G. E. (1981). Where do you want to go? *Journal of School Health, 57*(8), 529–531.

Nolte, A. (1976). The relevance of Abraham Maslow's work to health education. *Health Education, 1*(3), 25–27.

Oberteuffer, D. (1977). *Concepts and convictions.* Washington, DC: AAHPERD Publications.

O'Rourke, T. (1989). Reflections on directions in health education: Implications for policy and practice. *Health Education, 28*(6), 4–14.

Patton, M. Q. (1990). *Qualitative evaluation methods.* Beverly Hills, CA: SAGE.

Rash, J. K. (1985). Philosophical bases for health education. *Health Education, 16*(2), 48–49.

Russell, R. D. (1975). *Health education.* Washington, DC: National Education Association.

Russell, R. D. (1976). *There is no philosophy of health education! Rather . . . our strength and our weakness is in the many.* AAHE presentation, session on philosophy in Health Education, Milwaukee, WI.

Shirreffs, J. A. (1988). The nature and meaning of health education. In L. Rubinson & W. F. Alles (Eds.), *Health education: Foundations for the future* (pp. 35–62). Prospect Heights, IL: Waveland Press.

Timmreck, T. C., Cole, G. E., James, G., & Butterworth, D. D. (1987). The health education and health promotion movement: A theoretical jungle. *Health Education, 18*(5), 24–28.

Timmreck, T. C., Cole, G. E., James, G., & Butterworth, D. D. (1988). Health education and health promotion: A look at the jungle of supportive fields, philosophies and theoretical foundations. *Health Education, 18*(6), 23–28.

U.S. Department of Health and Human Services. (1991). *Healthy People 2000.* Washington, DC: Public Health Service.

# PART

3

# COGNITIVE APPROACHES IN HEALTH EDUCATION

*One major philosophical approach well represented in Health Education literature is the cognitive approach. In the past, health education frequently focused on information dissemination and the increase of knowledge regarding specific content areas of health. The cognitive-based philosophy has its roots in the hygiene health educational programs founded within schools at the turn of the twentieth century, and it remains still a prevailing philosophy. Health educators who espouse this philosophy define the purpose of health education informing by giving the best scientific health practices.*

*Creswell and Newman (1989) viewed the cognitive-based approach to learning in terms of objectives and quantifiable terms to be measured. They advocated the cognitive approach as a means of transferring a large base of knowledge relatively quickly. Cognitive-based philosophies of health education have been viewed as a foundation upon which other philosophies can be developed (Kolbe, 1982).*

*One limitation to the cognitive-based approach to health education is that this philosophy does not ensure the adaptation of healthy lifestyles. Also, the scientific base of health knowledge changes rapidly and the transfer of specific knowledge produces only short-term health effects. Yet, as the cognitive approach to health education continues to be researched and developed, additions to this philosophy have been made. The cognitive-based health education philosophical perspective includes strategies and approaches that focus on constructivism, critical thinking, and decision making. Critical thinking techniques enable learners to reason dialectically and to reach conclusions in an analytical and logical format. Critical thinking works with cognitive-based philosophy by emphasizing the ability to reason as a higher-order thinking skill and is foundational for the synthesis of cognitive information. Decision making is viewed as a systemic approach to education, designed to equip learners with skills that enable them to make self-satisfying decisions and appropriate choices based on up-to-date factual information.*

*The concept of health literacy (Joint Committee on National Health Education Standards, 1995; Tappe & Galer-Unti, 2001; American Association of Health Education, 2008) is a good example of a cognitive approach in health education that employs both the skill of critical thinking and decision making in practice. The American Association of Health Education's position statement on health literacy is reprinted in Appendix C.*

*In summation, the cognitive-based philosophy of health education is found to be strongly supported, with the school structure as the most effective way to affect the learner's health. Although the primary purpose of this philosophy is to impart knowledge, coupled with decision making and critical thinking skills, learners can be taught how to apply facts to real-life situations.*

## ARTICLES

The articles in Part 3 provide a sampling of applied cognitive-based health education philosophies. Ubbes, Black, and Ausherman (1999) tackle the issue of how to teach for understanding in health education with an emphasis on the inclusion of critical and creative thinking skills. In "The Paradigm Shift Toward Teaching for Thinking," Keyser and Broadbear (1999) challenge the health educator to think beyond the dispensing of factual health information to arming students with the skill of thinking by giving them opportunities for practice. Veselak (2001) provides an historical perspective of what he calls "modern" (1959) school health programs, the most common setting for encountering the cognitive-based philosophy of health education. Finally, the article by Oberteuffer, reprinted in 2001, was first published in 1953 and explains the philosophical underpinnings of the school health program by addressing the nature of the student, group development for program success, and the social/ political context within in the program. These four articles provide a sample of cognitive-based philosophical approaches within health education, its historical roots, and the critical additions that make this philosophy responsive and useful in today's world.

## CHALLENGE TO THE READER

As you read these articles, try to identify principles that you can apply in your practice and delivery of health education. Pay particular attention to the purpose, the role of the health educator, the role of the learner, and the strategies, techniques, and methods for delivery of health education.

# TEACHING FOR UNDERSTANDING IN HEALTH EDUCATION: THE ROLE OF CRITICAL AND CREATIVE THINKING SKILLS WITHIN CONSTRUCTIVISM THEORY

VALERIE A. UBBES

JILL M. BLACK

JUDITH A. AUSHERMAN

Health education literature is scattered throughout physical, biomedical, behavioral, educational, psychological, and social science journals (Frazer, Kukulka, & Richardson, 1988). To date, health education scholars have not fully outlined how critical and creative thinking skills can be used as cognitive tools for studying our behavioral science *and* educational theories as parallel, complementary processes. Educational theory, which encompasses curriculum, instruction, and assessment, needs further conceptualization in health education. Constructivism theory may be one viable lens for viewing teaching and learning in health education. In educational contexts where participants are engaged in critical and creative thinking, assumptions are open to question, divergent views are aggressively sought, and inquiry is not biased in favor of a particular outcome (Kurfiss, 1988). The depth of these discussions obviously depends on the cognitive development of the learners (Baxter Magolda, 1995; King & Baxter Magolda, 1996; Obeidallah et al., 1993; Piaget, 1952). However, all learners can be encouraged to be inquisitive and learn to generate questions about themselves and their world. Younger children will contextualize "their ways of knowing" from themselves, family, and friends, but adolescents will also expand their world views to more community and global concerns. For many learners, learning how to generate questions through problem posing and framing (Fernandez-Balboa, 1993; Freire & Faundez, 1989; Shor, 1992) can be just as instructive as knowing the answers.

When health educators query children and adolescents about their health needs and interests (Trucano, 1984), effective curriculum development can result. Inquiry-based curriculum and instruction can build on what learners already know and extend to what they want to know. Inquiry-based learning can also help academicians to refine our educational theories and models in health education. For example, this article will discuss constructivism theory as a basis for critical and creative thinking. We will address four key questions: (1) Why should we construct knowledge for understanding in health education? (2) How do we teach for understanding in health education? (3) What is the theoretical basis for critical thinking in health education? (4) Why should creative thinking be included in health education?

The main purpose of our article is to explore how critical and creative thinking can extend our understanding of health-related content. To help learners improve how they think, "teaching has changed from covering the content to ensuring that students understand and know what they have learned. The switch has been to a less-is-more philosophy" (Halpern & Nummedal, 1995). Our theoretical assumption is that learners who participate in both individual and collaborative processes can construct and reconstruct meanings about their health and educational status better than either process alone. When learners are encouraged to generate critical questions about self and others and to probe health content for underlying meanings and assumptions, they are better able to understand the hows and whys of health behavior.

## WHY SHOULD WE CONSTRUCT KNOWLEDGE FOR UNDERSTANDING IN HEALTH EDUCATION?

Health educators need to refine the cognitive domain of our profession. Knowledge acquisition is a needed component in health education pedagogy and has been recognized as one of five health education philosophies (Welle, Russell, & Kittleson, 1995). However, behavioral outcomes, namely health behaviors, have emerged as the predominate focus in much of the literature and as the leading philosophical preference in educational settings (Welle et al., 1995). We believe there is a continuing need for scholarly work that clarifies how knowledge is epistemologically and pedagogically define and established in health education.

Constructivist theory suggests that learners construct and reconstruct information to learn (Brooks & Brooks, 1993). These constructions (and understandings) evolve when learners actively gather, generate, process, and personalize health-related information rather than passively receive knowledge from teachers or health-related resources. We can explicitly teach learners to organize existent and new information by using concept organizers (Bellanca, 1992; Carter & Solmon, 1994; Maylath, 1989; Wooley, 1995). Wurman (1989) claims that "knowing how things are organized is the key to understanding them" (p. 8). He offers these guiding questions for consideration: "How can I look at this information? How would reorganizing the information change its meaning? How can I arrange the information to shed new light on the problem? How can I put the information in a different context?" When existing information is reorganized and connected in different ways, new patterns can lead to new meanings and interpretations. Consequently, a higher level of knowing results; this is called understanding.

In health education, we know that sharing of health-related information does not often enlighten our learners unless equal time is spent on reducing the misinformation and misconceptions that they bring to the lesson or session. When new information is disseminated in the form of basic information (facts), the depth of understanding is limited. Several variables need to be considered when sharing health-related content with participants: the developmental readiness of the learners (Bibace & Walsh, 1981); issues of age, race, ethnicity, socioeconomic status, and gender (Fernandez-Balboa, 1993); the declarative and procedural knowledge of the learner (Marzano, 1992); the declarative and procedural knowledge of the teacher (Rink, 1997); the declarative and procedural knowledge of the curriculum framework (Kendall & Marzano, 1996); the learning environment (Barr & Tagg, 1995); and a wide range of selected methodologies.

If we really intend to teach for understanding, we also need to teach toward concepts so that learners can see meaningful new patterns and relationships between the topics. One of the five principles of constructivist theory (Brooks & Brooks, 1993) includes the structuring of learning around "big ideas" or primary concepts. For example, the macro concept in the *National Health Education Standards* is health literacy. Other concepts in the seven broad standard statements include prevention, culture, behavior, risks, and communication.

King (1995) suggests that learners can exhibit "the habit of inquiry by learning to ask thoughtful questions—of themselves and of each other—about the material they read, hear in lectures, and encounter during class discussions." She states: "Good thinkers are always asking What does this mean? What is the nature of this? Is there another way to look at it? Why is this happening? What is the evidence for this? And How can I be sure? Asking questions such as these and using them to understand the world around us is what characterizes critical thinking."

The *National Health Education Standards* (Joint Committee on NHES, 1995) indicate that critical thinking and problem solving, along with creative thinking and decision making, are appropriate skills for learners in grades K–12. The standards document states that a health-literate person is a critical thinker and problem solver; a responsible, productive citizen; a self-directed learner; and an effective communicator. Five of the seven health education standards emphasize that students will demonstrate the ability to do behavioral outcomes. We believe that the use of cognitive psychology within pedagogy will help health educators to guide and facilitate learners to understand the reasons, that is, the "whys," for doing health-enhancing behaviors rather than simply knowing the "whats" and "hows" with minimal practice. Both the knowing and doing are important skills. Generation of health-related content based on the developmental readiness of the learners requires that both teachers and learners do the thinking. Within constructivist theory, this means that health educators do more than teach the content. When teaching for understanding, health educators must *facilitate* the students to work with the content. As such, when learners are challenged to go beyond facts into constructing personal meaning and understandings about health, their behavioral outcomes may be enhanced and extended as well.

We believe that behavior change theory must evolve simultaneously with the conceptualizations of the cognitive and affective domains so that people are treated as holistic learners. We especially need to emphasize the first step in educational planning in which the health needs and interests of learners are assessed initially and continually throughout the educational experience. This requires an assessment process of coming to know the learner from multiple perspectives, for instance, race, age, gender, culture, intellectual, developmental, and many others. It also supports another guiding principle of constructivism, which is to seek and value students' points of view.

Learners will demonstrate many *behaviors* when they have learned to think. Learners will demonstrate more persistence in problem solving, less impulsiveness when answering questions, increased ability to listen with empathy, acceptance of ambiguities, improved self-assessments, improved questioning ability, improved transfer of learning between different situations, and increased metacognition (thinking about thinking) (Costa & Lowery, 1989).

Constructivist approaches try not to view the learner's behaviors as objects of analyses that can be manipulated and controlled. Instead, constructivism assesses student learning in the context of teaching and adapts the curriculum to address students' suppositions (Brooks and Brooks, 1993). When learners (and teachers) construct their own knowledge and critique the received wisdom of their culture, an emancipator curriculum may evolve. Grundy and Henry (1995) describe an emancipatory interest in curriculum which "acknowledges the dynamic interrelationship of knowledge and power . . . . Emancipatory knowledge is thus concerned with confronting issues of power and domination, and with empowering individuals and groups to act with autonomy and responsibility." The intent of this curricular approach would not aim to control the production or application of knowledge. However, as the learner copes with the conflict of personal meaning within the curriculum, "a new form of knowledge emerges, one which is authentic, which is empowering and liberating" for the learner. This inquiry approach requires "an interactive process, in which teacher and students together determine the curriculum, in order to make meaning of the world" (Grundy & Henry, 1995). As we discuss in the next section, this speaks to the need for learner-centered lessons in health education *balanced* with the more traditional teacher-directed lessons. How this translates into comprehensive, categorical, and integrated curricula is the focus of a future article.

## HOW DO WE TEACH FOR UNDERSTANDING IN HEALTH EDUCATION?

This section will offer three suggestions on how to teach for understanding in health education: (1) the use of collaborative learning, (2) focus on the developmental needs and interests of the learners, and (3) the need for systems thinking in addition to linear thinking to develop multiple perspectives.

### Use of Collaborative Learning

First, we believe that an individual learns better when there is a balance between learner-centered lessons and teacher-directed lessons. Learner-centered lessons are often grounded in inquiry and facilitated by the teacher; in short, students help to determine the topics and questions for learning. When students and teachers collaborate as a team to determine some of the lessons, both students and teachers become the learners. As such, the curriculum becomes more learner-centered and less hierarchical (Arrendondo, Brody, Zimmerman, & Moffett, 1995). Collaborative approaches also help learners to draw out each other's ideas, enter into and elaborate on them, and build together a concept that none of them could have constructed alone (Clinchy, 1995). As one outcome to learner-centered lessons, students have the potential to learn more about health-related content that is relevant to them, and teachers learn more about their students' developmental needs, interests, and backgrounds within the context of a certain lesson. Marzano (1992) refers to learner-centered lessons as "workshop classes" and teacher-directed lessons as "presentation classes."

Constructivism places individuals in collaborative environments for learning. The *National Health Education Standards* recognize that learners need assistance in understanding personal, community, and global contexts about health. For example, the seventh standard states that "students will demonstrate the ability to advocate for personal, family, and community health" (Joint Committee on NHES, 1995). Learners often need help moving from individualistic, egocentric views of health to a community, sociocentric view of health. A more worldcentric view brings an "expanded self" with implications for optimal well-being and human potential (Fahlberg & Fahlberg, 1997). Warren (1994) states that "it is difficult, if not impossible, to consider seriously other points of view . . . if one is not aware that there *are* other points of view." Constructivism helps learners participate in cooperative learning activities so that "cognitive discrepancies" are exposed and reconciled. King (1995) states that "when we are engaged in peer interaction, we discover that our own perceptions, facts, assumptions, values, and general understandings of the material differ to a greater or lesser extent from those of others. When confronted with these conceptual discrepancies, we want to reconcile the conflicts. To do so, we must negotiate understanding and meaning. And this negotiation, this co-construction of meaning, occurs through explaining concepts and defending our own views to each other." According to Cobb (1988), when learners engage in reconciling differences and reaching negotiated meaning, they are continually restructuring their thinking—the basic tenet of constructivism.

## Focus on Developmental Needs, Interests, and Backgrounds

A second suggestion for teaching for understanding is to focus on the developmental needs, interests, and backgrounds of the learners. A developmental perspective focuses continually on how students learn, rather than focusing more typically on the content of the lesson, and/or the methodology for delivering the content. A focus on student outcomes rather than teacher outcomes is an important shift in educational theory and practice (Marzano, 1992, p. 179). Grundy and Henry (1995) remind us "to think of classroom interactions in terms of learning experiences rather than teaching strategies."

Grundy and Henry's suggestion can help us transform some of our health education practices. For example, teaching ideas are often shared for different topics, settings, and populations at professional conferences and in our health education literature. These teaching ideas can provide creative innovations for our curricula and programs and assist health educators who received minimal background in pedagogy. However, we caution that a particular methodology, technique, or strategy should be secondary to the developmental needs, interests, and background of the learner(s). Health educators who make ongoing assessments of their learners during a lesson will understand the amount and extent of health-related content needed for that situation. How that information is shared, whether in didactic and/or collaborative methodologies, requires critical and creative thinking on the part of the health educator. Since health-related information can be disseminated through a variety of methodologies and technologies (the science of health education), we believe that the art of health education is knowing *what* educational tool to use *when* and with *whom*. Nummedal and Halpern (1995) warn that "just as learning to think critically involves more than developing a repertoire of critical-thinking techniques (i.e., skills, strategies, heuristics, and models), so too learning to teach critical thinking involves more than developing a repertoire of instructional techniques." To be successful in both requires what Weimer (1993) describes as the "management of that repertoire—the ability to select from one's bag of tricks a technique relevant to the . . . moment."

## Need for Systems Thinking

A third way to teach for understanding is to assist learners to recognize the limitations of value dualisms that occur through linear, dichotomous thinking (Wheatley, 1994). Warren (1994) defines *value dualisms* as "either-or pairs in which the disjunctive terms are seen as exclusive (rather than inclusive) and oppositional (rather than complementary), and where higher value is attributed to one disjunct than the other." Some examples of value dualism are yes/no, white/black, head/heart, and mind/body. When value dualisms are extended to systems (relational) thinking, these same examples become yes, no, maybe; white, black, gray; head, heart, soul; and mind, body, spirit. The use of systems thinking in addition to dichotomous linear thinking can help learners develop multiple perspectives and ways of knowing.

Perry (1970) advocated moving learners from egocentric, dualistic thinking to more mature, relativistic thinking. Gilligan (1982) reminds us also to include the female critical perspective in developmental psychology models. Many of these psychological models are first disseminated to health education students in course work from departments of educational psychology and/or psychology. Consequently, if these developmental theories are not revisited and extended within health education course work (and developed at a higher sophistication in our professional literature), learner-centered models can be overshadowed by a teacher-directed curriculum or by instructional methods that may not be authentic or relevant for the learners. Systems thinking can broaden our understanding of health and education concepts by seeking relationships between and among different variables. This is very important for pre-service teachers during their professional development, and it is valuable for pre-K–12 learners who receive limited health instruction during their developmental years.

## WHAT IS THE THEORETICAL BASIS FOR CRITICAL THINKING IN HEALTH EDUCATION?

This section will expand on the theory of critical thinking within health education. Skill-based curricular approaches are preferred. For example, Fetro (1992) has advocated the understanding and integration of personal and social skills—for example, decision making, refusal skills, goal setting, stress management—across health curricula. These personal and social skills could also be labeled thinking skills (Ubbes, 1997), but we also hypothesize that they could be a combination of cognitive, affective, and psychomotor actions within personal and social contexts. Health educators should help learners understand how a personal or social skill used in one situation can transfer to a different situation or context. Critical thinking is a necessary component of this learning process (Scales, 1993). Rehearsal of personal and social skills within and across different situations and contexts is critical. Hostetler (1994) claims that "education aimed at critical thinking must be concerned with developing a particular content and context as opposed to focusing merely on skills. Skills certainly have their place. But while there may be techniques or skills *in* critical thinking there can be no technique of critical thinking." McPeck (1994) agrees that "critical thinking is not a content-free *general ability."* He criticizes the offering of critical thinking as a separate course, because learners need relevant knowledge about the types of problem within the context of a field or discipline.

The *National Health Education Standards* (Joint Committee on NHES, 1995) highlight the importance of critical thinking in the context of our field or discipline. The standards define a health-literate person as "a critical thinker and problem solver who uses decision making and goal setting in a health promotion context." The standards also define a health-literate person as a responsible, productive citizen, an effective communicator, and a self-directed learner. The latter characteristic fits nicely within Marzano's (1992) Dimensions of Learning model, which uses five types of thinking to promote learning.

Warren (1994, p. 171) believes that "critical thinking always takes place within *some* conceptual framework. In this respect, critical thinking must be understood as essentially contextual, that is, sensitive to the conceptual framework in which it is conceived, practiced and learned or taught." She reminds us that "at any given time, a conceptual framework functions for an individual as a finite lens, a 'field of vision,' in and through which information and experiences are filtered. As such, conceptual frameworks set boundaries on what one 'sees' " (p. 156).

In addition to the seven National Health Education Standards used as a framework for curriculum development in grades K–12, health educators in higher education also have a conceptual framework for the professional preparation of health educators. The *Competency-Based Framework for Professional Development of Certified Health Education Specialists* (NCHEC, 1996) provides guidelines for the development of multiple competencies and responsibilities in the profession, including thinking skills. Health educators might begin to assess which competencies require more explicit thinking skills.

In advocating a more sophisticated discussion of thinking skills in health education, we are not saying that we need to question everything. However, health educators should be moving learners beyond an initial knowledge of health-related content. Techniques like "Fat and Skinny Questions" (Fogarty & Bellanca, 1993). Bloom's taxonomy (Bloom, 1956), and KWL (Know, Want to Know, What You Learned; Marzano, 1992) can assist learners to understand health-related content. The use of questioning techniques and writing narratives (see Exhibit 11.1) are helpful techniques for probing what our learners know and understand about health-related topics, issues, and problems.

The move to include fewer topics and more concepts in health education curricula may be an advantage to our learners. This will require an explicit teaching of thinking skills through less content and more rehearsal time during pre-K–12 health education classes and our professional preparation courses. Critical thinkers are needed so we can solve the challenges of our profession, among them how to have more than twenty-two minutes per day (or about sixty hours per year) of K–12 health instruction. Consequently, problem solvers will need to employ creative thinking skills to such challenges as explained in the next section.

**EXHIBIT 11.1** **Suggested Questioning Techniques When Leading a Discussion**

Begin class with a problem or controversy.

Allow thinking time after the question.

Probe for completion of the response:

- Probe for assumptions (What are you assuming? What is underlying what you say?)
- Probe for reasons and evidence (How do you know? What are your reasons for saying that?)
- Probe for implications and consequences (What are you implying by that? What might happen?)
- Probe for clarification (What do you mean by . . .? Could you give an example?)

Ask for elaboration if the response is short.

Redirect responses to other students.

*Sources:* R. Paul, Socratic questioning, in R. Paul (Ed.), *Critical thinking* (Rohnert Park, CA: Sonoma State University, Center for Critical Thinking, 1990); W. Wilen, *Questions, questioning techniques, and effective teaching* (Washington, DC: National Education Association, 1987).

## WHY SHOULD CREATIVE THINKING BE INCLUDED IN HEALTH EDUCATION?

Trunnell, Evans, Richards, and Grosshans (1997) have explored the factors associated with creativity in health educators who have won university teaching awards. Participants in their study ($n = 10$) defined creativity as "the generating of something new and different . . . or taking something old and giving it a new direction or shaping it in a different way." Cinelli, Bechtel, Rose-Colley, and Nye (1995) have suggested the use of three types of questioning strategies in health instruction. One strategy is called "divergent questioning," which uses brainstorming for eliciting a variety of possible responses to a given situation. Brainstorming is one of the best creative thinking skills in health education.

When confronted with health-related challenges, learners can use critical thinking skills and both inductive (particular to general conclusions) and deductive (general to particular conclusions) reasoning to solve problems. However, reasoning and logic should not be used at the expense of thinking. Walters (1994) suggests that "thinking encourages wonder, while reasoning tends to stifle it by concentrating on immediately solvable problems" (p. 178). Wheatley (1994) talks about this process: "In our past explorations, the tradition was to discover something and then formulate it into answers and solutions that could be widely transferred. But now we are on a journey of mutual and simultaneous exploration. In my view, all we can expect from one another is new and interesting information. We cannot expect answers. Solutions . . . are a temporary event, specific to a context, developed through the relationship of persons and circumstances" (p. 151).

Antonietti (1997) states that "children should learn that, when trying to think creatively, they may have to deal with many confusing, conflicting, and ambiguous ideas." Children need to learn "to think past the obvious responses, search for more original ideas, and become aware of some mental strategies they can adopt in facing novel problems." Creativity is not needed in every situation; creativity is most needed when there is no single correct answer.

Learners in our health education classes should be encouraged to use logical, critical thinking with a willingness to take imaginative and intuitive risks. Imagination and intuition are two related and complementary processes. Walters (1994) reports that "intuitive insights often follow intensive reflection upon a particular problem within a specific context, but, when and if they arise, they are unexpected and not consciously premeditated. Characteristically they hit the subject with a sudden and comprehensive 'Aha!' impact" (p. 72). If intuitive insight is often unanticipated and spontaneous, then imagination is more planned and conscious. Barrow (1988) warns that imaginative thinking is not a mere generation of unusual ideas. As Walters (1994) states, "odd or unorthodox ideas can be nonconventional without necessarily being imaginative, particularly when they are absurd, incoherent, whimsical, or delusional" (p. 71). Hence, imaginative thinking must be effective in "extending cognitive comprehension and enriching practical utility." Walters reminds that "critical thinking and creative thinking, then, are not incompatible with one another nor are they mutually exclusive. Indeed, genuine success in one entails facility in the other. It follows that the education of good thinkers requires training in both . . . [We need to provide] students with pedagogical opportunities for enhancement in imagination as well as analysis, creativity alongside justification, problem construction in addition to problem solving" (pp. 69–70).

Gardner (1993) studied the creativity of famous individuals whom he called "Exemplary Creators" and their "defining works" to determine whether creativity is domain-specific. He investigated the "triangle of creativity" by observing the "dialectics among the individual person or talent; the domain in which the individual is working; and the field of knowledgeable experts who evaluate works in the domain. No matter how talented the individual is . . . unless he or she can connect with a domain and produce works that are valued by the relevant field, it is not possible to ascertain whether that person in fact merits the epithet creative" (p. 380). Perhaps these creativity guidelines can be further explored in the health education field.

## CONCLUSION

This article began with a discussion of why we should construct knowledge for understanding in health education. Suggestions on how to teach thinking were offered using constructivist theory as a foundation for teaching and learning. A balance between learner-centered lessons and teacher-directed lessons was suggested, including the use of a developmental perspective that focuses more on learner outcomes. The use of systems thinking can also help learners develop multiple perspectives and ways of knowing. The impact of critical and creative thinking skills needs additional discussion and development in the health education literature.

## REFERENCES

Antonietti, A. (1997). Unlocking creativity. *Educational Leadership*, *54*(6), 73–75.

Arredondo, D. E., Brody, J. L., Zimmerman, D. P., & Moffett, C. A. (1995). Pushing the envelope in supervision. *Educational Leadership*, *53*(3), 74–78.

Barr, R. B., & Tagg, J. (1995). From teaching to learning—A new paradigm for undergraduate education. *Change*, *27*(6), 13–25.

Barrow, R. (1988). Some observations on the concept of imagination. In K. Egan & D. Nadaner (Eds.), *Imagination and Education* (pp. 79–90). New York: Teacher College Press.

Baxter Magolda, M. B. (1995). The integration of relational and impersonal knowing in young adults' epistemological development. *Journal of College Student Development*, *36*(3), 205–216.

Bellanca, J. (1992). *The cooperative think tank II: Graphic organizers to teaching thinking in the cooperative classroom*. Palatine, IL: IRI Skylight Training and Publishing.

Bibace, R., & Walsh, M. E. (1981). *Children's conceptions of health, illness, and bodily functions*. San Francisco: Jossey-Bass.

Bloom, B. S. (1956). *Taxonomy of educational objectives. The cognitive domain*. New York: David McKay.

Brooks, J. G., & Brooks, M. G. (1993). *In search of understanding: The case for constructivist classrooms*. Alexandria, VA: Association for Supervision and Curriculum Development.

Carter, J. A., & Solmon, M. A. (1994). Cognitive mapping: An activity for health education. *Journal of Health Education*, *25*(2), 108–109.

Cinelli, B., Bechtel, L. J., Rose-Colley, M., & Nye, R. (1995). Critical thinking skills in health education. *Journal of Health Education*, *26*(2), 119–120.

Clinchy, B. M. (1995). A connected approach to the teaching of developmental psychology. *Teaching of Psychology*, *22*(2), 100–104.

Cobb, P. (1988). The tensions between theories of learning and instruction in mathematics education. *Educational Psychologist*, *23*, 78–103.

Costa, A., & Lowery, L. (1989). *Techniques for teaching thinking*. Pacific Grove, CA: Midwest.

Fahlberg, L. L., & Fahlberg, L. A. (1997). Wellness re-examined: A cross-cultural perspective. *American Journal of Health Studies*, *13*(1), 8–16.

Fernandez-Balboa, J. M. (1993). Critical pedagogy: Making critical thinking really critical. *Analytic Teaching*, *13*(2), 61–72.

Fetro, J. V. (1992). *Personal and social skills: Understanding and integrating competencies across health content*. Santa Cruz, CA: ETR Associates.

Fogarty, R., & Bellanca, J. (1993). *Patterns for thinking, patterns for transfer: A cooperative team approach for critical and creative thinking in the classroom* (2nd ed.). Palatine, IL: IRI/Skylight Publishing.

Frazer, G. H., Kukulka, G., & Richardson, C. E. (1988). An assessment of professional opinion concerning critical research issues in health education. *Advances in Health Education*, *1*, 27–42.

Freire, P., & Faundez, A. (1989). *Learning to question*. New York: Pantheon.

Gardner, H. (1993). *Creating minds: An anatomy of creativity seen through the lives of Freud, Einstein, Picasso, Stravinsky, Eliot, Graham, and Gandhi*. New York: HarperCollins.

Gilligan, C. (1982). *In a different voice: Psychological theory and women's development*. Cambridge, MA: Harvard University Press.

Grundy, S., & Henry, M. (1995). Which way home economics? An examination of the conceptual orientation of home economics curricula. *Journal of Curriculum Studies, 27*(3), 281–297.

Halpern, D. F., & Nummedal, S. G. (1995). Closing thoughts about helping students improve how they think. *Teaching of Psychology, 22*(1), 82–83.

Hostetler, K. (1994). Community and neutrality in critical thought: A nonobjectivist view on the conduct and teaching of critical thinking. In K. S. Walters (Ed.), *Re-thinking reason: New perspectives in critical thinking* (pp. 135–154). Albany, NY: State University of New York Press.

Joint Committee on National Health Education Standards (1995). *National health education standards: Achieving health literacy.* Atlanta, GA: American Cancer Society.

Kendall, J. S., & Marzano, R. J. (1996). *Content knowledge: a compendium of standards and benchmarks for K–12 education.* Aurora, CO: Mid-Continent Regional Educational Laboratory.

King, A. (1995). Inquiring minds really do want to know: Using questioning to teach critical thinking. *Teaching of Psychology, 22*(1), 13–17.

King, P. M., & Baxter Magolda, M. B. (1996). A developmental perspective on learning. *Journal of College Student Development, 37*(2), 163–173.

Kurfiss, J. G. (1988). *Critical thinking: Theory, research, practice, and possibilities* (ASHE-ERIC Higher Education Report No. 2). Washington, DC: Association for the Study of Higher Education.

Marzano, R. J. (1992). *A different kind of classroom: Teaching with dimensions of learning.* Alexandria, VA: Association for Supervision and Curriculum Development.

Maylath, N. S. (1989). Constructing concept maps for health instruction. *Journal of School Health, 59*(6), 269–270.

McPeck, J. E. (1994). Critical thinking and the "trivial pursuit" theory of knowledge. In K. S. Walters (Ed.), *Re-thinking reason: New perspectives in critical thinking* (pp. 101–117). Albany, NY: State University of New York Press.

National Commission for Health Education Credentialing (NCHEC) (1996). *The competency-based framework for professional development of certified health education specialist.* Allentown, PA: NCHEC.

Nummedal, S. G., & Halpern, D. F. (1995). Introduction: Making the case for "Psychologists Teach Critical Thinking." *Teaching of Psychology, 22*(1), 1–5.

Obeidallah, D., Turner, P., Iannotti, R. J., O'Brien, R. W., Haynie, D., & Galper, D. (1993). Investigating children's knowledge and understanding of AIDS. *Journal of School Health, 63*(3), 125–129.

Paul, R. (1990). Socratic questioning. In R. Paul (Ed.), *Critical thinking: What every person needs to survive in a rapidly changing world.* Rohnert Park, CA: Sonoma State University, Center for Critical Thinking.

Perry, W. (1970). *Form of intellectual and ethical development in the college years: A scheme.* New York: Holt, Rinehart & Winston.

Piaget, J. (1952). *The origins of intelligence in children.* New York: International Universities Press.

Rink, J. E. (1997). Teacher education programs: The role of context in learning how to teach. *Journal of Physical Education, Recreation, and Dance, 68*(1), 17–24.

Scales, P. C. (1993). The centrality of health education to developing young adolescents' critical thinking. *Journal of Health Education, 24*(6), S10–S14.

Shor, I. (1992). *Empowering education: Critical thinking for social change.* Chicago: University of Chicago Press.

Trucano, L. (1984). *Students speak: A survey of health interests and concerns (Kindergarten through twelfth grade).* Seattle, WA: Comprehensive Health Education Foundation.

Trunnell, E. P., Evans, C., Richards, B., & Grosshans, O. (1997). Factors associated with creativity in health educators who have won university teaching awards. *Journal of Health Education, 28*(1), 35–41.

Ubbes, V. A. (1997). Transforming individuals and organizations for the 21st century. *Journal of Health Education, 28*(3), 187–191.

Walters, K. S. (1994). Critical thinking, rationality, and the vulcanization of students. In K. S. Walters (Ed.), *Re-thinking reason: New perspectives in critical thinking* (pp. 61–80). Albany, NY: State University of New York Press.

Warren, K. J. (1994). Critical thinking and feminism. In K. S. Walters (Ed.), *Re-thinking reason: New perspectives in critical thinking* (pp. 155–176). Albany, NY: State University of New York Press.

Weimer, M. (1993). The disciplinary journals on pedagogy. *Change, 25*(6), 44–51.

Welle, H. M., Russell, R. D., & Kittleson, M. J. (1995). Philosophical trends in health education: Implications for the 21st century. *Journal of Health Education, 26*(6), 326–332.

Wheatley, M. J. (1994). *Leadership and the new science: Learning about organization from an orderly universe.* San Francisco, CA: Berrett-Koehler.

Wilen, W. (1987). *Questions, questioning techniques, and effective teaching.* Washington, DC: National Education Association.

Wooley, S. E. (1995). Behavior mapping: A tool for identifying priorities for health education curricula and instruction. *Journal of Health Education, 26*(4), 200–206.

Wurman, R. S. (1989). *Information anxiety.* New York: Doubleday.

# CHAPTER

## 12

# THE PARADIGM SHIFT TOWARD TEACHING FOR THINKING: PERSPECTIVES, BARRIERS, SOLUTIONS, AND ACCOUNTABILITY

BETTE B. KEYSER

JAMES T. BROADBEAR

A continuing educational concern in the United States is the need to teach thinking skills at all educational levels from primary grades through college (Costa & Lowery, 1989; Halpern, 1998; Meyers, 1987). According to Haycock (1996), even students who arrive at college with high school grades reflecting an A or B average cannot think critically. A review of educational literature indicates a plethora of information has been available for several decades on the issues of thinking in schooling.

Throughout the history of health education, primary emphasis has been on content transmission and teacher-centered instruction. This type of approach limited opportunity to develop critical thinking in students and contributed to minimal interest by health educators toward issues relevant to teaching thinking. However, current guidelines for health education professional preparation and the recent National Health Education Standards indicate a growing concern by health educators toward teaching skills of thinking. In addition, many initiatives undertaken as part of the current U.S. educational reform demonstrate efforts to restructure America's schools to prepare students for high thinking work rather than low skilled tasks. Reform strategies to develop this kind of schooling have direct impact on teacher educators, the structure of professional preparation programs, and entering teachers of all disciplines. Meagerness of discussion in the health education literature on the topic of teaching for thinking provides minimal guidance to the teacher educator and others desiring to be more fully informed or to become an active, effective participant of the paradigm shift toward teaching for thinking.

To address the paucity of our own professional literature, this article serves as a concise discussion highlighting past and recent educational literature most relevant to critical thinking. Within this overview the classroom practitioner will be introduced to four areas that are predominant in the educational literature. The first area focuses on perspectives regarding teaching for thinking expressed in the literature. Second, barriers to teaching for thinking will be described. Third, a discussion will follow on specific suggestions identified in the literature on how to reduce some of the barriers impeding the present paradigm shift toward developing student thinking in educational practice. Last, accountability factors for teaching thinking in health education will be identified.

## PERSPECTIVES ON THE NEED FOR TEACHING THINKING

Meyers (1987) points out that it is evident in the literature there is a need to address critical thinking at all levels of education in this country. While there are various terms and definitions related to thinking, educational theorists, philosophers, cognitive psychologists, and researchers of pedagogy generally agree that thinking is a skill learned through opportunities for practice and coaching by others, and it should have a more important role in the learning process (deBono, 1994; French & Rhoder, 1992; Hester, 1994; Howard, 1990; Paul, 1995). Although theorists provide different definitions for thinking and believe their definition best conveys the basic concept of thinking, they do not view other definitions as wrong or not useful. The proposed definitions are more similar than different and should not allow an educator to dismiss the importance of teaching for thinking because the experts do not seem to find agreement on a definition among themselves (Paul, Binker, Martin, Vetrano, & Kreklau, 1989). Even writers whose definitions of thinking differ share consensus that it is an essential skill needed for success in a rapidly changing world.

The historical roots of critical thinking that most educators agree upon originate in the era of ancient Greece with the teachings and treatises of Socrates, Plato, and Aristotle. The term "critical thinking" is commonly used in education today. According to deBono (1994), this term perpetuates the view of teaching engaged in by the "Greek Gang of Three" which emphasized the skills of analysis, judgment, and argument through a dialogue involving continuous questioning. The word *critical* comes from the Greek word *kritikos*, which means "judge," while "Socratic questioning" is a method of asking deep questions to probe one's thinking for rationality to claims of knowledge. Socrates demonstrated over 2,500 years ago that even persons with power or in a high position representing authority could not always be depended upon for sound knowledge and insight, hence the need for critical thought.

Although teaching for thinking began hundreds of years ago, it continues to be of concern for today's society. According to Hester (1994), beginning in the twentieth century, U.S. schools had a major goal of mastery of thinking or reasoning yet the achievement of this goal is still lacking. For example, concern over content vs. process was expressed by Alfred North Whitehead in 1929 who advocated for a needed change in education and suggested that the "real fruits of education are the thought processes that result from the study of a discipline, not the information accumulated" (Meyers, 1987, p. 2). This early concern described by Whitehead as separation of content from process has been a point of concern and clarification continuing into current educational discussions.

Several experts on thinking, such as deBono (1994), Howard (1990), and Costa and Lowery (1989) clarify that thinking skills are needed in addition to content, but not at the expense of eliminating the disciplines' major concepts and key information. Salient to these individuals is the idea that thinking skills need to be taught directly as a part of classroom time. Advocates of this approach offer evidence, which demonstrates increases in student performance, and further suggest that this method shows students that thinking skills are a key component of education. Such an approach is based on a philosophy that thinking can be taught separately as process-based instruction, then taught in a meaningful context with deliberate teaching for skill transfer through repeated practice (Costa & Lowery, 1989). However, within this field of thought differences abound as to how thinking skills should be taught, that is, step by step or in a holistic manner (Paul et al., 1989).

Others, most notably Richard Paul (1995), a leader on critical thinking from Sonoma State University, espouses infusion of thinking and content as a single educational endeavor. From this perspective it is believed that thinking can only occur in the presence of content thereby producing contextualization and indivisibility between thought and its subject. This represents a direct contrast to those advocating thinking skill instruction separate from teaching content Sternberg (1987) cautions educators to not be subject to binary choices, such as separate instruction for teaching thinking versus instruction with infusion of content and thinking. He advises careful deliberation of such artificial dichotomies and suggests teachers seek a third option better than the two presented, namely, a combination of these approaches.

Regardless of differences in how experts view the relationship of content and thinking and approaches to teaching thinking, they enumerate a variety of valid reasons for teachers to engender needed changes in teaching for thinking. A reason often providing support for a paradigm shift toward teaching for thinking is frequent reference to the latest educational reform movement.

The impetus for the most recent reform movement in this century began over fifteen years ago with a federal publication identifying the poor status of American education as shown through student achievement scores (Levine, 1996). Steinberg (1996) cites the significance of the 1983 federal report *A Nation at Risk: The Imperative for Educational Reform* and the trends indicated by data gathered from the National Assessment of Educational Progress (NAEP). The NAEP is a federally administered assessment of students' proficiency in mathematics, reading, writing, and science. Steinberg points out that scoring on the NAEP relies less on rote memory of facts known by students than their general skills, such as writing a coherent, persuasive argument or solving a problem using scientific information rather than demonstrating possession of the knowledge alone. French & Rhoder (1992) further elaborate on the importance of the early 1980s results of the NAEP, often referred to as the "Nation's Report Card," as evidence that American students do not do well with thinking. The same authors also report following the publication of *A Nation at Risk* that the Harvard School of Education in 1984 recommended adoption of critical thinking as a basic skill along with reading, writing and math. Today, the movement for teaching for thinking is viewed as an integral part of school improvement and efforts to improve student learning (Hester, 1994).

A second reason cited by experts on thinking is that we are living in an information age with complex demands on people for organizing information in order to benefit from it (deBono, 1994; French & Rhoder, 1992; Hester, 1994). According to deBono (1994) who is a leading authority in cognitive studies, our current thinking which is inherently non-critical is not adequate for the rapidly changing world in which we live and the attended demands.

Closely related to the "information age" rationale is yet another argument, which focuses on the role of schooling in preparing students to enter today's society and the new century. Education needs to provide students with the thinking skills essential to becoming autonomous, self-reliant citizens (French & Rhoder, 1992) who, as independent and creative thinkers, problem-solvers and effective decision-makers, can make positive impacts upon their environment through innovation, invention, and discovery (Hester, 1994). According to economists, the future of our country's success is dependent upon the academic achievement of students fostering their ability to succeed in a highly competitive international economy (Steinberg, 1996). Perhaps, deBono (1994) summarizes it best by stating, "Thinking is the ultimate human resource. The quality of our future will depend entirely on the quality of our thinking" (p. xi).

A fourth reason is a growing body of knowledge related to the thinking processes offered in the literature and available to practitioners. Many authors comment that teachers do not use teaching methods or pedagogy to encourage and develop thinking in students, but are teaching just factual knowledge (French & Rhoder, 1992; Meyers, 1987; Raths, Wassermann, Jonas, & Rothstein, 1986). The range and depth of this literature requires educators to do considerable reading to become familiar with descriptive information on differentiation in thinking, such as creative, reflective, analytical, and lateral, coupled with pedagogy appropriate to develop each type of thinking. Continuous and careful review of the literature will assist educators to better understand their role in nurturing thinking in ways, perhaps, that were neither addressed nor taught in their undergraduate professional education courses.

## BARRIERS TO TEACHING FOR THINKING

Realities of present day schooling and the educational world present a variety of barriers that interfere with attempts by teachers to create a learning environment for teaching thinking. The type of barrier fluctuates according to the level of education as well as specific educational setting. However, each barrier serves as a reminder of typical restraints impinging upon the practitioner who is making a serious attempt at teaching for thinking.

Within the school environment are several identifiable barriers impeding teachers' progress toward participating in the paradigm shift toward teaching for thinking. Factors such as large class size, faculty reward structures that work against a critical thinking emphasis, and the time and effort required to shift one's teaching orientation are cited as possible barriers by Haas and Keeley (1998). Teaching to tests which are based on recall of what has been read and heard serves as an obstacle to developing student competence as thinkers (Raths et al., 1986). Another barrier identified by Meyers (1987) are the 50-to-60-minute class times which allow little time for students to adequately process or interact with subject matter and to reflect upon what has occurred in a learning activity.

Even if time were not a factor, Meyers characterizes teachers as products of the way they were taught so they continue to rely upon assignments, methods, and objective tests that emphasize recall of information rather than offer potential for higher order thinking skills. Teachers seldom engage students in dialogical (thinking that involves dialogue or extended exchange between different points of view or frames of reference) or dialectical reasoning (thinking that tests the strengths and weaknesses of opposing points of view), but rather require no more thought than recall (Paul et al., 1989).

Stated more strongly than being a product of the past experiences, Haas and Keeley (1998) describe faculty resistance to teaching for thinking in higher education as a common problem. According to the authors, although college instructors purport to acknowledge critical thinking as an educational outcome for their students, it is evident many faculty fail to make critical thinking a reality in their classrooms. Reasons cited for this failure are: critical thinking was not included as part of their own educational experiences, their mentors exhibited only teaching methods of lecture and served primarily as dispensers of information, a lack of confidence in teaching what they have not been trained to do, and belief that attention to critical thinking is incongruent with content coverage and interferes with content transmission. Meyers (1987) adds that few opportunities to learn about teaching critical thinking are available through professional development, disciplinary conferences and everyday collegial dialogue.

Another barrier to teaching for thinking is the limitation of most textbook writers to incorporate consistent aspects of critical thinking terminology and use of thinking skills by students (Raths et al., 1986). When there is some effort to include checklists for evaluating reasoning or analysis of an argument, there is an overall avoidance of asking the textbook reader to view the argument as a whole and evaluate it as a whole. Frequently arguments are not presented as complete arguments and students receive only portions of the issue. Many texts suggest debates as extensions of teaching, but do not emphasize the need for students to rationally evaluate their views, assess arguments, or justify their conclusion. Likewise, many texts only ask students to either agree or disagree with the conclusion, again without providing reasoned evaluation (Paul et al., 1989).

A final obstacle to teacher engagement in teaching for thinking cited in the literature is the attitude of intellectual passivity or disengagement of students in classrooms that replaces the sense of wonder or inquisitiveness exhibited in them as children. Natural curiosity can be thwarted as early as the middle grades in elementary school creating a challenging situation for those teaching higher order thinking in subsequent grades (Meyers, 1987).

Steinberg (1996), author of *Beyond the Classroom*, offers an interesting view on the evolving student disengagement displayed in schools. He first proposes students perform according to the method of evaluation, thus any attempts to teach for thinking is resisted by students who continue their passivity because they know involvement in thinking skills is not requisite to evaluation activities. His second explanation is based on his studies on forces outside of the school affecting students' interest and performance in school. Their findings suggest that schools are not alone accountable for the poor performance of students, lack of motivation, and general disengagement. Contributors to these latter problems include parents who display serious disengagement regarding interest in the child's performance and progress in school, peer culture which affects students from trying as hard as they can for fear of what friends will say, and students' activity schedules that interfere with any energy directed to schooling beyond the classroom. Thus, student disengagement is more likely to result from external forces such as parents and employers who contribute to the devaluing of education which is then transferred and reflected in the students' attitudes and values about education.

## SOLUTIONS TO OVERCOMING BARRIERS

Writers in the educational literature spend little time in providing ideas or solutions on how to overcome the barriers facing teachers in the move away from didactic teaching recognized as counterproductive to teaching for thinking. Most ideas can be narrowed to two areas of concern. First, a concern is expressed to provide training related to those preparing to become teachers, and second, proactive strategies are needed to address the resistance by current educational practitioners to teach for thinking.

Although often there is a lack of courses in teacher preparation that give systematic instructional training in how to implement teaching for thinking (Raths et al.,

1986), some authors in the educational literature mention increased resources available to those who desire to participate in training future teachers differently. Consensus for recommendations of specific resources to use in teacher education programs is not clear. Likewise there is a lack of discussion of approaches or models employed by university and college teacher education units to successfully prepare individuals to teach for thinking.

Some writers with an interest in higher education do provide information regarding opportunities for resisting change by faculty at colleges and universities who often do little more than embrace thinking as a major teaching goal. For example, Meyers (1987) offers hope for such college and university professors by stating, "Happily, things are beginning to change" (p. 102). In his opinion, more resources are available to these educators, and there is increasing interest in a number of professional organizations to include workshops to exchange teaching ideas. National conferences, interdisciplinary in nature, are being offered that focus on critical thinking.

According to Haas & Keeley (1998), the right incentives and a supportive environment encourage educators to attempt to make changes in teaching. Specifics described by the authors are teaching philosophy changes to show emphasis on development of thinking skills with follow-up changes to reflect the change in emphasis in forms of evaluation used by administrators, peers, and students. Individual exploration and group meetings to discuss teaching concerns in initiating changes for teaching thinking are staff development strategies advocated for overcoming resistance by faculty. Group discussions with leaders who have experimented with critical thinking approaches offer structure and focus to collegial exchange. At least one faculty member needs to be knowledgeable, thereby garnering the respect and interest of colleagues. In a similar fashion students who began as resisters but developed into enthusiastic critical thinkers can share their experiences with student resisters.

## ACCOUNTABILITY FOR TEACHING THINKING IN HEALTH EDUCATION

Current national education standards and national health education guidelines demonstrate the significance of performance-based standards articulating what both students and teachers should know and be able to do. A review of these standards and guidelines revealed frequent references to thinking skills as an outcome-based goal. Being aware of documents providing such references is especially pertinent to the health educator redesigning the health education professional preparation curriculum to meet recent standards, to the teacher educator preparing school health teachers, and to the veteran teacher incorporating new practices to provide high quality education for all students.

The *National Standards for Quality Teaching* are specific to licensing new teachers. These standards articulated by the Interstate New Teachers Assessment and Support Consortium (INTASC) redirect the focus from student completion of courses and credits offered to descriptions of what entering teachers should possess as qualities, know, and be able to do in order to teach diverse learners. INTASC is a program of the

Council of Chief State School Officers. Specifically, these standards identify ten principles that reflect the knowledge, dispositions, and performances deemed essential for new teachers regardless of their specialty area. One principle describes the new teacher as a reflective practitioner, one who continually evaluates the effects of choices and actions on others, and actively seeks out opportunities to grow professionally. One disposition related to this standard is the teacher who values critical thinking and self-directed learning as habits of the mind (Interstate New Teachers Assessment and Support Consortium, 1995).

Another set of national standards, the *Standards for Teacher Educators*, is the work of the Association of Teacher Educators, which is solely interested in improvement of teacher education for both the school and campus-based educator. The first of the seven standards describes the master teacher as modeling teaching practices that reflect the best available practices in teacher education. One indicator the campus-based teacher is proficient in meeting the first standard is by demonstrating and encouraging critical thinking and problem solving to prospective teachers. For example, videotapes of students engaging in critical thinking can be included in a teaching portfolio (Association of Teacher Educators, 1996).

In addition to national standards related to the performance of beginning and experienced teachers, *A Framework for the Development of Competency-Based Curricula for Entry-Level Health Educators* published by the National Commission for Health Education Credentialing (1985) supports development of critical thinking skills in students during their undergraduate education. Although not explicitly labeled as critical thinking in the guidelines that identify the seven responsibilities and competencies of an entry-level health educator, many aspects of the critical thinking and reasoning process are evident. Competencies such as interpreting concepts, purposes and theories of health education, selecting valid sources of information, seeking ideas of others, applying criteria for effectiveness, and inferring implications are traits common to the critical thinking process. These seven responsibilities and competencies serve as the standards used in the American Association for Health Education and the National Council for Accreditation of Teacher Education (AAHE/NCATE) portfolio process conducted during the NCATE accreditation of professional teacher education programs.

A decade later, the *National Health Education Standards* were released by the Joint Committee on National Health Education Standards (1995). This document was intended to reform health education by emphasizing the essential knowledge and skills elementary and secondary students need to be healthy. School health educators are charged with the responsibility to develop health literate individuals. Within this document, one of the four characteristics identifying the health literate individual is being a critical thinker and problem solver. The national standards serve as a framework for state and local curriculum revision and fundamentally alter ways in which health instruction is planned, delivered, and evaluated.

Another set of standards that accompanies the *National Health Education Standards* document is the *Opportunity to Learn Standards for Health Education*. These standards have direct implications for those instructing future school health educators. For example, undergraduate students should develop the ability to design K–12 curriculum, instruction and authentic assessment for both health content and health related skills. Beginning school health educators should feel competent to develop in their students the skill of critical thinking as requisite to selecting and adopting health-enhancing practices (Joint Committee on National Health Education Standards, 1995).

Previously discussed national education standards and the professional health education guidelines and national standards have direct implications for health educators. It is evident health educators have several responsibilities specific to teaching thinking. Responsibilities include health educators as

■ Planners and implementers of professional preparation programs, to structure curriculum, instruction and assessment that enable students to be critical thinkers during undergraduate education and as entry-level health educators;

■ Instructors and mentors, to regularly role model the process of reasoning and critical thinking to students;

■ Teacher educators, to prepare beginning school health educators to provide regular opportunities for their students to practice and assess their own thinking skills;

■ Master teachers in health education, to demonstrate and encourage critical thinking among those with whom we work, including our colleagues and other teacher educators.

## SUMMARY

As evident by a review of the educational literature, most writers challenge the U.S. classroom tradition of didactic teaching characterized by an emphasis on lecture, passive student learning, and lower cognitive skill development, such as memorization and recall of information through assignments, activities, discussion, and testing. They provide sufficient reasons supporting the need to teach for thinking at all levels of schooling in this country. However, many of the same writers admit to the difficulties and variety of barriers encountered in shifting to an emphasis on teaching for higher order thinking.

Salient to a successful paradigm shift are major changes in undergraduate preparation of new teaching professionals and strategies to overcome practitioners' resistance to teaching students skills of thinking. Although both of these changes are identified and advocated for in the literature reviewed, discussion on how to proceed with making changes in the way teachers are prepared for teaching thinking in the classroom is extremely limited to nonexistent in sources reviewed by authors of this article. More evident are proactive strategies intended to provide encouragement to current educational practitioners who resist the current paradigm shift toward teaching for thinking.

Health educators are directly affected by current educational reform initiatives involving adoption of education standards, national or discipline specific, to guide reforms of preparing and licensing teachers, accrediting teacher education institutions and professional preparation programs, and recognizing master teachers with advance certifications. Health educators should review the current national education standards and more specific health-related standards and guidelines to clarify their role and responsibilities in teaching thinking. The literature on teaching thinking, current national education standards, and recent health education documents on professional standards and guidelines should prompt health educators to engage in serious thought about active commitment to and participation in teaching for thinking.

## REFERENCES

Association of Teacher Educators. (1996). *Standards for teacher educators*. Reston, VA: Author.

Costa, A. L., & Lowery, L. E. (1989). *Tec hniques for teaching thinking*. Pacific Grove, CA: Critical Thinking Press & Software.

deBono, E. (1994). *deBono's thinking course* (rev ed.). New York: Facts on File.

French, J. N., & Rhoder, C. (1992). *Teaching thinking skills: Theory and practice*. New York: Garland.

Halpern, D. F. (1998). Teaching critical thinking for transfer across domains: Disposition, skills, structure training, and metacognitive monitoring. *The American Psychologist 53*(4), 449–455.

Haas, P. F., & Keeley, S. M. (1998). Coping with faculty resistance to teaching critical thinking. *College Teaching, 46*(2), 63–68.

Haycock, K. (1996). Thinking differently about school reform: College and university leadership for the big changes we need. *Change 28*(1), 13–18.

Hester, J. P. (1994). *Teaching for thinking: A program for school improvement through teaching critical thinking across the curriculum*. Durham, NC: Carolina Academic.

Howard, V. A. (Ed.). (1990). *Varieties of thinking: Essays from Harvard's philosophy of education research center*. New York: Routledge.

Interstate New Teachers Assessment and Support Consortium (INTASC). (1995). *Next steps: Moving toward performance-based licensing in teaching*. Washington, DC: Council of Chief State School Officers.

Joint Committee on National Health Education Standards. (1995). *National health education standards: Achieving health literacy*. Reston, VA: American Association for Health Education.

Levine, A. (1996). Educational reform: Designing the end game. *Change 28*(1), 4.

Meyers, C. (1987). *Teaching students to think critically: A guide for faculty in all disciplines*. San Francisco: Jossey-Bass.

National Commission for Health Education Credentialing. (1985). *A framework for the development of competency-based curricula for entry level health educators*. New York: Author.

Paul, R. W. (1995). *Critical thinking: How to prepare students for a rapidly changing world*. Santa Rosa, CA: Foundation for Critical Thinking.

Paul, R., Binker, A. J., Martin, D., Vetrano, C., & Kreklau, H. (1989). *Critical thinking handbook: 6th–9th grades*. Rohnert Park, CA: Sonoma State University.

Raths, L. E., Wasserman, S., Jonas, A., & Rothstein, A. (1986). *Teaching for thinking: Theory, strategies, and activities for the classroom* (2nd ed.). New York: Teachers College, Columbia University.

Steinberg, L. (1996). *Beyond the classroom: Why school reform has failed and what parents need to do*. New York: Simon & Schuster.

Sternberg, R. J. (1987). Teaching critical thinking: Eight easy ways to fail before you begin. *Phi Delta Kappan*, 456–459.

# CHAPTER

## 13

# HISTORICAL STEPS IN THE DEVELOPMENT OF THE MODERN SCHOOL HEALTH PROGRAM

### KENNETH E. VESELAK

The three phases of the modern school health program, namely, healthful school living, health education, and health services had their conception during the nineteenth century (American Child Health Association, 1929, p. 31).

## HEALTHFUL SCHOOL LIVING

The first phase of the school health program that received attention was that of healthful school living. During the nineteenth century the term "school hygiene" was used to describe this phase of the program (Van Dalen, Mitchell, & Bennett, 1953, p. 374). Several publications produced at this time indicate that school hygiene was primarily concerned with problems of school sanitation and construction. In 1829, William A. Alcott expressed the need for improving school buildings in his publication *Construction*

Note: This article is intended to be read for its pholosophical perspective. Originally published in 1959, it may contain factual material or examples that are dated.

*of School Houses*. In the year 1837 Horace Mann discussed the problem of school hygiene in his *First Annual Report*. In the same year Henry Barnard's *An Essay on School Architecture* was published which contained a discussion of school housing. After the Civil War and up to the beginning of the twentieth century, progress in this area of the school health program continued to be made at a slow pace. Undoubtedly the developments in physical education, health instruction, and health services in the public schools at this time must have given some impetus to this phase of the program.

It wasn't until after the year 1908 that growth in school hygiene really began to be noticed(Van Dalen et al., 1953, p. 491). At this time the public began to realize the value of utilizing the public schools as social centers. As a result of the pressure exerted by various community groups and the desire of the educational leaders to meet the needs of the people, many improvements were made in the architectural structure of school buildings and many new facilities were added, including gymnasiums, shower rooms, swimming pools, health service suites, auditoriums, and lecture rooms. Increased emphasis was also placed on more effective lighting, heating, ventilating, and humidifying of school plants; providing a safe water supply and adequate waste disposal facilities; beautifying the school buildings and grounds; and preventing the spread of communicable disease.

In New York City in the year 1910, the first formal lunch program was installed in the public schools (Bryant, 1913, pp. 147–183). This marked the beginning of the installation and maintenance of kitchens and cafeterias in public schools, making it possible for children and school personnel to have warm and nutritious lunches daily. The National School Lunch Act (Public Law 396), passed by Congress in the year 1946, served as an impetus for the development of kitchens and cafeteria facilities and services in public schools throughout the country.

This act made available Federal funds

> to safeguard the health and well-being of the Nation's children, and to encourage the domestic consumption of nutritious agricultural commodities and other foods, by assisting the states, through grant-in-aids and other means, in providing adequate supply of food, and other facilities for the establishment, maintenance, operation, and expansion of nonprofit school lunch programs. (U.S. Department of Health, Education, and Welfare, 1954, p. 74)

The installation of kitchens and cafeterias in the public schools led to an increased emphasis on the maintenance of sanitary and safe cooking and eating facilities and equipment. The importance of hiring healthy food-handlers was also stressed.

Toward the middle of the twentieth century, in addition to providing healthy and safe school buildings and grounds as well as adequate kitchen and cafeteria facilities, emphasis began to be placed on providing a healthy staff to work in the public schools, good teacher-pupil and staff relationships, and the development of a school program that was not harmful to the physical and mental health of the students as well as the staff. In addition to having healthy food-handlers, it was recognized that since teachers and other school personnel came in daily contact with the students, any abnormal health condition that they might have would be detrimental to the health of the pupils. Many school systems therefore took steps to protect the health of students by giving all new teachers and other employees pre-employment examinations, yearly tuberculosis checkups, and in some instances, yearly physical examinations.

Wholesome teacher-pupil and staff relationships were also stressed at this time. It became increasingly recognized that the mental health of students as well as school employees was greatly affected by the human relationships that existed within the schools. The results of the Lewin experiments with autocratic, laissez-faire, and democratic groups, and the Hawthorne industrial studies convinced educators that the mental health of students and school personnel could best be maintained when a democratic atmosphere and democratic leadership were provided. (For an excellent review of these experiments, read James A. Brown, *The Social Psychology of Industry: Human Relations in the Factory* [Harmondsworth, Middlesex: Penguin, 1954], 69–96, 219–244.)

Educators also recognized that the mental and physical health of children were greatly affected by the educational program to which they were exposed. Providing educational programs that did not meet the needs of children, were too burdensome, or were no challenge to the abilities of children was considered to be detrimental to the health of all pupils. School authorities therefore tried to provide educational programs that were conducive to good health. Many schools began to revise their curriculums and teaching loads so that they would not be detrimental to the health of the pupils as well as the teachers. Several schools began to develop modified programs in order to meet the needs of handicapped children, mentally retarded children, and exceptionally brilliant children (the term used to designate this program is now known as Special Education). All of these new developments led to the introduction of a new term to describe this phase of the school health program. The term "healthful school living," being broader in scope than the term "school hygiene," is now used to describe this phase of the program.

## HEALTH EDUCATION

The health education phase of the school health program, which consists primarily of health and safety instruction, had its conception during the second half of the nineteenth century. Horace Mann indicated the need for health instruction in the public schools in the year 1842 (Turner, 1939, p. 9). Physicians were also active in advocating the teaching of physiology in the public schools at this time. Elementary facts of physiology were combined to form textbooks which were used to teach the subject in many of the public schools throughout the country (Rice & Hutchison, 1952, p. 247). "Hygiene" was the name that was given to this new subject. Between 1850 and 1880 physiology was the main topic that was discussed in hygiene courses. It wasn't until after 1880 that the interest in teaching health in the public schools really began to grow. Pressure groups, one of the most significant of which was the Woman's Christian Temperance Union, led by Mrs. Mary Hunt, began to pressure state legislatures to enact laws which would require schools to teach the effects of alcohol and narcotics (Brownell, 1949, p. 235). Between 1880 and 1890 practically every state in the country passed a law requiring instruction concerning the effects of alcohol and narcotics (Turner, 1939, p. 9). In forty of the states these laws specified that the instruction should be part of a broader program of instruction in physiology and hygiene (Rogers, 1930, p. 2). Some of these laws specified the grades at which these topics were to be presented and whether or not a textbook was to be used.

Several years after the passage of state laws requiring the teaching of the effects of alcohol and narcotics to all pupils there occurred a widespread movement to introduce physical education into the school curriculum. The first state to pass a law making physical education a required subject in all public schools was North Dakota in the year 1899 (Rogers, 1930, p. 4). By 1910 most of the states throughout the country passed laws requiring that physical education be made part of the public school curriculum (Grout, 1953, p. 14). Many of these laws specified that health habits should be taught to children as well as physical education activities. It should be noted that the American Physical Education Association, formed in the year 1885 and now known as the American Association for Health, Physical Education and Recreation, played a vital role in advancing the development of both physical education and health education programs in public schools throughout the country.

Several other developments during the first half of the twentieth century helped to strengthen the foothold of health education in the public school curriculum. The American Child Hygiene Association, formed in the year 1909 under the name of the American Association for the Study and Prevention of Infant Mortality, made significant contributions to the advancement of health education in schools through the educational programs it conducted for the better care of children (Grout, 1953, p. 15). In 1915, the National Tuberculosis Association, which was formed in the year 1904, initiated the "Modern Health Crusade" (Grout, 1953, p. 15). This movement was the first recognition of the importance of enlisting child interest as an important factor in modifying child health behavior (Paterson, 1950, p. 143).

The results of the medical examinations of draftees in World War I also gave impetus to the development of health education programs in the public schools. Soon after the war, in the year 1918, the Child Health Organization was formed. It was this organization that coined the phrase "health education," a new name for hygiene, at one of its conferences in the year 1919 (Lucas, 1946, p. 4). The Joint Committee on Health Problems in Education of the National Education Association and the American Medical Association, which was formed in the year 1911, began in 1922, under the able leadership of Dr. Thomas Wood, to pioneer in the formulation of plans, objectives, curriculum content, materials, teacher training requirements, and other essentials for an adequate program of school health education (Conrad, 1935). This committee has been and still is one of the most powerful groups influencing the development of all phases of the school health program. The American Child Health Association, formed in 1923 with the merging of the American Child Health Association and the Child Health Organization, did a great deal to promote school health until its dissolution in the year 1935 (Grout, 1953, p. 15).

In the year 1925, the health education programs conducted in many of the public schools broadened in scope to include safety instruction (Van Dalen et al., 1953, p. 468). School health demonstrations conducted between the years 1914 and 1938 with the aid of the American Red Cross, the Massachusetts Institute of Technology, the Commonwealth Fund, and the Milbank Memorial Fund played a significant role in proving that health education could change behavior and therefore was of extreme value in improving the health of children and adults (Grout, 1953, p. 16). The National Conference for Cooperation in Health Education, formed in 1938, has also played an important role in stimulating the development of health education in public schools. Many of its publications, including *Suggested School Health Policies*, have been used in guiding the development of school health programs throughout the country (Grout, 1953, p. 16). The American Public Health Association established qualifications for school health educators in the year 1938 (Grout, 1953, p. 19). These qualifications helped to elevate the quality of health instruction that was being conducted in public schools as well as communities.

The findings of the physical examinations of World War II draftees also had a stimulating effect on the development of school health education programs. In 1948 the National Conference on Undergraduate Professional Preparation in Health Education, Physical Education, and Recreation established desirable qualifications and training for health teachers working in the public schools. The mid-century White House Conference on Children and Youth held in 1950, as well as the previous conferences (1909, Conference on the Care of Dependent Children; 1930, Conference on Child Health and Protection; and 1940, Conference on Children in a Democracy) all played a significant role in the advancement of health education (National Conference on Undergraduate Professional Preparation, 1948, p. 17). In 1950 the National Conference on Graduate Study in Health Education, Physical Education, and Recreation established desirable graduate training and qualifications for health education teachers working in the public schools.

As a result of Kilander's report published in 1951, it was discovered that thirty-three states required health education in the secondary schools. Of these thirty-three states, twenty-seven required health education as a result of a state law and six required it as a result of a regulation by the state department of education. Of the thirty-three states requiring health education in the secondary schools, twenty-five reported that health instruction was included in the curriculum as a required subject; the other eight states reported that it was integrated with other subjects. Of the fifteen states without laws or regulations regarding health education, only four reported that health instruction was available in no school either as a required or an elective subject. Thirty states reported having special legislation requiring the teaching of the affects of alcohol and narcotics (Kilander, 1951, p. 19).

At the present time [1959] many of the public schools throughout the country have highly developed health education programs. In addition to giving instruction in physiology, the effect of alcohol and narcotics, and safety, the modern school also provides instruction on such topics as growth and development, food, rest, exercise, personality, personal appearance, mental hygiene, family life, disease, and public health (Wilson, 1948, pp. 237–238). There is no doubt that in the future many more new topics will be added to enrich the school health education program.

## HEALTH SERVICES

The health service phase of the school health program had its conception near the end of the nineteenth century. With the increasing prevalence of disease and illness during this period the value of carrying on health services in the schools, especially medical inspection, began to be realized. In the year 1872, because of the prevalence of smallpox, a "sanitary superintendent" was employed by the board of education in Elmira, New York (Rogers, 1942, pp. 1–2). In San Antonio, Texas, in the year 1890, a school medical inspection service was established (Van Dalen et al., 1953, p. 402). In 1890, following a series of epidemics among school children, Dr. Samuel Durgin, health commissioner of Boston, established a system of medical inspection in the schools (Turner, 1939, p. 10). Fifty "medical visitors" were appointed to carry on health work in the schools of Boston. The primary responsibility of these physicians was to visit the schools daily and to examine those children who were suspected of having a communicable disease. Pupils found to be infected were taken out of school and quarantined (Turner, 1939, p. 10).

Similar programs of medical inspection developed in other large cities of the country including Chicago in 1895, New York in 1897, and Philadelphia in 1898 (Turner, 1939, p. 10). In 1899 the first state law relating to the medical inspection of school children was passed in Connecticut (Wood & Rowell, 1928, p. 19). This law also required teachers to test the eyesight of their pupils once every three years. In 1902, with the aid of Miss Lillian Wald, twenty-five nurses were appointed to work in the public schools of New York City (Turner, 1939, p. 10). In 1903 the first school dentist was appointed in Reading, Pennsylvania (Turner, 1939, p. 10). In 1904 ear, eye, and throat examinations of school children were made compulsory in Vermont (Turner, 1939, p. 11). In the year 1914, with the aid of Dr. Alfred Fones, ten dental hygienists were employed in the schools of Bridgeport, Connecticut (Turner, 1939, p. 11).

Some of the greatest gains in the school health service phase of the health program began to be made after World War I. As a result of draft examinations of inductees, it was realized that over half of the defects detected could have been corrected during the school years, thereby challenging the school to inaugurate a remedial program for young children (Van Dalen et al., 1953, p. 445). Many schools began to improve and broaden the scope of health services provided to their pupils. During the 1920s the term "health service" came into use to describe the broader responsibilities of the school toward the student (Van Dalen et al., 1953, p. 445). Between 1930 and 1951 the contributions of the previously mentioned organizations, educational institutions, and world events gave additional impetus to the development of a superior program of health services for school children.

Kilander's report published in the year 1952 indicated that school health services were in operation in ninety-one percent of all school systems in cities with a population of 2,500 or more. The health services provided in these cities included at least a medical and a dental examination or inspection (Kilander, 1952, p. 36). At the present time the health service program of the more advanced schools includes daily health observations, periodic screening examinations, periodic dental and medical examinations, health counseling, immunization and vaccination procedures, and first aid (Wilson, 1953, p. 486).

## CONCLUSION

Although the field of school health is in its infancy, it is growing rapidly. The improvements made in healthful school living, health education, and health services during the past century have made the public schools a healthier place in which to work and study. There is no doubt that future improvements made in the school health program will lead to the development of better schools which will provide better educational programs for their students.

Originally printed in the *Journal of School Health Education* in 1959.

## REFERENCES

American Child Health Association. (1929). *Teamwork for child health*. New York: Author.

Brownell, C. L. (1949). *Principles of health education applied*. New York: McGraw-Hill.

Bryant, L. S. (1913). *School feeding*. Philadelphia: Lippincott.

Conrad, H. L. (1935, May). Historical steps in the development of health education, *Mind and Body, 42*, 81–82.

Grout, R. E. (1953). *Health teaching in schools: For teachers in elementary and secondary schools* (2nd ed.). Philadelphia: Saunders.

Jean, S. L. (1946, June). *Health education—Some factors in its development* (newsletter). Ann Arbor, MI: School of Public Health, University of Michigan.

Kilander, H. F. (1951). *Health instruction in the secondary schools: An inquiry into its organization and administration* (Office of Education Pamphlet 1951, No. 110). Washington, DC: U.S. Government Printing Office.

Kilander, H. F. (1952). *Health services in city schools* (Office of Education Bulletin 1952, No. 20). Washington, DC: U.S. Government Printing Office.

National Conference on Undergraduate Professional Preparation in Health Education, Physical Education, and Recreation (held at Jackson's Mill, Weston, WV, May 16–27, 1948). (1948). *A Report*. Chicago: The Athletic Institute. 40 pp.

National Conference on Graduate Study in Health Education, Physical Education, and Recreation (held at Père Marquette State Park, IL, January 1950). (1950). *A Report*. Chicago: The Athletic Institute. 31 pp.

Paterson, R. G. (1950). *Foundations of community health education*. New York: McGraw-Hill.

Rice, E. A., & Hutchison, J. L. (1952). *A brief history of physical education* (3rd ed.). New York: A. S. Barnes.

Rogers, J. F. (1930, May). *State-wide trends in school hygiene and physical education as indicated by laws, regulations, and courses of study* (Pamphlet No. 5). Washington, DC: U.S. Government Printing Office.

Rogers, J. F. (1942). *Health services in city schools: Biennial survey of education in the United States, 1908–40*, Vol. 1. Washington, DC: U.S. Government Printing Office.

Turner, C. E. (1939). *Principles of health education* (2nd ed.). New York: Heath.

U. S. Department of Health, Education, and Welfare. (1954). *Federal funds for education 1952–53 and 1953–54* (Office of Education Bulletin 1954, No. 14). Washington, DC: U.S. Government Printing Office.

Van Dalen, D. B., Mitchell, E. D., & Bennett, B. L. (1953). *A world history of physical education: Cultural-philosophical-comparative*. New York: Prentice Hall.

Wilson, C. C. (Ed.). (1948). *Health education* (4th ed.). Washington, DC: Joint Committee on Health Problems in Education of the National Education Association and the American Medical Association.

Wilson, C. C. (Ed.). (1953). *School Health Services*. Washington, DC: Joint Committee on Health Problems in Education of the National Education Association and the American Medical Association.

Wood, T. D., & Rowell, H. G. (1928). *Health supervision and medical inspection of schools*. Philadelphia: Saunders.

# CHAPTER

## 14

# PHILOSOPHY AND PRINCIPLES OF THE SCHOOL HEALTH PROGRAM

**DELBERT OBERTEUFFER**

The program of health education in schools has come a long way in the twenty-five years of the existence of this Association [the American School Health Association, founded in 1927]. The evolution of practice and principle has been strong, sure, and constructive. From humble beginnings the program has become a giant—a giant whose scope is broad, whose activities are legion, and, more important, whose results are everywhere around us.

But does it have a body of principle—and is it guided by any philosophical considerations? The answer is obvious. It does. Let us look at at least three of these basic considerations to see if we can find any agreement as to their essentiality and any common understanding as to their application.

*Note:* This article is intended to be read for its pholosophical perspective. Originally published in 1953, it may contain factual material or examples that are dated.

## WE ARE DEALING WITH THE HUMAN ENTITY

**First: With whom are we dealing? What is the essential nature of this child, this pupil, this student? What is he like?** Actually, we do not know much about him yet, but what little we do know makes it perfectly clear that he is one, an entity, a being indivisible and whole, and one who retains his integrated character as long as possible in the face of an adverse environment. This beneficiary of our handiwork is no segmented animal. He cannot be divided into mental and physical, muscle and mind, emotion and intellect, psyche and soma. There is no substantial thread of evidence which permits us to believe the contrary, but only recently are we beginning to understand this unity and to act in accordance with its meaning. The essential truth of man's unity has caused us to re-cast our concept of health and to re-appraise the effects of all we do for its sake.

Health is no physical thing. It is no "state of physical well-being." It cannot be measured by pounds or feet, by dynamometers or audiometers. We cannot go around appraising the healthiest boy or girl by measuring the strength of muscles or testing vital capacity. Even counting carious teeth will not describe the status, the quality, the nature of the particular organization of tissue which is a given child. We are coming to know that "health" is a word, a descriptive word, not used to describe status but to measure the degree to which the aggregate powers of an individual are able to function. "Good" health thus becomes an expression of function; so does bad health; and the function is not the function of the liver or the leg or the eyes or ears but the function of the totality which is a person. We must come to understand as quickly as we can that to study, or test, or treat the parts of an individual will throw little light on the whole because the whole is something different from and greater than the parts.

Properly to understand and to approach the contribution of health education to the developing child and to the adult requires the study of what Angyal (1941) describes as a science of the person, "a science over and above disciplines merely related to the person." One could not profitably study the relation of a health experience to the development of behavior, for example, without knowing fully the physiological, anatomical, social, and psychological causes of acceptable or unacceptable behavior. Whatever is done in health education, whether it is the teaching of an activity for endurance, examining the mouth for dental decay, or requiring knowledge of immune processes—must be done in relation to the problem presented by that whole and individual organism, Once the organism is assumed to be a unity and not a plurality, then, one applies a formulation of S. Howard Hartley and Eloise Chute (1947), "as psychology is not rightfully handled except with the light of physiology, physiology cannot be all it ought except in the light of psychology or whatever discipline it is that provides for the personal in its logic. Operationism [in this instance health education] cannot rightly be used to justify the excursion onto tangents of interest that leave the organism fragmented into a plurality." Health education is essentially an operation, a means of producing something, and thus it may neither employ, rely upon, nor use any "tangent of interest" which assumes the individual to be a "plurality," that is, made up of several separate and unrelated systems or parts. The full measurement of value in health education is its production of good for "me," not for "my eyes" or "my weight" or "my body." In modern health education the concept of "body" disappears. So does the concept of health education as good for any fragmented part. In its place is the evaluation of the effect of health education upon the individual as a person.

What meaning does this have in our daily operations in school health programs? Well, Thomas Shaffer found it when he described his conception of how to judge the fitness of athletes for competition. His were neither quantitative nor numerical standards. Dr. Shaffer wants us to see each boy as a boy, as a whole, and to judge his fitness by readiness, readiness of *all* the boy for the tests he will meet in athletics. The Joint Committee understands it when they advocate student counselors who can bring *all* the evidence from examinations, *all* the experiences from group living, *all* the intelligence from the genetic background into a collated story understandable by the child as he seeks to understand himself and not just his hearing problem. A. S. Daniels understands it when he sees his program of physical education for the atypical student, the handicapped, not as productive merely of an improved tonus in an afflicted limb, or a skill to be proud of, but as having a bearing upon all of the life of that student, his acceptance of self and others, of organic, social and psychological improvement so inextricably involved as to defy segregation and measurement. Derryberry understands it when he seeks motives for behavior which belie the knowledge which can be proven present. And Nyswander knows there is something yet undiscovered which will help us produce social or group action. Dr. Francis D. Moore, the Harvard surgeon, is motivated by this concept in his research on the relation of hormones and of water, fat, and muscle to recovery from surgery. His investigations, like others in the making, are revealing new relationships of body elements.

These are all more or less related to the oneness of man. The modern health educator is not merely screening for vision or caries or tuberculosis. While he manipulates his Snellen chart or any other device, he is gathering evidence, to be sure, but he is potentially exploring for personality variations, related, for example, to vision, and if glasses are fitted they may do vastly more for the pupil-patient than restore 20/20 eyesight. "Mind" and "body" disappear as recognizable realities and in their stead comes the acknowledgment that a boy, a whole being, stands before you to be dealt with in accordance with whatever contribution you can make to him.

## COOPERATIVE EFFORT IS NEEDED

**Second: Slowly and not without some pain we are coming to understand the necessity for cooperative group effort in the development of the program.** Time is helping us develop a professional confidence in and respect for one another. There are so many of us involved that for years we have straggled with the curious element of protocol that seems to surround us when educators, physicians, nurses, dentists, and others try to work cooperatively in a cooperative program. We have been bothered by uncertain boundaries, by overlapping responsibilities, and sometimes by professional jealousies. We have raised questions of administrative jurisdiction. Who shall be the boss? Who shall "head the department?" Who is best qualified to express judgment on procedure or to assume responsibility for administration?

For example, one picks up a recent (1951) publication of a state medical association (Ohio) and one is astonished to find the statement that "so far as possible, the administration and coordination of health and medical services, and *health education activities in each school* [sic] should be under the leadership and control of a doctor of medicine." A well-read book in the field makes just the opposite recommendation. This argument has been going on for years and there are those of us who are veterans of the guerrilla warfare which has been waged over this matter of who shall be in charge! When will the question become old hat? Must we forever go about ever so carefully trying not to step on sensitive toes and making sure that so-and-so is chief regardless of his personal and professional abilities?

Let us look the thing squarely in the face for a moment. The school health program requires many people to make it operate successfully. It is not a one-man job. Responsibility for the health of youngsters belongs to all who deal with them. Many talents are needed—medical, educational, nursing, administrative, psychiatric and more. Why argue about which talent is the most important? What we have to realize is that we are all important to the welfare of the child and if any one of us bogs down then no one suffers particularly except the child who may have contracted tuberculosis while we argued over who shall sign the payroll!

## UNDERSTANDINGS NEEDED

May I be bold enough to suggest that in the next twenty-five years of the American School Health Association we strive together to bring about certain understandings? And these are

a.  The educator must realize that because he read a hygiene book once or took a three-hour hygiene course in college he is not fully prepared to teach youngsters in that area. He must be richly prepared in the life sciences, and the scientific accuracy of his teachings must be unquestioned.

b.  The educator must accept wholly and fully the idea that he needs and can get help from other professionals in the development of his school health program if he will ask for it, but he need not sell out his professional interest in nor administrative responsibility for the program merely because he has received this help.

c.  The physical education teacher, who for so many years has carried a heavy load of instruction in the program and who has been thanked less and ridiculed more, must study harder and give more time to health education or relinquish his equity in the program.

It must be constantly remembered that personnel in physical education were among the pioneers in the development of school health education. Their efforts were bearing fruit long before the recent upsurge of interest which marks our current development. And there are thousands of schools today whose health programs, of instruction particularly, are dependent upon the zeal of these teachers for its support. Criticism of the physical education group is hardly gracious as we seek cooperative development.

d. Nurses are becoming more important to this program all the time. And they are becoming better educated, better prepared, and better qualified, to do a responsible job in school health. They need a helping hand to lift them beyond the peonage which traditionally has been their lot. The idea that a nurse, because she is a nurse, is vastly inferior in every respect to physicians and educators is tommyrot, and we ought to recognize it as such. Deference when it is paid, should be paid to superior judgment and wisdom and to nothing else.

e. Local physicians are to be welcomed into this program warmly and fully. It is a cooperative venture. It took local and state medical associations a long time to wake up to what was going on. Now they are in action with state and local, committees, and their zeal should be appreciated. We should understand fully that the school health program lives not in isolation from but is a part of the entire community problem of healthful living. In such a relationship community talent, both official and unofficial, should be used.

f. Boards of health and boards of education must learn to work together by agreement or contract or both in the school health program. However, it must be appreciated by everyone involved that boards of education and their appointed administrative officers, the superintendents of schools, have no desire to relinquish administrative control over any phase of school life. They are held responsible by the public for everything that goes on in the schools. If they let out a concession for the school lunch or contract for repairs on a building, they still retain the right to final decision relative to acceptance. One could not expect them to do otherwise on any phase of the school health program. Health officers, therefore, cannot simply move in and take over, no matter how broad is their concept of the community and its health problems.

## THE PROGRAM MUST FIT OUR SOCIAL PHILOSOPHY

**Third: We must examine the relationship between school health education and the social and political philosophy of our people.** It is basic to any phase of education that its operation must reflect and demonstrate the democratic way and have no aims or practices at variance from that culture. Now where do we stand? What are we doing? What is the end effect of the school health program upon those who come through it? Are we developing a kind of health care for our people which is only one step short of that found in a welfare state? Is school health education merely a respectable form of state medical practice—or is it truly an educational experience leading its beneficiaries into self-sufficient, intelligent behavior seeking medical and dental assistance on the voluntary basis?

We have been at this business of teaching about health for a long time now. We have discussed medical care in our classrooms, given free patch tests to millions, discovered dental hazards, given free lunches, screened for vision handicaps, given countless physical examinations, and dispersed volumes of advice. By so doing are we teaching our people to expect something for nothing, to live on the taxes of the other fellow, or are we teaching people to stand on their own feet?

This is a problem we have to meet head on and with full intelligence and insight. We have invested millions of dollars in school health work, and anyone has a right to ask us about the relationship between what we are doing and the popular or unpopular political doctrines of the day.

Whatever we do in the name of school health education must meet the needs of the people. But in meeting those needs for medical care or for health advice, or for anything else, we must not destroy the capacity for self-direction and the will of the individual to look after himself and his family. The great moral virtue of our free life is to be found in our independence, in our freedom from indigency, in the greater sacredness of the individual over the state. To preserve our choices, to pay our own way, to buy and sell as we choose, to retain the honor of paying our own bills—these are some of the values to be preserved within a free society.

We simply cannot afford to develop school health education without giving thought to the moral values within it. If we run a low cost dental clinic for indigent people and a well-to-do person patronizes it because there he can have his teeth fixed more cheaply, then we have failed to develop an essential morality in that person's background! If we teach youngsters to run to their school physician for every diagnosis and treatment because it will be free, then we are destroying something important in our culture. We simply cannot put on vision demonstrations, test thousands for hearing, do mass tuberculosis screening, immunize people by the millions at public expense unless these are justifiable measures in the interest of protecting the public health and without dealing at the same time with the orientation of what we are doing with the private free-enterprise type of medical practice.

We do these things in school not for clinical or reparative reasons, but primarily to demonstrate and to educate. In some instances we can justify our activities on the grounds of public protection and in others because education cannot go on economically unless they are done. But the practices we undertake in school health education should never undermine our evolving conception of medical and dental care. On the contrary they should be undertaken in such form and with such discipline as to support it. But the great effort, regardless of this relationship, must be made to meet the needs of the people.

These then are three suggested principles or basic considerations which must underlie our thinking and planning in school health education. The development of practice stemming from these principles will be varied, but such variations will not matter if the basic direction is maintained.

## REFERENCES

Angyal, A. (1941). *Foundations for a science of personality* (Chapter 1). New York: Commonwealth Fund.

Bartley, S. H., & Chute, E. (1947). *Fatigue and impairment in man.* New York: McGraw-Hill, p. 47. (Bracketed material the author's.)

Originally presented at the General Session on the 25th Anniversary of the American School Health Association, October 20, 1952, and published in the *Journal of School Health Education* in 1953.

# PART

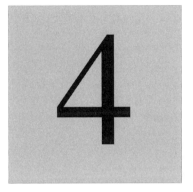

# CHANGING BEHAVIOR IN HEALTH EDUCATION

*Health educators have the unique opportunity to shape and influence behavioral health. Health educators who espouse the behavior change philosophy believe that while the cognitive and affective domains are important parts of the process, the psychomotor domain is the ultimate objective. Green, Kreuter, Deeds, and Partridge (1980) brought this philosophy to the forefront of the profession by defining health education as "any combination of learning experiences designed to facilitate adaptations of behavior conducive to health" (p. 7). Key tenets in the methodology of behavior change are motivation programs, behavior modification, goal setting and attainment, positive reinforcement, behavior contracting, and self-monitoring/man-agement skills. Modeling behavior of the health educator is an essential component to successful health education behavior change programs (Brennan & Galli, 1985; Blomquist, 1986). Modeling has been found to aid in the educational processes of attention, retention, motor performance, and motivation.*

*Advantages of behavior change philosophy in health education include its versa-tility; it can be applied to various health content areas in a variety of health education settings. Behavior change philosophy can produce changes in lifestyles in a relatively short period of time, and behaviorally based programs are easy to evaluate.*

*Critiques of this philosophical approach to health education cite limitation of individual choice, unnecessarily pessimistic approach, and ethical limitations to appropriate intervention, among others (Russell, 1983; Paul, 1984; Greenberg, 1978). Despite criticism, behavior change philosophers contend that successful health edu-cation is rooted in the ability to develop and maintain or change behaviors (King, 1982). Knowledge, theories, values, and critical thinking skills mean little if a person continues behavioral choices that create harm. The role of health educators is to assist their clientele in the acquisition of health behaviors conducive to a healthy lifestyle.*

## ARTICLES

The articles in Part 4 touch on the importance of behavior change philosophy in health education and challenge professionals to expand their understanding of behavior change as it relates to health education. Fertman (2002) encourages health educators to use their unique skills to push behavioral health toward care and promotion. The concept of psychoneuroimmunology is examined in relation to the effect of nutrition, exercise, drugs, emotions, and environmental influences on the bodymind relationship and behavioral health (Read & Stoll, 1998). Garman, Teske, and Crider (2001) approach behavior change in health education from a problem-based learning model. Finally, Labonte (1994) contrasts three approaches in health education—medical, behavioral, and socioenvironmental—as they relate to empowerment. Each article addresses an aspect of using health education to produce behavior change and acknowl-edges the challenges in doing so.

## CHALLENGE TO THE READER

As you read these articles, try to better define the philosophy of behavior change. This philosophy of health education can reflect experiences, training, and beliefs. Perhaps these readings will help you understand the place of behavior change philosophy within the health education profession.

# CHAPTER

## 15

# BEHAVIORAL HEALTH AND HEALTH EDUCATION: AN EMERGING OPPORTUNITY

**CARL I. FERTMAN**

I think the report of the 2000 Joint Committee on Health Education and Promotion Terminology (2001) is missing a term. The term is *behavioral health*. The roots of the term *behavioral health* can be traced directly to the managed health care industry. "Behavioral health" in the early 1990s became the managed health care industry name for services to individuals with mental health and substance abuse disorders that often required specialized knowledge and skills different from those needed to manage general medical care (Freeman & Trabin, 1994). However, somewhere along the way from the early 1990s to today, the term *behavioral health* has taken on new meanings; and although I cannot be sure, it does seem that behavioral health is here to stay and with it is an opportunity for health education and health educators to become more involved in helping formulate the structure and function of this arena.

At one time I might have been the first to argue that health education and health educators do not need to know about or be bothered by a term coined from the managed health care industry. I have been involved with promoting health and wellness for children and teenagers. My concern has been keeping youths drug free and mentally healthy. Yes, I knew about health insurance. I had my own insurance for me and my family. But as a professional, I was not involved with treating youths or providing any type of mental health or substance abuse counseling services that required fee collection or health insurance reimbursements. I was busy enough just trying to figure out how to fund projects to develop school health curricula and community health education programs designed to prevent substance abuse and promote mental health among teenagers. I often argued that money should be taken from treatment services to fund prevention programs.

It was as if, in my mind, a schism existed between prevention and treatment, between health education and health care—to some degree between health and medicine. Even if I was willing to accept that having such limited vision was not helpful and perhaps even harmful, I surely did not need to know how health insurance worked—especially in the current case of behavioral health, which had promulgated its own idiosyncratic jargon and terms. "Risk sharing," "gatekeeping," "utilization management," "contracts for administrative services," "full risk contracts," "carve-outs," and "product lines" are examples of such terms and jargon that seemed very far from the reality of most health educators, including myself.

At some point I changed my mind about wanting to know more about behavioral health: what the term meant, what it was. As a health educator, I began to see changes in the health arena, medicine, and public health that forced me as a stakeholder to reexamine health educators' present and future roles. Somehow the line was blurring between medicine and public health. The schism in my mind was closing. I found myself agreeing with the Committee on Medicine and Public Health (Lasker, 1997), which concluded that an imperative exists to address the health needs of people from a collaborative paradigm with two distinct perspectives: one looking out for the health needs of individual patients, the other committed to improving the health of the entire population. The fact is, health educators already span the medicine and public health sectors. Health educators work in clinical care, with its focus on individual patients—diagnosing symptoms, preventing and treating disease, providing comfort, relieving pain and suffering, and enhancing the capacity to function. Health educators work in public health, with its focus on populations—assessing and monitoring health behaviors, designing, implementing, and evaluating programs. Health educators also work across multiple areas such as public, private, and volunteer sectors of the economy. Health educators work in the public sector in schools and health departments, voluntary sectors in community agencies and national organizations, and increasingly, health educators can be found in the private sector in businesses and consulting.

Working in public health, clinical care, and other sectors of the economy, health educators stand at the intersection of many very different arenas. Each arena operates on different principles (Morone, Kilbreth, & Langwell, 2000). Each has its own assumptions, rules, actors, funding sources, policy debates, and patterns of power. For example, public health runs on federal and state funds guided by federal and state rules. The chain of command runs through the state capitol. Public education, in contrast, inverts all that. Local taxes (sometimes mixed with state money) fund the schools; local boards make the important decisions. In public health the state Medicaid agency is a major player, in education, there is rarely a state agency with comparable muscle (or money).

The common alarming thread for health educators, regardless of where they work, is managed care and, in particular, its application of the term *behavioral health* to define mental health and substance abuse programs and services without the voice of health educators. Our effort for evidence-based education, programs, and services to promote health for individuals, families, and communities seemed threatened in the push for cost containment, utilization review, and quality assurance. Another reason that I changed my mind about behavioral health was because I realized that all of my work in trying to prevent substance abuse and to promote mental health among teenagers seemed for naught, if most children and teenagers in need of services never receive them (U.S. Department of Health and Human Services, 2001). I wondered how I was doing as an educator if the people I served lacked the information, attitudes, and skills necessary to access programs and services. It was even more distressing to consider that the environment could be so hostile to allow such misery to continue. In my exploration of behavioral health, I now find myself grappling to understand current behavioral health practices and to determine what, if any, opportunity lies ahead for the field of health education to shape and refine the behavioral health arena.

What I found as I began to explore behavioral health and managed care is that the managed care industry is now well established in the United States and continues to grow at a rapid pace. It is no longer an experiment, an emerging trend, or an anomaly distinguishing certain regions of the country. Managed care is the primary mode of insuring Americans in the twenty-first century. Health professionals, including health educators, now work in an environment that is radically different from that of just ten years ago. There are new rules, new funding mechanisms, and new incentives for health professionals—incentives that have many health professionals angry, or at least confused.

In the year 2002, the mental health and substance abuse benefit packages that cover most privately insured Americans involve some form of managed behavioral health care. Likewise, the public sector mental health and substance abuse programs and services are in the midst of a dramatic revolution. Virtually all states are implementing managed behavioral health programs. Most uncertain is how managed care is providing services for people with the most severe illnesses and how managed care and the privatization of public mental health affect people with serious mental health problems. The private sector experience of behavioral health is very different from the public sector experience of behavioral health (Sturm, 1999).

My exploration of behavioral health left me excited about the potential of health educators to shape and refine what is meant by the term *behavioral health*. Standing at the intersection of so many arenas, health educators need to be poised for action, to seize the opportunity to shape and refine the concept of behavioral health.

## OPPORTUNITY FOR HEALTH EDUCATION AND HEALTH EDUCATORS

The opportunity for health educators to shape and refine the concept of behavioral health springs from the breadth of their field. As mentioned previously, health education spans many areas. Health educators function everywhere behavioral health reaches and operates: school, health care, criminal justice, community, workplace; they encompass public, private, and voluntary sectors. The opportunity for health educators lies in the fact that the promise of behavioral health has not yet met the reality of behavioral health. It has not produced a seamless system of care to meet the mental health needs of people (Mechanic & McAlpine, 1999; Ross, 2000). As a concept, behavioral health is still in its formative stage.

Motivating me to action is the health education socio-ecological model (McLeroy, Bibeau, Steckler, & Glanz, 1988), which supports and mandates health educator efforts at multiple levels, from programs and services for individuals to organizational and community change, to media campaigns, to advocacy for policy initiatives. Working at these different levels can help to ensure mental health and substance abuse education, programs, and services share equity with other areas of clinical care. The model suggests that health educators move beyond their own settings to bring our broad set of health education skills and expertise to bear on shaping what is behavioral health. In particular, health educators' efforts in three areas can influence the ultimate practice of behavioral health.

Health educators can work to help define behavioral health as a system of care that spans prevention to treatment to promotion and wellness for all people, communities, and organizations. To a large degree, behavioral health continues to focus on individuals with severe mental health and substance abuse illnesses. Only recently have models been put forth that reflect more expansive practice that focuses on health behavior assessment, health promotion and wellness, families, and communities (Altman, 2001). Such models open the doors to reducing stigma, achieving parity in mental health and substance abuse programs with those provided for physical health needs, and meeting people's mental health needs (prevention to treatment to promotion and wellness). By not joining the discussion but choosing to stay within our own settings, be they schools, public health agencies, hospitals, clinics, or businesses, and trying to address the mental health needs of those we serve, we potentially miss the larger debates about how to finance and shape the arena to meet these needs. Health educators need to be part of this dialogue. We can help to shift the behavioral health paradigm from being synonymous with treatment and payment to being synonymous with care and promotion.

We need to demand accountability. A shift has occurred. Evaluation and public accountability of mental health and substance abuse education, programs, and services under behavioral health have changed. Lumping together mental health and substance abuse prevention, intervention, and treatment under the banner of behavioral health may make sense in the long term. However, in discussions about behavioral health, one often hears concerns related to ongoing business and management practices by managed care providers. Discussed less frequently are topics such as positive individual outcomes, consumer satisfaction, management innovation, and comprehensive service delivery networks. A paradigm shift is being proposed in the arena of mental health and substance abuse needs and problems, which could include efforts to prevent them. More public accountability is needed. If, as health educators, we are going to prepare and support individuals to access and utilize education, programs, and services to address mental health and substance abuse needs and problems, we need more information. We need to be involved with the evaluation of behavioral health as it evolves. Health educators have the expertise to lead the evaluation efforts. In doing so, we can advocate for systems and organizations to be accountable for the provision of high quality comprehensive care.

As health educators we want to promote individual, family, and community participation in planning, implementing, and evaluating behavioral health. Start by investigating your own behavioral health plan offered as part of your personal health insurance. Talk with family members, colleagues, and friends about behavioral health. Help them to investigate their options and benefits. Hold community forums on the impact of behavioral health on community health education, programs, and services. Work to have communities hold accountable behavioral health care providers for their programs and services. Behavioral health is a commodity being purchased for people by businesses and state governments. An entity or intermediary in the form of the managed behavioral health organization now exists in health and medicine, in the public, private, and voluntary sectors to address mental health and substance abuse needs and problems. Individual consumers, their families, and com munities are distant from the decision-making process that affects what is available to them. Educating individuals, their families, and communities about behavioral health and its implications for care is a priority if they are to be informed consumers. I worry that my own attitude—that I did not need to know about behavioral health—is more common than I would hope.

In my daily work in schools and communities, I continue to work to prevent substance abuse problems and promote mental health among teenagers. My work is with mental health and substance abuse education, programs, services, and systems. At the same time, I am aware of bigger struggles being waged under the banner of behavioral health to shape and deliver mental health and substance abuse education, programs, and services to meet my own needs as well as the needs of the individuals, families, and communities I serve.

## REFERENCES

Altman, L. (2001). *Large employer trends in EAPs and managed behavioral care*. Washington, DC: U.S. Center for Mental Health Services.

Freeman, M. A., & Trabin, T. (1994). *Managed behavioral healthcare: History, models, key issues, and future course*. Rockville, MD: U.S. Center for Mental Health Services.

Joint Committee on Health Education and Promotion Terminology. (2001, March–April). Report of the 2000 Joint Committee on Health Education and Promotion Terminology. *American Journal of Health Education, 32*(2), 89–104.

Lasker, R. D. (1997). *Medicine and public health: The power of collaboration.* New York: Academy of Medicine.

McLeroy, K., Bibeau, D., Steckler, A., & Glanz, K. (1988). An ecological perspective on health promotion programs. *Health Education Quarterly,* 15, 351–377.

Mechanic, D., & McAlpine, D. (1999). Mission unfulfilled: Potholes on the road to mental health parity. *Health Affairs, 18,* 7–21.

Morone, J., Kilbreth, E., & Langwell, K. (2000). Back to school: A health care strategy for youth. *Health Affairs, 20,*122–136.

Ross, E. C. (2000). The promise and reality of managed behavioral health care. In R. W. Manderscheid & M. J. Henderson (Eds.), *Center for Mental Health Services: Mental health, United States, 2000* (DHHS Publication no. SMA 01-3537). Washington, DC: U.S. Government Printing Office.

Sturm, R. (1999). Tracking changes in behavioral health services: How have carve-outs changed care? *Journal of Behavioral Health Services & Research, 26,* 360–371.

U.S. Department of Health and Human Services. (2001). *U.S. Public Health Service report of the Surgeon General's conference on children's mental: A national agenda.* Washington, DC: Author.

# CHAPTER

## 16

# HEALTHY BEHAVIOR: THE IMPLICATIONS OF A HOLISTIC PARADIGM OF THINKING THROUGH BODYMIND RESEARCH

**DON READ**

**WALT STOLL**

It seems not so long ago (1985) that one of the authors of this article and Robert D. Russell debated "Is Behavior Change an Acceptable Objective for Health Educators?" The debate, if held today [1998], would most certainly be focused on a transcendent step beyond into causation: "Is Behavior Determined on a 'Physical' or 'Mental' Basis, or a Combination of Both?"

It is only now that global communication and technological process have begun to bring East and West together, while substantiating the unexplained observations from both East and West, that we are beginning to glimpse that "undiscovered country" and "the astonishing hypothesis" so well stated by the wise men of our age.

Just a glimpse of the wonders to come has been enough to vastly expand what we, as health educators, can do. It is as though we have been trying to do our jobs blind-folded and the blindfold has begun to slip ever so slightly.

The purpose of this paper is to encourage readers to open their eyes and peek past the blindfold to a wondrous new world of potential for helping those we can't help today. Even beyond that: we would help *our-selves* to be healthier and thus have more to offer those with whom we work (health educator heal thyself).

*The results of sci-entific research very often force a change in the philosophical view of problems which extend far beyond the restricted domain of science itself.*

—ALBERT EINSTEIN

From our viewpoint health education needs to either take hold of bodymind concepts, as they apply to health promotion, or other profes-sions will take the lead. The American Holistic Nurses Association is a perfect example of a profession that already has a twenty-year head start.

It appears that the health education profession continues to focus on an outdated "theory" about motives of and influences on health behavior. We feel it is urgently necessary for health educators to explore a closer cooperation between the empirical findings of psychoneuroimmunology (the evidence that thought and emotion affect the immune system at cel-lular and subcellular levels), and the logical, analytical concepts and rea-soning expressed in current holistic thinking as it applies to healthy behavior. We intend within this paper, in this charter issue of the *International Electronic Journal for Health Education*, to expand the old paradigm of health behavior into one suggested by these divergent mind sciences. This can only be done by exploring, and bringing together, a wide variety of disciplines to form a holistic concept of what the authors now choose to call healthy behavior.

We elect to promote the term "healthy behavior" to supplant the conventionally uti-lized term "health behavior" for several reasons: *Health* is a noun which—as defined by Webster—connotes a static definition. *Healthy* is defined as a state of *being* and, as such, is a dynamic and ever-changing state of bodymind—just as it must be in any individual. Few of us in the health education profession would have any argument with that. The profession of health education must become more dynamic. Calling our goal "healthy behavior" is one more step in the direction of this necessary development.

Today, these divergent disciplines are forming a science of the bodymind and "environment" (see Ferguson, 1980) that promises a major advance in our understand-ing of behavior and mental phenomena. What is emerging from this confluent effort is a conception of the bodymind that has been called "the astonishing hypothesis" by Nobel laureate Francis Crick, co-discoverer of the DNA double helix. The identity of the bodymind connection to healthy behavior has been underlined for years; from Kenneth Pelletier's classical work *Mind as Healer, Mind as Slayer* (1977) to the pro-vocative findings of current bodymind research.

Research and theory, as we explore them here, from such fields of psychoneuroimmu-nology, Eastern and Western philosophy, cognitive psychology, nutritional biochemistry, quantum physics, computer science, endocrinology, molecular/neurobiology—to name but a few—are converging to provide a vast new paradigm. The conclusions of bodymind research are truly being accepted as a physical (and non-physical) component of the natural world, subject to scientific laws, accessible to experimentation, and therefore open to understanding, prediction, and control. Bodymind concepts, in essence, are not the elusive, fuzzy—restricted to brain activity—entities we have considered them to be but rather an indivisible and interconnected (holographic) property of every cell. (See Joseph Chilton Pearce, 1992.) The brain is but a switchboard—albeit a powerful and complex one—of the bodymind gestaltic processes.

Besides that, there is now incontrovertible evidence that we do not end with our skin. This indivisible entity we call a human being physically, emotionally, socially and spiritually extends out to, and interacts with, the rest of the universe in ways not yet fully explored within the profession (Dossey, 1993; "Cardiologist studies effect of prayer," 1986).

As an example, in a 1994 report released by the Carnegie Council on Adolescent Development, *Starting Points: Meeting the Needs of Young Children*, which concluded that "how children function from the preschool years all the way through adolescence, and even adulthood, hinges in large part on their experience before the age of 3."

What makes this fact important is that most recently, dramatic technological advances have produced sophisticated scanning equipment such as positron-emission tomography, or PET, scanning that allows researchers to get incredibly detailed images and insights about the brain's functioning. Using PET scans, researchers can watch a baby's brain continue to form long after birth.

Advanced brain research such as PET addresses the longstanding "nature vs. nurture" debate that posits either a genetically "done deal" or a "clean slate" at birth. We believe it is *both* and does not begin at birth.

What this and other bodymind research is showing is that we must not be confined by our present out-of-date beliefs inside and outside of our own field of health education. We must gain the emerging and transcending insights, now being illuminated by other scientific fields, to open our minds to a paradigm that will transform our currently one sided approach to the complex field of healthy behavior. Health education has essentially been static and resistant to change—a characteristic of all professions. Health educators still have an opportunity to expand their knowledge by being sensitive to the widely divergent issues involved in the current paradigm shift in healthy behavior.

Should anyone doubt the critical importance of the health educator, s/he has but to view Kenneth Pelletier's videotape (*Health and Your Whole Being*, 1988) to begin understanding the political/economic factors inhibiting the incorporation of this vital data into our system of health promotion. It can be argued that the health educator is the most important professional in this system since only public awareness and pressure can bypass these political and economic roadblocks. It is the health educator who is perfectly positioned to influence public opinion.

A *Journal of the American Medical Association* paper reported, more than ten years ago, that most all of the leading causes of death prior to the age of 65 are caused by personal behavior and can be prevented. All of the causal factors are lifestyle and all changes are learnable. (See Ken Pelletier's videotape, 1988.)

The monopoly given the allopathic paradigm, in 1911, has given the AMA more than eighty years to mold public opinion to consider medical-care and health promotion identical when in fact it is far from that. Medical/health-care, as it is practiced in this country, is disease-management, just as health insurance is really illness insurance and life insurance is death insurance. Calling what we do in this country "health-care" is but one way we keep our current medical monopoly in power. If it was working, we would not need to change it. Health promotion explores the many ways to healthy behavior. Who would be interested in buying "death insurance"?

*Never utter these words: "I do not know this, therefore it is false." One must study to know: Know to understand: Understand to judge.*

*—Apothegm of Narada*

Until health educators clearly see that distinction, they are part of the problem. The sections of this paper that discuss the medical model of health care are designed to lead the reader from the viewpoint of the fiction of medical/health-care to the fact of medical/disease-care. Only then can we rationally discuss healthy behavior.

## THE POSSIBILITY FOR DEFINITIONS?

The authors have chosen to define certain terms such as *psychoneuroimmunology*, *holism*, and *emotional intelligence* for clarity only. Other terms such as *health*, *bodymind* have never been clearly defined precisely within our Western culture. As an example, there is not single word that can be used to link the body and mind together. The authors use the term *bodymind*, but this term cannot be found in any dictionary. What the authors do stress is that every human being *not* be considered as a composite of several levels, such as body, mind, spirit, but as a multidimensional unity.

One good opportunity for appreciating this fact can be this: often when the term *health* is defined, it is reduced to some static, biological, physiological concept that has no correlate in the real world. It is entirely appropriate, here, to recommend to those who hunger for a "scientific" basis for a more useful definition of these necessary transformative concepts, to look at Bohm's videotape (*Interview with David Bohm*, 1994) for insights into the indivisibility of all nature. Using Bohm's theory, in order to understand health, one must understand all the dimensions of life in the cosmos. (See Paul Tillich, *The Meaning of Health*, 1981.)

A comprehensive definition of *health* is impossible from the perspective of a purely Cartesian (Rene Descartes) philosophy—the "gold standard" of Western philosophy—whereas it is routinely defined from an empirical (from the holistic concept that the functional definition of all systems is that they are more than, and different from, any possible summation of their parts) viewpoint. Until we stop defining *health* in terms of circumstantial evidence, we will forever be held to the old paradigm. (See video *The Meaning of Health with Bill Moyers*, 1993.)

Larry Dossey, MD, in his book *Beyond Illness: Discovering The Experience of Health* (1984) moves as close as we feel one can get to defining the term health by constructing a powerful case for the deeply causative role of the mind in health. His concept of health includes such thoughts as these:

- We can learn to participate in grief and pain from an utterly new perspective, a perspective that modifies the meaning we impart to experience.

- Spirit is radically beyond health. No-Health is beyond body and mind.

- People who attain it move beyond illness.

- There is the most elegant ordinariness to persons who go beyond illness.

This is the "nothing special" quality of the world that is sensed by those who know it deepest. It is the stage where once again mountains become mountains and rivers become rivers. It is the awareness wherein suffering and illness becomes, once again, illness.

The Ken Pelletier videotape (1988) reminds us that, as the present system of medical care exists: "We know a lot about disease. We know practically nothing about health." Is it any wonder that our system of "health care" is in trouble?

Ken Pelletier is one of the pioneers in the concept of consciousness being the basic factor of our Western approach that has been excluded from the equation. When consciousness is factored in, suddenly all observed phenomena of healing and health promotion are explainable. (See Pelletier's 1988 video *Health and Your Whole Being*.)

The problem lies in the fact that in all too many instances, our modern view of healthy behavior has outgrown the expressions we habitually use—outdated words, concepts, and beliefs which were created long ago to convey Cartesian (Descartes' basis for our reductionistic/mechanistic Western paradigm) beliefs. We must grow beyond the concept of health being static. We must open ourselves to the dynamically changing definition that acknowledges the implications of a new holistic paradigm of thinking through bodymind research—all leading to a more holistic understanding of healthy behavioral response. Part of the problem is that these antiquated words, concepts and beliefs about the bodymind connection are major factors holding back the field of healthy behavior. (See Dossey, 1993, video *Recovering the Soul: A Scientific and Spiritual Search*.)

Psychoneuroimmunology offers us many exciting insights into not only the roots of how healthy behavior is materially influenced by bodymind, but also the factors that influence bodymind functioning. It is this process that opens into the details of the effects of those necessary changes in consciousness.

Mathematician Charles Muses proclaimed about the future direction of our discussion: "The potentials of consciousness remain well nigh the last reachable domain for man not yet explored—The Undiscovered Country." The authors suggest this statement is properly followed up by French neurologist Frederic Tilney's prediction that we will "by conscious command evolve cerebral centers which will permit us to use powers that we now are not even capable of imagining." One of the authors of this paper had, for many years, used as the postmark on his postage meter: "You Are More Than You Think!" The technology of the West (biofeedback) has already brought us a long way toward realizing Tilney's prediction.

Biofeedback research has also finally laid to rest our narrow Western viewpoint that used to reject, out of hand, the now reproducible observations of cognitive control of physiological systems common in eastern philosophical traditions.

## THE REVOLUTION

From the classic nineteenth-century case study of Phineas Gage, the railroad worker whose frontal lobe was pierced by a metal rod, to the enchanting glimpses of brain functioning expanded by modern positron emission tomography and neuromagnetometry—among other newly developed systems of mind function analysis—mind research has provided increasingly remarkable insights into the mysteries of behavior and mental phenomena. Gage showed behavioral and personality changes which may have been mysterious and unexpected in 1848 but today are recognized as the typical results of damage to the frontal lobe. His and similar case studies initiated the development of new research into the physical representation of personality and emotions in the bodymind which is only now reaching fruition. (See Daniel Goleman, Chapter 11, "Mind and Medicine," in *Emotional Intelligence*, 1995.) The concept of "emotional intelligence," as Goleman uses it, includes the abilities to rein in emotional impulses, to read another's innermost feelings, to handle relationships smoothly and to motivate oneself. "These are the capabilities that are going to determine our success in family life, in careers, with friends, as citizens," he says. "These are the abilities that make us people." The foundations of healthy behavior most certainly require these positive attributes.

In an analogous fashion, Norman Cousins' work has been grossly simplified. His "Anatomy of an Illness (as Perceived by the Patient)," first published in the *New England Journal of Medicine* (1976), and his statements and thoughts concerning the complex relationship between mental attitude and physical health have been reduced in some quarters to the apparently absurd notion that laughter can cure cancer.

Cousins used laughter as a metaphor for the foil range of the positive emotions, including hope, love, faith, a strong will to live, determination and purpose.

What we are discussing here is a vital additional step toward the health promotion for the twenty-first century. Up to now, we have followed the conventional medical penchant for ignoring the observed and documented happenings in the world of "anecdotal health behavior." However, we cannot afford to continue doing that when the bases or the validity of these "happenings" have already been well established by fields outside health education. Thus, the most common way we have protected ourselves from changing our paradigm has been for us to just ignore those happenings we could not explain with our old Cartesian philosophy. A wise man once said: "The appearance of one sparrow proves the existence of birds." Research, in the current age, has tended to throw out the anomalous findings in favor of the "mean." It is time to be brave enough to look at *all* the evidence and not just what is considered "convenient." (See Stoll, 1996; Grossinger, 1980; and Coulter, 1973–1994.)

The 1990s are already being viewed as the decade of behavioral medicine and the bodymind connection. In an introduction to the Ninth International Conference, "The Psychology of Health, Immunity, and Disease," sponsored by the National Institute for the Clinical Application of Behavioral Medicine (NICABM; 1997), it was stated:

> Today, in America and throughout the world, we are witnessing a cultural transformation in health care. This change is emerging at a time when mind/body therapies and approaches to healing are clearly taking shape. As practitioners, we have achieved a new level of credibility among the conventional medical community by demonstrating behavioral medicine as a viable healing methodology that can not only control costs, but increase overall quality of life.

It can be said that more has been learned about the science of the bodymind in the last fifteen years than in all the previous years of research. Although these newly discovered (by our Western scientific method) mechanisms and interactions have been applied empirically for the last ten thousand years, it has only been recently that bodymind has been included in the scientific research as a holistic entity. The most important qualification for the proposal of any new theory of "reality" is that it explain *all* of the observable phenomena. The ideas presented in this paper, so far, describe the only theory that meets that criterion: *everything* in the cosmos is connected holographically.

Moreover, modern researchers are not restricted to case studies. In addition, they are using technically advanced methods that can even probe individual brain cells or map neural circuits in a project similar to the Human Genome Project (the mapping of the "addresses" of each gene on all forty-six human chromosomes). The present goal is to construct a detailed map of the human brain, chart its intricate webbing of cells, and identify the corresponding mental, cognitive, emotional, and biobehavioral experience. However, these studies only involve the brain which we now know may be but a major *part* of the total bodymind interactions of healthy behavior. Already, psychoneuroimmunologists have pieced together an impressive (albeit still incomplete) understanding of bodymind anatomy and functioning and, in the process, have stimulated widespread collateral research and speculation in related fields. Biofeedback research quickly established that one could learn (in a few hours) to consciously control one single muscle (or nerve) cell.

Cognitive psychologists have developed new technologies for research and, consequently, have made cognitive psychology an integral component of the new bodymind science. These and related efforts remind us that bodymind research is developing an ever-increasing diversity of branches and that the new science of bodymind is truly multidisciplinary. This most certainly includes health education—which, undoubtedly, *can* be the most important single cog in the wheel of the health-promotion system to come.

Our professional need for this new science, as we enter the twenty-first century, is of crucial importance to health educators, especially in professional preparation and most certainly in programs promoting healthy behavior. This potential—together with the fact that study of bodymind issues is so fascinating—probably accounts for the attention that the new bodymind science has received from the popular media.

## WAYS TO FACILITATE THE PSYCHOSOCIAL APPROACHES TO HEALTH EDUCATION

Most people find it hard to work on their health from a psychosocial approach alone. All health educators have had personal experience with that fact. Frequently, simply improving the quality of the function of the physical bodymind (nutrition, exercise and skilled relaxation [Davis, Eshelman, & McKay, 1988])—the three basic approaches recommended by all holistic health practitioners—brings a more energetic individual to the professional suggesting healthy behavioral changes. (See video: Andrew Weil, *8 Weeks to Optimal Health*, 1997.) *We health professionals know, from our personal experiences, that most people start their learning (healing) journey exhausted, depressed and sick and that we wish that we had seen the person sooner in her/his slide into illness.* One of the ways to bring them back toward this more energetic level of function, where our psychosocial skills in health education will be so much more effective, is to consider the Orthomolecular Psychiatric Association's discoveries over the past forty years.

We suggest that people radically changing their nutritional habits for a 2–4 week trial period, while observing the effect on their well-being, is an often more efficient and effective alternative to a purely psychosocial health education approach. Of course, the recommendations for this change need to be based on the personal knowledge of the health educator doing the evaluation. *We say* trial *since the science of nutrition is still too complex for anyone to be sure of choosing the perfect diet for that person the first time.* There are some basic rules for anyone although the quickest, and most dramatic, changes are individually determined (Stoll, 1996). Even the regular practice of any effective approach to skilled relaxation or aerobic exercise—or better yet, the combination of them together, will eventually produce similar results in a few months. (Note: The concept of stress management includes skilled relaxation techniques (Davis et al., 1988), strategies for engagement and involvement, as well as mechanisms for increased "internal locus of control"(Hafen, Karren, Frandsen, & Smith, 1996, pp. 473–484). Who among us can say that we can reach similar effects in the average person we counsel—when we use psychosocial methods alone? (See Reed, 1983, and Schauss, 1980.)

When the nutritional approach is used alone, the results are more predictable and within two weeks the individual would experience sufficient benefits that they would want to continue it indefinitely. With the nutritional approach, done correctly, results seem to happen much faster than with any other single modality. Besides, as the individual experiences more and more energy, they become more and more interested in more healthy behaviors: "If I can feel this much better, this soon, by just doing this, what could I feel like by doing more?" (See Reed, 1983.)

Personally observing this one eye-opener, alone, creates many professional converts who become truly committed to looking at the problems of health education through a much wider lens. Of course the health educator personally experiencing these changes is an even more effective way.

Table 16.1 reports data that has been well established for twenty years. We offer it as one example of the difficulty of changing one's paradigm of reality. Nearly all professionals in the field of health promotion were educated without being privy to this information. Why? Is it really true that only high tech, and very expensive, therapeutic approaches are taught? Besides, a medical license is not required to share these approaches with the public. They do not even require testing of any kind. All that is needed is that the information be available to the caring parents and concerned child. As such, this information is seen by the medical professionals in charge of the "system," as competition. This is opposed to what we have experienced in our practices: which is that they are complementary to the current allopathic monopoly.

The feet that this twenty-year-old knowledge is not commonly applied testifies to the difficulty of shifting our approaches to dealing with these difficult problems. Perhaps the reader has noted that most of our references are ten to twenty years old. This is not new stuff. It is just that it takes a generation for radical new discoveries to become part of the common consciousness. We have had our generation. It is now past time to move forward.

For more than twenty years it has been known that various very simple changes in diet create dramatic improvements in bodymind function in a short period of time—this without any evaluation at all. (See Table 16.1.) The reluctance of the medical profession to make these simple, safe and inexpensive approaches at least part of the "treatment of choice" is based primarily upon economics and the fear by the professional of being ostracized by her/his colleagues. The only protection the public has, against this non-health-related delay in "what is best for the person," is to become knowledgeable in the area which concerns their own particular problems and so become more active participants in their own health promotion (internal locus of control). Who would be better than the health educator to facilitate this process in any individual?

## TRANSPERSONAL PSYCHOLOGY: A VEHICLE FOR CHANGE

Joan Borysenko, PhD, is one who understands the new paradigm and practices it in her profession. Her tapes graphically describe and explain its powerful and practical application to change to healthy behavior, *receptivity to health education* and the individual empowerment produced by these freeing concepts. These ideas make it much more practical for the individual to firmly establish an "internal locus of control" (Hafen et al., 1996, pp. 473–484)—an essential first step toward healthy behavioral change.

## TABLE 16.1 Effects of Treatment on Children's Behavior

| Treatment Option | Percentage Improved | Percentage Worsened |
|---|---|---|
| Removing milk | 32.0 | 1.0 |
| Removing wheat | 50.0 | 2.0 |
| Removing sugar | 51.0 | 3.0 |
| Psychotherapy | 9.0 | 1.0 |
| Patterning | 38.0 | 3.0 |
| Exercise | 44.0 | 7.0 |
| Day School | 6.0 | 3.0 |
| Residential School | 31.0 | 4.0 |
| Operant Conditioning | 20.0 | 5.0 |
| All drugs combined | 1.6 | 1.0 |
| Mellaril (best drug) | 12.0 | 5.0 |
| Vitamins | 45.0 | 1.5 |

*Source:* Walt Stoll, Saving yourself from the disease-care crisis (Panama City, FL: Sunrise Health Coach, 1996); reprinted from Bernard Rimland (1977, June), Comparative effects of treatment on child's behavior (Drugs, therapies, schooling, and several non-treatment events), Publication 34, Institute for Child Behavior Research (San Diego, CA).

Gerald Jonas, in his book *Visceral Learning: Toward a Science of Self-Control* (1972), discusses human behavior and individual control in this way: "Our personal experience, supported by a cultural heritage of several millennia, assures us that somewhere inside the person seen by others there is an invisible core of being—a purely private self that observes, if it cannot always control, our public actions and is ultimately free of all controls imposed on the organism from outside. Whether it makes any sense or not, that is what it *feels* like to be conscious, and any definition of 'conscious control' that fails to mention such a feeling is like a weather report that fails to mention whether it is raining or sunny."

The question of which must come first in behavior change—the individual or the society—is neatly laid to rest by Dr. Borysenko's facility with the genre: "Inner transformation *does* change the world."

She tells the story of her friend, Peter Russell's (author of *A White Hole in Time*) answering machine message: "This is not an answering machine. It is a questioning machine. Who are you? What do you want?"

The fact is that the vast majority of us, of the Western Cartesian philosophy, come into this life and finally leave it without ever answering either of those questions. Is it any wonder that we are inundated with chronic diseases (Borysenko video, 1996)?!

It is the function of health education to be the opening wedge into resolving this unhealthy societal condition. How can we, as health educators, be more than a part of the problem until we, personally, can make the transcendent leap into a more holistic paradigm of health?

## THE PROBLEM OF TRANSCENDENCE

This "problem" is probably due to the fact that our Western culture has had more than two hundred years to become fixed in the concrete of a Cartesian (rationalistic) paradigm of reality as being the *only* valid approach to health promotion. This "seeing the trees and not the forest" kind of reductionism is a powerful philosophy for dealing with many things—*just not everything*. For thousands of years, before this modern era of reductionism, the holistic paradigm was the only practical way we *had* to approach complex health problems: "Seeing the forest and not the trees."

One of the basic arguments, at the time of the acceptance of the Flexner Report by the U.S. Congress (1911)—thus ushering in the present allopathic monopoly over health-care thinking in this century—was that empirical thinking methods of research and application were too difficult and could not yet be proven in the laboratories of the time.

William James, MD, who has been called the father of American psychology, tried to stop the stampede by the national legislature toward accepting this report feat promised a much simpler way to approach medicine. He suggested that we still didn't know everything and there was a real possibility that we could be shutting off the very research most needed to improve our concepts of effective health-care. The law that passed (based completely on the Flexner Report—sponsored by the AMA of the time) refused any government money for research in any field other than allopathy. From that grew our present disease-care crisis. This was the most recent "victory" of rationalism over empiricism. Now, of course, we are proving those empirical concepts every day in our advanced laboratories—and still barely scratching the surface. The acceptance of the Flexner Report just put off by more than eighty years this essential research effort. (Grossinger, 1980, and Coulter, 1973–1994)

Reductionistic (rationalistic) thinking *was* (and is) easier but has proven to be of insufficient scope to cope with the chronic diseases of civilization—all of which are multi-factorial in causation. The current disease-care crisis can be directly attributed to our desperately clinging to the idea that, if we just threw enough money into it, *we could force the health-care camel through the eye of the allopathic needle*.

All of the non-allopathic systems of health-care, practiced over the entire world today, are based on empiricism. The allopathic philosophy, based on rationalism alone, has not the depth to deal with the chronic illnesses of civilization—empiricism does. By combining rationalistic thinking (for acute care) with empirical thinking (for chronic conditions) we have a blueprint for the health care of the twenty-first century. That involves, however, our willingness to transcend the current narrow views of reality *and to* create a level playing field (at least so far as insurance coverage and licensing laws are concerned), in this country, for all major global approaches to health promotion. There are citizens' committees, who understand what is needed, functioning in thirty states already. Any of them could be contacted by anyone wanting to understand the problem—or even join into lobbying for change. Until health educators make this leap of transcendent thinking, how can we expect the public to do so? A wise man once said: "If you always do what you have always done, you will always get what you have always gotten" (source unknown). If you are not part of the solution, you are a part of the problem. A definition of "insanity": Doing the same thing over and over while expecting different results.

Recall the half century of acrimonious controversy in the field of physics during which half of the world's top physicists insisted light behaved as a wave and half insisted that it behaved as a particle. Each side could set up experiments that would prove their theory was correct. It was only when they finally came to the realization that light behaved *both* as a particle *and* a wave that they could progress to the modern quantum physics theory—the logjam was broken.

The method of this seemingly paradoxical conclusion in physics can be directly applied to the fact that rationalism and empiricism are both "correct." We will not progress in health promotion until that 4,000-year-old "divided legacy" is resolved (Coulter, 1973–1994).

There is already far more than enough scientific data upon which to base a firm paradigm of everything being holographically related. The effectiveness of auricular acupuncture, reflexology and iridology as well as the functional reality of the holographic brain (Karl Pribram, 1978, 1979) are but a few examples within the human alone. Healing by prayer at a distance (San Francisco Cardiology Study is but one of many such studies) takes us beyond the human structure into the cosmos. The only understandable reason for the reticence by professional health educators, for not accepting this impressive array of new scientific ideas into an ingenious and optimistic portrait of healthy behavior for the twenty-first century, is a reluctance on the part of health educators to give up cherished paradigms which have served us all so well for so long. Why do you think there is a disease-care *crisis* worldwide today?

In her book *Neurophilosophy* (1986), philosopher Patricia Smith Churchland proposes the sensible idea that a satisfactory understanding of bodymind and behavior would be much facilitated by—and perhaps even requires—a closer cooperation between the empirical findings of neurophilosophy and the logical, analytical concepts and reasoning of traditional philosophies. It would behoove brain researchers to become familiar with philosophy, Churchland argues. She also suggests that philosophers could ground their propositions more firmly in scientific research. A hallmark of our age is that modern scientific discoveries are substantiating traditional philosophies. And, we can add here, it would also behoove health educators to become more familiar with both.

*I know that most men, including those at ease with problems of the greatest complexity, can seldom accept even the simplest and most obvious truth if it be such as would oblige them to admit the falsity of conclusions which they have delighted in explaining to colleagues, which they have proudly taught to others, and which they have woven, thread by thread, into the fabric of their lives.*

*—Leo Tolstoy*

The firefighter climbing the ladder must let go of the current rung in order to reach for the next one. We are fortunate in our profession that we at least can bring the old rung along with us. All we have to admit to ourselves is that there is more than one rung on the ladder! Both/and is another hallmark of our era.

## WHERE IN THE BODY IS THE "HOUSE OF THE MIND"?

The title for this section came from one author's memory of an ancient similarity of mystical knowing represented by the well known idea of "the Cave of Brahmin." This fourth ventricle of the brain was known by many ancient disciplines to be the "house of God" where everything seemed to center. Our most competent technology is just now proving that their ancient, vitalistic (empirical) knowing was correct without resorting to "science." The only difference is that now we are advanced enough to recognize that the Cave of Brahmin is but the clearing house for the mind of the *rest* of the body. (See Joy Brugh's 1988 video, *Healing and the Unconscious*.)

Perhaps the most far-reaching blank spot in the thinking of many professionals in the field of healthy behavior is the persistent idea that our emotions, as well as certain properties of our minds such as *will, feelings* and *attitudes*, are qualities which are wholly explained by brain operations. A common idea in the ancient world was that mind and emotions emanated from the heart, not the head. Even today, we commonly see references to this notion in such phrases as "I have this gut feeling," or "My heart tells me." We now know that heart muscle creates the same endorphins manufactured by the brain. The white blood cells have receptors for the endorphins made in the brain. The intestinal lining also makes the endorphins which were originally considered the unique province of the brain.

Unfortunately, a similar error has persisted in the field of healthy behavior, and in which wants and feelings as related to health issues are treated as if they exist in a separate, transcendent reality that can magically interact with brain neurochemistry. "Wants" and "feelings" are *not* pure and simple brain processes but are influenced by the same forces that intermingle with other brain processes—namely, the internal biochemical/electromagnetic environment of the rest of the body—as well as experiences from the external world.

It is very disconcerting to hear experts speak of, and textbooks bind themselves to, a very narrow and disjointed approach to such a complex field as healthy behavior. In this vein it is disquieting to note that the *American Journal of Health Behavior*, in its wonderfully stated objectives, suggests a holistic and comprehensive view but instead only publishes papers that persist in expanding an unconnected, one-sided view of body and mind. The same can be said of *Health Behavior and Health Education* (Glanz, Lewis, & Rimer, 1997) in which the focus is one dimensional by totally ignoring the influence of bodymind possibilities that truly matter in terms of healthy behavior. We attribute this "narrow" focus to either an unwillingness on the part of the editors (and thus acceded by the writers) to publish research/ideas discussing these transcendent subjects, or a lack of understanding and/or acceptance of these ideas. It is our contention that the evolution of bodymind research will *soon* lead to a new kind of healthy behavior and health education thinking *only* if it is so viewed by a wide segment of the members of the health education profession; although it will eventually happen without us if we don't participate.

There will be a new kind of thinking for the twenty-first century which includes the fact that everything interacts with, and is wholly influenced by, everything else— no exclusions. (See George Leonard, *The Silent Pulse*, 1978.) This concept seems difficult only until the individual achieves the transcendence of perspective always necessary before a paradigm shift is possible—then, suddenly, it is easy. And so it is with the term "holistic." Breaking with our promise that we will not define specific terms, let us take liberties by doing so again. For the benefits of understanding, the term *holistic* refers to the fact that any functioning system of parts creates something *in addition to, and separate from*, any possible summation of the parts. All of the body is in the mind, and all of the mind is in the body. (See video *Interview with David Bohm*, 1994, and the San Francisco Cardiology study of the effects of distant prayer, *Recovering the Soul* with Larry Dossey, 1993.)

The single most important ingredient for healthy behavioral change is the individual's desire to change. Toward that end, developing an "internal locus of control" (Hafen et al., 1996, pp. 473–484) is the first, and absolutely essential, step toward the effectiveness of any approach to health education. One of the aims of this paper is to bring to the total equation of behavioral change the holistic procedures that would improve the quality of the *tissue* (the entire body) making the decisions and implementing the lifestyle changes needed. *Attitudes, personalities, healthy behavior, even the mind itself—all are produced by bodymind processes and should not be viewed as somehow separate or apart from them. Healthy/unhealthy behaviors are bodymind processes, pure and simple, and are influenced by the same forces that influence other bodymind processes—namely, the biochemical/electromagnetic environment and experiences from the internal and external world.* It is therefore disconcerting to hear health educators talk about social change as if it were some mystical essence to be imposed on the mind from *without*. The fact is that healthy behavior and the mind are not all produced by brain processes and must have been seen as encompassing the holographic bodymind/environment.

## TO THE POINT

"Mind" truly matters when it comes to healthy behavior. It is our contention that health education continues to assume that mind is truly not a part of the body, and thus is treated as a sort of side dish to the main meal. As an example of the indivisibility of mind from the environment, we offer Table 16.2.

In 1980, William Philpott, MD, published his landmark book *Brain Allergies*, which is still a classic in the field. Many substances from the environment can influence brain chemistry.

So too, are healthy behaviors conceived as states produced by, but not a part of, the bodymind. Thus we in health education conceive of healthy behaviors as some of the most elusive and nebulous concepts separate from the physicalness of the bodymind. This concept is gradually being debunked by the new bodymind research. It makes sense within the field of health education to look seriously and closely at a bodymind paradigm for the healthy behaviors needed to go beyond our present crisis in health-care. Doing that will require significant changes in our popular ideas.

TABLE 16.2    **Nervous System Manifestations of Allergy-causing Substances**

| | Percentage of Effect | | | | |
|---|---|---|---|---|---|
| Changes | Food | Pollens & Dust | Mold | Bacteria | Drugs & Misc. |
| Mood changes | 84 | 33 | 28 | 20 | 24 |
| Minimal brain dysfunction | 45 | 23 | 0 | 0 | 32 |
| Mental & neurological syndrome | 89 | 35 | 3 | 16 | 22 |

*Source:* M. B. Campbell. (1973, October). Neurologic manifestations of allergic disease. Annals of Allergy, *31*(10):489. Reprinted by permission of Robert Anderson, MD (Anderson, 1993).

## TOWARD A HEALTHY BEHAVIOR PARADIGM

Modern neuroscience has offered us many exciting insights into the mechanics of how mental states, emotions, and healthy behavior are produced by the mind, as well as what factors influence mind functioning and the details of such psychological processes. It is not helpful or useful, therefore, to pass over bodymind research vis-à-vis professional journals, conferences, text books, and the like without serious consideration and thought. We need to learn to rely more heavily on clear, sound, scientific understandings and interpretations from many fields of endeavor which are presently considered outside our own profession. More constructive patterns of healthy behavior; enhancement of emotional sensitivity; greater control of one's life: These are the primary and secondary outcomes of all effective health education. Far from being vague or elusive, these outcomes have been shown by the overwhelming weight of empirical evidence to be as objectively verifiable as they are personally meaningful. The individual's development of new and more constructive patterns of healthy behavior is reflected in his or her ability to reach previously unattainable goals. Effective health education and healthy behavioral change, then, result in meaningful and measurable outcomes.

## THE ROLE OF HEALTH EDUCATION

Health education has published accounts of this mindbody science which has appeared in numerous professional journals. At the same time these academic endeavors are often reported to the general public via the popular media: television, magazines, newspapers, best-seller list, and so on—often as quasi "new age." Herein lies what we perceive as another major problem. While new bodymind science is receiving more popular attention than any other academic research, it would appear that the majority of the profession itself remains skeptical. Even when addressed in journals and/or professional conferences; holistic, bodymind, spirituality issues are treated as an addition—as parts rather than whole. The real reason for, and thesis of, this article is the magnificent open-ended possibility of how our concept of healthy behavior is predicated by the magnificent open-ended possibilities our higher structures of bodymind offer for changing behavior. Since professionals are usually the last to make transformative leaps within their own professions, it is imperative that the readers of this paper understand that it is *more difficult* for them than it is for the lay person to understand and accept new truths.

Professionals frequently excuse their personal reluctance to change their paradigm by choosing instead to believe it is only media exploitation; which more often than not reflects and interprets these scientific ideas through a lens clouded by erroneous assumptions. By blaming the media's frequent pandering to a "natural" quick fix about mind and behavior, professionals can avoid the painful process of taking seriously the true meaning and implications of the intellectual revolution we are now experiencing.

This attitude is not shared by all, though. Blair Justice, who is a professor of psychology in the School of Public Health at the University of Texas at Houston, addresses this revolution in his book *Who Gets Sick: Thinking and Health* (1995):

*No one factor determines who gets sick and who does not. Whether we are talking about heart attacks, cancer or AIDS, "cofactors"—not single causes—are responsible. And a key cofactor, now intensely researched as part of the new science of biological and molecular psychology, is the cognitive—how our heads affect our health.*

*Since it is now known that the brain has power to regulate all bodily functions, disregulation of the central nervous system is increasingly being implicated as a contributing factor in disease. What goes on in our heads, then, has far-reaching influence on not only our nervous system but also the immune system, the hormone system and our health.*

*Most health professionals…concede that the mind has something to do with physical illness, but few know how the two affect each other or what the evidence is that they are related. Even fewer can keep up with the mushrooming research, from the molecular to the behavioral effect of the brain on the body.*

The growing field of psychoneuroimmunology is based on a system that examines the ways in which psychological processes are intertwined with both the nervous and immune system.

## THE WAVE TO COME

If we in health education do not take a leadership role in the coming paradigm, we believe the profession will be swept along in these changes by other professional fields within the health care field. Holistic nursing (American Holistic Nurses Association) is a good example of a profession doing an outstanding and imaginative job already.

One of the major changes that must take place within health education, in order to take a leadership role, is the transcendent commitment to do what is best for the individual and society and not, primarily, what is best for the profession. The best example of the antithesis of this attitude lies in what the AMA is doing right now to protect its monopoly.

As Fred Polak has so eloquently pointed out in his *Images of the Future*, if we are to survive we must begin to invent viable images and discover the best ways to utilize them.

There are grave difficulties involved in talking about paradigm shifts for they often take on a life force of their own and are always a threat to the status quo. Health education needs to move decisively into a growing consciousness that healthy behavior (and health promotion) requires a form of ecological, bodymind and holistic thinking that up till now has been sorely missing.

What can be done to help the twenty-first century become the century of the integration of the bodymind into a comprehensive approach to healthy behavior? Remember, this is going to happen with or without us. This is our opportunity to have some influence on the direction it will go. We can start by reversing all of the negatives we have stated above and focusing on totally integrating bodymind thinking and research into all aspects of health education, and including

- professional journals
- professional conferences
- professional programs in healthy behavior

## A PROGRAM IN HEALTHY BEHAVIOR

It is the authors' contention that a graduate career devoted to purely intellectual development is no longer an adequate preparation for becoming a Health Educator who is focusing on the area of healthy behavior. The core of our suggested program is an experientially *balanced* development of the individual—the integration of the physical, intellectual, spiritual and bodymind aspects of the personality. Our goal is to explore and experience behavior in an environment that provides opportunities for intensive personal growth and integration of one's own bodymind self.

Five areas of study are emphasized. Each area involves intensive personal participation, academic study, and an emphasis on professional training related to counseling, teaching, and research. Tools for communication will be taught in each area.

### 1. Bodymind Work

Students are expected to develop competence sufficient to teach an introductory course in Healthy Behavior or to practice professionally in any number of health education settings. Some bodymind disciplines may include breathing, T'ai-Chi, Aikido, Bioenergetics, among many others.

Academic study would include work in anatomy, physiology, psychology, philosophy, clinical holistic nutrition (*not* dietetics), health promotion, stress management, behavioral health and bodymind course work. Basic information would include personal familiarity with centering, stress reduction and movement techniques. Stress would be placed on new ways of integrating bodymind experience and health education, with a focus on techniques for maintaining, improving health and preventing illness among people who are currently healthy (see Matarazzo, 1980; Matarazzo, Herd, & Weiss, 1984).

### 2. Group Work

Extensive use of group techniques will allow students to work on communication skills and to develop a transpersonal orientation to group work, facilitating what Jon Kabat-Zinn calls "heightened awareness." Instead of competition and grade-orientation we strongly emphasize the building of a sense of shared goals and developing a supportive group community within the program. Specific systems would include Rogerian group work, problem-oriented group work, gestalt therapy, and the like.

### 3. Individual Work

Exposure to various techniques and systems of healthy behavior and health education will be available, in a clinical setting, in order to facilitate personal development and clarification of individual goals, as well as professional training.

### 4. Intellectual Work

At the core of the academic program is an in-depth study of a single system of philosophy, or research in healthy behavior, chosen by each student. Students read and research what they are most interested in, teach each other what they have learned, and evaluate each other's work.

### 5. Spiritual Work

Emphasis is placed on a personal commitment to a specific path which will help to actualize each student's individual goals. We would stress integration of one's spiritual discipline and perspective in daily life. Emphasis would be on such works as Herbert Benson's book *Timeless Healing* (1996) and Larry Dossey's *Healing Words: The Power of Prayer and the Practice of Medicine* (1993).

## SYNTHESIS

To a certain extent the general acceptance of an approach to healthy behavior has been the result of shifting public/professional perceptions of traditional medicine and the conventional medical establishment. Certainly in the past two decades there has been growing interest in traditional forms of intervention (as contrasted with conventional forms), with a resulting burgeoning of approaches to and kinds of health care. The problem within health education is that the notion of a lived condition of healthy behavior gets lost. Instead, an opposition is set up between the process of realizing a potential and a static concept of "health" behavior. Until healthy behavior is seen as a personal possession for which the individual must take responsibility (internal locus of control), health education will forever live in the mold of "conventional medicine."

We would like to conclude by raising some questions one of the authors of this article brought up in his book *Health Education: A Cognitive/Behavioral Approach* (1997). We hope the readers will think about and discuss these questions in their classes on healthy behavior:

■ Must we choose between a scientific and an unscientific definition of health, or can the two coexist?

■ How are mind and body connected? Is mind part of soul, and if so, can it exist apart from the body?

■ How do we know how healthy we are? Are our perceptions built into our minds, or do we develop them from our external perceptions and experiences?

■ How does perception work? Are our impressions of health and illness true representations of what we are? How can someone know whether or not s/he is healthy?

■ Which is the right road to true health: pure knowledge from the outside, data gathered from the inside, or a combination of both?

■ Does the mind rule the body, or vice versa? Or, do they play an equal role?

■ Can we present not only the analytical and logical but also the intuitive in health education?

The authors would like to add one more question: What is the true potential of the human construct? Remember what the wise man said, "The appearance of one sparrow proves the existence of birds."

We hope that we have answered some of these questions. Others need to be explored more closely in the field of healthy behavior. *We intended this article to create an opportunity for the health educator to see what is coming in time to participate in the direction it will go.* Since everybody knows more than anybody, we hope this will serve as an opening for more fruitful discussion.

The improvement in both *personal* health and human relations, that we argue for in this article is an understanding of healthy behavior through a bodymind awareness of its behavioral consequences.

We really love a quote by Ram Dass, in an article entitled "De-Crystallizing the New Age" by David Spangler (1997): "I think there is a paradigm shift going on in our civilization. It's a slow, big, deep, rhythmic, oceanic process. I think it's very delicious, and I want to encourage it. But I don't want to label it, because I think any label is reductionistic. The problem with calling something "New Age" is that it polarizes you from the old age. I'm not a revolutionary; I'm much more of an evolutionist. I find the word "new" partly exciting, like the good news in Christianity, but also partly offensive, because it's not new at all; it's just a remembering of what we have collectively forgotten."

## REFERENCES

### Books, Articles, and Journals

*American Journal of Health Behavior.* Star City, WV: PNG Publications.

Anderson, R. (1993). *Dr. Anderson's guide to wellness medicine.* CT: Keats.

Baker, B. (1997, July–August). Herbert Benson: The faith factor. *Common Boundary.*

Benson, H. (1984). *Beyond the relaxation response.* New York: Times Books.

Benson, H. (1985). *The relaxation response.* New York: Morrow.

Benson, H. (1996). *Timeless healing: The power and biology of belief.* New York: Scribner.

Bishop, G. D. (1994). *Health psychology: Integrating mind and body*. Boston: Allyn and Bacon.

Black, D. (1993). *Pigs in the dirt*. Springfield, UT: Tapestry Press.

Black, D. (1994). *Health at the crossroads*. Springfield, UT: Tapestry Press.

Borysenko, J. (1987). *Minding the body, Mending the mind*. New York: Bantam.

Borysenko, J., & Borysenko, M. (1994). *The power of the mind to heal: Renewing body, mind, and spirit*. Carson, CA: Hay House.

Brown, B. (1980). *Supermind*. New York: Harper & Row.

Chugani, H. (1997, November). Brain development implications for children's health, safety, and learning. Keynote address, New England School Development Council (NES-DEC) in cooperation with Education Commission of the States, Families, and Work Institute, and the New England Board of Higher Education, Worcester, MA.

Churchland, P. S. (1986). *Neurophilosophy: Toward a unified science of the mind/brain*. Cambridge, MA: MIT Press.

Colbin, A. (1990). *Food and healing*. New York: Ballantine.

Coulter, H. (1973–1994). *David legacy* (4 vol.). Washington, DC: Center for Empirical Medicine (4221 45th Street, NW, Washington, DC 20016).

Cousins, N. (1976, 23 December). Anatomy of an illness (as perceived by the patient). *New England Journal of Medicine, 295*, 1458–1463.

Dossey, L. (1984). *Beyond illness: Discovering the experience of health*. Boulder, CO: Shambhala.

Dossey, L. (1993). *Healing words: The power of prayer and the practice of medicine*. New York: HarperCollins.

Ferguson, M. (1980). *The Aquarian conspiracy: Personal and social transformation in the 1980s*. Los Angeles: J. P. Tarcher.

Frank, J. (1973). *Persuasion and healing*. New York: Schocken.

Gerber, R. (1988). *Vibrational medicine*. New Mexico: Bear & Company.

Glanz, K., Lewis, F. M., and Rimer, B. K. (Eds.). (1997). *Health behavior and health education: Theory, research, and practice*. San Francisco: Jossey-Bass.

Goleman, D. (1995). *Emotional intelligence: Why it can matter more than IQ*. New York: Bantam.

Grossinger, R. (1980). *Planet medicine*. New York: Anchor Books.

Hafen, B. Q., Karren, K. J., Frandsen, K. J., & Smith, N. L. (1996). *Mind/body health: The effects of attitudes, emotions, and relationships*. Boston: Allyn and Bacon.

Hills, C. (1968). *Nuclear evolution*. Boulder Creek, CA: University of the Trees Press.

Hills, C. (Ed.). (1975). *Energy matter and form: Toward a science of consciousness*. Boulder Creek, CA: University of the Trees Press.

Hutchinson, M. (1986). *Megabrain*. New York: Beechtree Books.

Illich, I. (1975). *Medical nemesis: The expropriation of health*. London: Marion Boyars.

Is behavior change an acceptable objective for health education? (1985). *Eta Sigma Gamma* (National Professional Health Science/Education Honorary).

Jonas, G. (1972). *Visceral learning: Toward a science of self-control*. New York: Viking.

Justice, B. (1995). *Who gets sick: Thinking and health*. Houston, TX: Peak Press.

Karagulla, S. (1967). *Breakthrough to creativity*. CA: DeVorss.

Kuhn, T. (1962). *The structure of scientific revolutions*. Chicago: University of Chicago Press.

Leonard, G. (1978). *The silent pulse: A search for the perfect rhythm that exists in each of us*. New York: Bantam.

Locke, S. (1986). *The healer within*. New York: Dutton.

Matarazzo, J. D. (1980). Behavioral health and behavioral medicine: Frontiers for a new health psychology. *American Psychologist*.

Matarazzo, J. D., Herd, A. J., & Weiss, S. M. (Eds.). (1984). *Behavioral health: A handbook of health enhancement and disease prevention*. New York: Wiley.

Mishlove, J. (1975). *The roots of consciousness: Psychic liberations through history, science and experience*. Berkeley, CA: The Bookwords.

Murphy, M. (1992). *The future of the body: Explorations into the future evolution of human nature*. New York: Putnam.

Nuland, S. B. (1997). *The wisdom of the body*. New York: Knopf.

Pearce, J. C. (1992). *Evolution's end: Claiming the potential of our intelligence*. New York: HarperCollins.

Peele, S. (1989). *Diseasing of America: Addiction treatment out of control*. Boston: Houghton Mifflin.

Pelletier, K. (1977). *Mind as healer, Mind as slayer*. New York: Delacorte.

Pelletier, K. (1979). *Holistic medicine: From stress to optimum health*. New York: Dell.

Pribram, K. (1978, 1979). Synthesis of Karl Pribram's holographic brain model with David Bohm's view of the physical universe were taken from lectures, conference proceedings and interviews in *Human Behavior*, May 1978, and *Psychology Today*, February 1979.

The psychology of health, immunity, and disease. (1997). Ninth international conference, National Institute for the Clinical Application of Behavioral Medicine, Mansfield Center, CT.

Read, D. (1997). *Health education: A cognitive/behavioral approach*. Sudbury, MA: Jones and Bartlett.

Reed, B. (1983). *Food, teens and behavior*. Manitowoc, WI: Natural Press.

Schauss, A. (1980). *Diet, crime and delinquency*. Berkeley, CA: Parker House.

Serinus, J. (Ed.). (1986). *Psychoimmunity and the healing process*. Berkeley, CA: Celestial Arts.

Spangler, D. (1997, February). De-crystallizing the new age. *New Age Journal*.

Stoll, W. (1996) *Saving yourself from the disease-care crisis*. Panama City, FL: Sunrise Health Coach.

Tansley, D. (1982). *Radionics: Science or magic?* England: C. W. Daniel.

Tillich, P. (1981). *The meaning of health*. Richmond, CA: North Atlantic Books.

Wilber, K. (Ed.). (1982). The holographic paradigm: And other paradoxes. Boulder, CO: Shambhala.

## Videotapes

Borysenko, J. (1996). *An evening with Joan Borysenko*. Cos Cob, CT: Hartley Film Foundation (59 Cat Rock Road, Cos Cob, CT 06807).

Brugh, J. (1988). *Healing and the unconscious*. Thinking Allowed Productions (5966 Zinn Drive, Oakland, CA 94611).

Dossey, L. (1993). *Recovering the soul: A scientific and spiritual search*. New York: Mystic Fire Video (P.O. Box 422, Prince Street Station, New York 10012).

*Interview with David Bohm: Quantum physicist and philosopher*. (1994). New York: Mystic Fire Video (P.O. Box 422, Prince Street Station, New York 10012).

*Meaning of Health with Bill Moyers*. (1993). New York: Mystic Fire Video (P.O. Box 422, Prince Street Station, New York, NY 10012).

Moyers, B. (n.d.). *Healing and the mind* (series of 6). New York: Ambrose Video Publishers (1290 Avenue of the Americas, Suite 2245, NYC 10104). Also distributed by Parabola.

Moyers, B. (n.d.). *Joseph Campbell and the power of myth*. New York: Mystic Fire Video, Inc. (Series of six.)

Pelletier, K. (1988). *Health and your whole being*. Oakland, CA: Thinking Allowed Productions (5966 Zinn Drive, Oakland, CA 94611).

Weil, A. (1996). *Spontaneous healing*. New York: Inner Dimension (200 Madison Ave., 24th Fl., NY 10016).

Weil, A. (1997). *8 weeks to optimal health*. New York: Inner Dimension (200 Madison Ave., 24th Fl., NY 10016).

*Who am I? Why am I here?* (featuring Thomas Moore). (1996). New York: Wellspring Media (65 Bleecker Street, New York).

## Conferences and Organizations

American Holistic Nurses Association. Website: http://www.ahna.org

*Brain/Mind Bulletin.* P.O. Box 42247, Los Angeles, CA 90042

Brain/Mind Collections. (1991). *Personality & Health. New Sense Bulletin.* (Los Angeles, CA)

Orthomolecular Psychiatric Association. The Huxley Institute for Biosocial Research, American Academy of Orthomolecular Medicine, 16 Florence Avenue, Toronto, Ontario, Canada M2N 1E9, (416-733-2117) and (800) 841-3802.

## Books That Offer Exercises, Experiments, Ideas, and Instruction

Benson, H. (1975). *The relaxation response.* New York: Morrow.

Benson, H. (1984). *Beyond the relaxation response.* New York: Times Books.

Davis, M., Eshelman, E. R., & McKay, M. (1988). *The relaxation and stress reduction workbook* (2nd ed.). Oakland, CA: New Harbinger.

Emery, R., & Travis, J. (1988). *Wellness workbook.* Berkeley, CA: Ten Speed Press.

Gendlin, E. (1973). *Focusing.* New York: Schocken.

Ornstein, R., & Sobel, S. (1989). *Healthy pleasures.* Reading, MA: Addison-Wesley.

Payne, B. (1974). *Getting there without drugs.* New York: Ballantine.

# CHAPTER

17

# PROBLEM-BASED LEARNING: CATALYST FOR BEHAVIORAL CHANGE

J. FREDERICK GARMAN
CAROL J. TESKE
DUANE A. CRIDER

Post-secondary education has recently been challenged to embrace new pedagogical paradigms that are intended to move professionals away from simply "teaching" toward strategies that actively promote "learning." Commentary (Barr & Tagg, 1995) has sounded a call to revaluate and revise classroom instructional methodologies so greater emphasis is placed on actively engaging students' in the learning process rather than simply transferring knowledge. Resulting comparisons of old versus new instructional strategies (Cox, 1999) suggest there are advantages to these approaches. However, does the movement away from the traditional, lecture recitation format of instruction, toward more pervasive use of active learning methodologies, have a favorable impact on the ability to change health behavior? With lifestyle decisions and habits continuing to be a significant contributor to morbidity and mortality (Johansson & Sundquist, 1999; Liebson & Amsterdam, 1999), this remains a salient question. The efficacy of promoting behavioral change among students in a post-secondary health education curriculum, through the use of problem-based learning, was compared to traditional, lecture recitation instructional methodologies and the development and extensive use of reflective, student portfolios in curricular offerings presented in Web-based formats. It was hypothesized that active curricular incorporation and use of problem-based learning methodologies would result in increased "readiness" for positive behavioral change.

## METHOD

Participants for this investigation were voluntarily recruited from students enrolled in a required health education course at a regional university located in eastern Pennsylvania. The multiple cohorts, as a group, demonstrated characteristics consistent with the enrollment demographics of the university (Kutztown University, 1999), that is, reflected an age of $20.68 \pm 0.437$ years (mean $\pm$ sem), were 62.70 percent female, and 91.89 percent were under the age of 25 years. Additionally, participants had completed $1.96 \pm 0.657$ (mean $\pm$ sem) years of university study. The course, Personal Health Management, was intended to provide a survey of diverse health topics relevant to a college-aged population and focused on expanding cognitive foundations, promoting the desirability of informed decision making, expanding repertoires of strategies enabling positive behavioral alterations, and, ultimately, promoting successful lifestyle modification. The survey course, offered by established faculty, followed uniform curricular content and was offered in three formats: lecture recitation (LR), problem-based learning (PBL), and interactive distance learning (DL). The lecture recitation approach followed an historically traditional format in which faculty were the primary disseminators of information, experiential learning activities were minimal, and faculty made all classroom decisions.

Problem-based learning, a modification of the use of case study, required students to take a much greater role in their learning. Through student initiated, faculty facilitated exploration of age and gender relevant, open-ended "health situations," participants were positioned, not only to expand their topical knowledge, but to refine higher order learning skills such as critical thinking, creative problem solving, quantitative analysis and database access and retrieval to the point where they could easily acquire relevant information and make knowledgeable informed decisions about their lifestyle habits and strategies for positive change. Interactive distance learning was a Web-based seminar course that required students to complete extensive readings, to participate in collective discussions, and to maintain a personal portfolio which provided an opportunity for on-going self-assessment, reflection, and analysis of lifestyle and change strategies. Though approaches to instruction differed, all courses covered similar curricular content, allocated similar time to varying instructional topics and provided students with both a rationale for lifestyle alterations and varied processes and strategies that can contribute to positive behavioral change.

The efficacy of these multiple instructional strategies in promoting lifestyle modification was assessed, over the course of a fifteen-week academic semester, through the evaluation of student position within Prochaska, DiClemente, and Norcross's

**EXHIBIT 17.1**  **Transtheoretical Model "Stages of Change"**

**1.** PRECONTEMPLATION—not interested in change. May deny a need exists.

**2.** CONTEMPLATION—recognizes a need. Begins to consider altering behavior.

**3.** PREPARATION—makes plans. May initiate small changes.

**4.** ACTION—makes commitment and undertakes action.

**5.** MAINTENANCE—alterations continue, stabilize and become ingrained.

(1994) "transtheoretical" model. This construct, also known as the "stage of change" model, suggests that behavioral alterations follow a continuum that begins with "precontemplation" and concludes, as seen in Exhibit 17.1, with "maintenance" (Robbins, Powers, & Burgess, 1997).

Additionally, the model demonstrates the ability to reliably apply to diverse habits including, but not limited to, smoking cessation, weight control and exercise acquisition, found within the college-aged population (Prochaska, Velicer et al., 1994). Ability to modify behavior can result from identifying position within the continuum as well as engaging in activities and experiences that expand knowledge, provide a rationale for change and explore diverse processes and strategies enabling transition between various stages (Prochaska, DiClemente et al., 1994; Robbins et al., 1997). This investigation focused on students initially positioned in "precontemplation" (stage 1) and "contemplation" (stage 2) and assessed the effectiveness of the multiple instructional approaches in moving them further along the continuum. Contrary to stages 1 and 2, stage 3, "preparation," while not demonstrating overt, ongoing commitment to lifestyle modification frequently included small alterations in existing behavior (Prochaska, DiClemente et al., 1994) and was eliminated from experimental consideration for that reason. The instrument utilized for evaluating student "stage" was a modification of an algorithm developed by Curry, Kristal, and Bowen (1992) which utilized self-reported responses to a series of questions designed to determine position within the model (Exhibit 17.2 and Table 17.1). Algorithmic assessment of position within the "stage of change" model has demonstrated acceptable validity and reliability between multiple samples (Green, Rossi, Reed, Wiley, & Prochaska, 1994).

Additionally, the instrument used in this investigation included questions that identified the behavior that was the foci of student change efforts. This was undertaken in order to determine whether behaviors being addressed by the study's samples were consistent with those reliably evaluated with the stage of change model (Prochaska, Velicer et al., 1994) and were similar between groups. Student behaviors, subjected to change efforts, were arbitrarily, numerically coded for statistical evaluation. Statistical evaluation of group characteristics, between group differences and change over a fifteen-week academic semester utilized accepted methodologies (Remington & Schork, 1970). Results were considered statistically significant at $p \leq 0.050$.

# EXHIBIT 17.2 **Stage of Change Assessment Questionnaire**

Please provide the following information.

Age _____ Gender _____ Height _____ Weight _____

Year in college _____ Date _____

Please answer the following questions.

1. In the past 6 months, have you ever changed your "lifestyle habits" in an attempt to improve your health?

   Yes

   No (If "no," skip to question #6)

2. What "lifestyle habit(s)" have you changed in the past 6 months?

3. IF YES (#1), are you currently making those efforts?

   Yes

   No (If "no," skip to question #6)

4. IF YES (#1), how long have you been successfully able to alter your "lifestyle habits"?

   Less than 30 days

   1–6 months

   7–12 months

   Over a year

5. IF YES (#1), would you say you are currently "healthier" as a result of your "lifestyle habit" changes?

   Yes

   No

6. In the past month, have you thought about changes you could make to improve your health?

   Yes

   No

7. How confident are you that you will make some of these changes (#6) during the next month?

   Very confident

   Somewhat confident

   Mildly confident

   Not at all confident

8. What affects your confidence that you will be able/not be able to make some of these changes during the next month?

TABLE 17.1 **Stage of Change Scoring Algorithm**

| Stage | Question(s) | Answer(s) |
|---|---|---|
| Precontemplation | 1 or 3 | No |
| | 6 | No |
| Contemplation | 1 or 3 | No |
| | 6 | Yes |
| | 7 | Mildly or not at all confident |
| Decision | 1 or 3 | No |
| | 6 | Yes |
| | 7 | Somewhat or very confident |
| Action | 1 and 3 | Yes |
| | 4 | 6 months or less |
| Maintenance | 1 and 3 | Yes |
| | 4 | 7 months or more |

## RESULTS

Measures of central tendency (Table 17.2) indicated a predominantly young adult, female sample at the close of their first, post-secondary academic year. The majority of participants, across all three pedagogical styles, appeared to be engaged in some type of positive lifestyle management with 82.8 percent (LR), 82.4 percent (PBL), and 71.4 percent (DL), at minimum, in the "preparation" stage (stage 3) of the "transtheoretical" model. The most frequent lifestyle foci of students at "stage 3" or beyond, initially, were 33.3 percent addressing physical activity patterns (LR), 47.1 percent addressing alcohol consumption habits (PBL), and 35.7 percent equally committed to focusing on activity patterns and nutritional concerns (DL).

## TABLE 17.2 Characteristics and Between-Group Differences

| | Lecture | Problem-Based Learning | Distance Learning | Significance |
|---|---|---|---|---|
| $N$ | 96 | 68 | 21 | |
| Age (mean ± sem) | 19.93 | 21.85 | 20.29 | 0.2012 |
| | ±0.229 | ±1.024 | ±1.624 | |
| College Year[1] | 1.99 | 1.90 | 2.00 | 0.2345 |
| (mean ± sem) | ±0.082 | ±0.121 | ±0.207 | |
| Age < 25 yrs. (%) | 95.83 | 88.24 | 85.71 | 0.0465* |
| Female (%) | 59.38 | 61.76 | 80.95 | 0.9137 |
| < "stage 3" – pre (%) | 17.17 | 17.65 | 28.57 | <0.0001* |
| < "stage 3" – post (%) | 9.80 | 9.26 | 14.29 | 0.0113* |
| Focus – pre[2] | 3.96 | 3.16 | 3.21 | 0.1122 |
| (mean ± sem) | ±0.255 | ±0.199 | ±0.422 | |
| Focus – post[2] | 3.67 | 2.98 | 3.46 | 0.2638 |
| (mean ± sem) | ±0.289 | ±0.188 | ±0.475 | |

[1]Freshman = 1, Sophomore = 2, Junior = 3, Senior = 4
[2]Behavioral focus coded numerically: 1 = weight management, 2 = exercise, 3 = nutrition, 4 = tobacco, 5 = alcohol, 6 = other drugs, 7 = stress, 8 = other
*Significance level: $p \leq 0.050$

Analysis of variance identified three statistically significant ($p < 0.050$) between group differences: percent "< age 25," percent "< stage 3" at the beginning of the inquiry and percent "< stage 3" at its conclusion. Though casual observation of the data would suggest that the significant difference in "age < 25" could be found within the

TABLE 17.3   **Instructional Methodologies' Impact on Stages 1 and 2, Pre/Post Analysis-*t*-test for Dependent Samples, All Groups***

| Group | t | df | p |
|---|---|---|---|
| Lecture | −2.204 | 17 | 0.0416** |
| Problem-Based Learning | −3.051 | 8 | 0.0158** |
| Distance Learning | −1.732 | 3 | 0.1817 |

*missing data pairwise deleted
**significance level $p < 0.050$

lecture group and variations in pre and post membership in "< stage 3" groups lay within the distance learning sample, post hoc analysis utilizing Scheffe's Test for multiple comparisons identified no clear indication of where the differences in "age < 25" arose. However, the post hoc analysis relevant to percent "< stage 3" seemed to confirm that, in both pre and post intervention cases, the differences originated from within the distance learning sample.

With the lack of statistical significance in other demographic variables, the rationale for these variations is difficult to identify and may be only due to the randomness of student course selection chronology. Speculatively, however, the attractiveness and/or convenience of non-traditional instructional methodologies to older students might contribute to these results and be worthy of additional investigation. A pre/post comparison of instructional methodology's impact on students' identified as initially in stages 1 or 2 (Table 17.3) demonstrated a mean percent change reduction of 88.58 percent of students in "precontemplation" and "contemplation" and resulted in statistically significant changes with both the lecture recitation and problem-based learning methodologies.

These findings appear to result from the impact of varied activities and strategies comprising the "processes of change" (Prochaska, DiClemente et al., 1994). Successful transition through differing stages results from engaging in activities appropriate to position (Bowen, Meischke, and Tomoyasu, 1994; Green et al., 1994). For example, providing awareness expanding information about the frequency and impact of health issues, in "precontemplation," may be a more appropriate approach than focusing on behavioral strategies for implementing and sustaining alterations. Conversely, for individuals in "action" or "maintenance," activities focusing on behavioral needs such as controlling environment and/or stimuli should yield greater success than efforts directed toward expanding cognitive foundations (Bowen et al., 1994; Green et al., 1994). While all processes are important, the initial need in altering behavior is to gain an understanding of the challenge and its impact. Stated more simply, the need is to become aware and informed. Both methodological approaches, demonstrating statistical significance, addressed and emphasized both the "why" and "how" of lifestyle issues. In doing so, they seemed to have provided relevant and adequate information to raise the awareness of participants initially in stages 1 and 2. This, by itself, may have precipitated the observed alterations (Robbins et al., 1997). However, comparatively, problem-based learning places a greater emphasis for learning on the student, has the instructor function as a facilitator rather than a provider of knowledge, and requires the student to develop and refine critical thinking, creative problem-solving, analytical skills and other desirable learning characteristics (Garman, 1999). By working through the process of problem-based learning and refining these aforementioned straits, students may develop a better understanding of issues, of available resources supporting enhanced behavior, and may have greater opportunities for self-evaluation and reflection. Consequently, by engaging in more numerous elements of the "processes of change" (Prochaska, DiClemente et al., 1994), effectiveness of the instructional methodology may be comparatively stronger. With the growing emphasis, in higher education, on "learning" rather than simply "teaching" (Barr & Tagg, 1995), this may warrant additional investigation.

While these data suggest both lecture recitation and problem-based methodological approaches to instruction can influence early stage of change position, the presence of several confounding factors necessitates a conservative approach to conclusions. While the use of self reported data has been supported in similar research (Curry et al., 1992; Mhurchu, Margetts, & Speller, 1997), the recognition that its use may interject a bias into the findings cannot be discounted. Also potentially influencing results may be the impact of unacknowledged personal exposure to evolving or active lifestyle related illness, which served as a major catharsis for change. Data (Burton, Shapiro, & German, 1999) suggested that these experiences frequently provide significant impetus for behavioral change. These variables were not assessed within the scope of the investigation. Though not acknowledged by any of the subjects, the potential influence of these occurrences can't be ignored as a strong impetus for altering behavior. Additionally, concluding that "distance learning" lacks the ability to impact position in the initial levels of the "stage of change" model needs to be viewed cautiously due to the small number of participants ($n = 21$) engaged with that instructional approach. While conventional practice frequently accepts an experimental cell of 20 (Bruning & Kintz, 1977), reduced numbers will affect the power of the statistical tests to a degree that differences may not be detected (Bruning & Kintz, 1977). A post hoc evaluation of the sample size within the distance learning cell, utilizing a desired power of 0.95 and both a moderate (0.50) and conservative (0.80) estimation of the "standard effect size" (Cohen, 1988) suggests a cautious approach to interpreting distance learning ineffectiveness may be warranted. Finally, the most frequently occurring post intervention foci differed from initial data with 75.9 percent (PBL) and 78.6 percent (DL) concluding the inquiry by addressing tobacco usage habits. Though not statistically significant, these changes suggest two possible occurrences: either participants engaged in change activities at the beginning of the investigation moved to a different behavior or they relapsed back to stages 1 or 2 and different individuals moved into or beyond stage 3. A retrospective assessment of respondents, within these two groups, indicated that of the participants initially at or beyond stage 3, 53.8 percent engaged with problem-based learning and 66.7 percent involved with distance learning remained committed to lifestyle change but altered the focus of their individual efforts. These results, while not as desirable as an ongoing commitment to a singular behavioral alteration, are consistent with the cyclic nature of the "stage of change" process (Robbins et al., 1997). However, they do raise concerns about the effectiveness of these instructional strategies in promoting sustainable change.

## CONCLUSIONS

Within the limits of this investigation, the following conclusion seems justified. Problem-based learning and lecture recitation appear to offer statistically superior methodological approaches to distance learning instructional strategies in promoting movement away from the "precontemplation" and "contemplation" phase of the "stage of change" continuum. However, with the presence of several potentially confounding factors, additional investigation is necessary to further evaluate and/or confirm the effectiveness of both these methodologies on initiating sustainable behavioral alterations.

## REFERENCES

Barr, R., & Tagg, J. (1995). From teaching to learning: A new paradigm for undergraduate education. *Change, 27,* 12–24.

Bowen, D. J., Meischke, H., & Tomoyasu, N. (1994). Preliminary evaluation of the process of changing to a low-fat diet. *Health Education Research, 9,* 85–94.

Bruning, J. L., & Kintz, B. L. (1977). *Computational handbook of statistics.* New York: Longman.

Burton, L. C., Shapiro, S., & German, P. S. (1999). Determinants of physical activity initiation and maintenance among community-dwelling older persons. *Preventive Medicine, 29,* 422–430.

Cohen, J. (1988). *Statistical power analysis for the behavioral sciences.* New York: Academic Press.

Cox, M. (1999, January). A focus on learning: Adapting and adopting bit by bit. In J. P. Schellenberg (Chair), *The learning paradigm: Impact on college teaching,* symposium conducted at the Kutztown University Center for the Enhancement of Teaching, Kutztown, PA.

Curry, S., Kristal, A., & Bowen, D. (1992). An application of the stage of change model of behavior change to dietary fat reduction. *Health Education Research, 7,* 97–105.

Garman, J. F. (1999). *Exploring health: A problem based inquiry.* New York: McGraw-Hill.

Green, G., Rossi, S., Reed, G., Wiley, C., & Prochaska, J. (1994). Stages of change for reducing dietary fat to 30% of energy or less. *Journal of the American Dietetics Association, 94,* 1105–1110.

Johansson, S. E., & Sundquist, J. (1999). Changes in lifestyle factors and their influence in health status and all cause mortality. *International Journal of Epidemiology, 28,* 1073–1080.

Kutztown University of Pennsylvania. (1999). *Fact book for fall 1999.* Kutztown, PA: Kutztown University of Pennsylvania.

Liebson, P. R., & Amsterdam, E. A. (1999). Prevention of coronary heart disease. Part I primary prevention. *Disease Monthly, 45,* 497–571.

Mhurchu, C., Margetts, B., & Speller, V. (1997). Applying the stages-of-change model to dietary change. *Nutrition Reviews, 55*, 10–16.

Prochaska, J., DiClemente, C., & Norcross, J. (1994). *Changing for good.* New York: Morrow.

Prochaska, J., Velicer, W., Rossi, J., Goldstein, M., Marcus, B., Rakowski, W., et al. (1994). Stages of change and decisional balance for 12 problem behaviors. *Health Psychology, 13*, 39–46.

Remington, R. D., & Schork, M. S. (1970). *Statistics with application to the biological and health sciences.* Englewood Cliffs, NJ: Prentice-Hall.

Robbins, G., Powers, D., & Burgess, S. (1997). *A wellness way of life* (4th ed.). New York: McGraw-Hill.

# HEALTH PROMOTION AND EMPOWERMENT: REFLECTIONS ON PROFESSIONAL PRACTICE

**RONALD LABONTE**

Recent reformulations of health promotion imply the notion of empowerment (WHO, 1986; Epp, 1986). Health promotion as "the process of enabling people to increase control over, and improve, their health" (p. 1) shares a similar ethos with empowerment as "the process by which people, organizations and communities gain mastery over their lives" (Rappaport, 1981, p. 3). Both notions, however, are rarely unpacked for their assumptions about social change processes. This article attends to some of these assumptions. It expresses ideas generated during six years of professional training workshops (1986–1992), involving over 2,500 community health practitioners in Canada, New Zealand, and Australia. These workshops asked, and answered, one question only: How could professionals, under the rubric of health promotion, engage in new practice styles that reduce or ameliorate inequitable social conditions?

## HEALTH PROMOTION, EMPOWERMENT, AND SOCIAL MOVEMENTS

Implicit in this question is a belief that professionals and their employing institutions might play an important role in challenging oppressive and health-threatening political and economic structures. At times, this potential role is accorded an almost revolutionary status. Health promoters in Europe and in the three countries in which the workshops were conducted often describe health promotion as a social movement, concerned with health "prerequisites" such as "peace, shelter, food, income, a stable ecosystem, social justice and equity" (WHO, 1986, p. 1). This mimics the manner in which community development was described in the 1960s and 1970s, and how empowerment was described by the mental health literature in the 1980s. Stevenson and Burke (1991) argue that, in doing so, health promotion conceptualizers have usurped the discourse of social movements, emphasizing the empowering capacity of "the community" but failing to address the role of the state (governments and their bureaucratic institutions) or macrosocial power structures in creating unhealthy conditions. Health promotion, particularly in countries like Canada where it has been embraced by government policy, is "a bureaucratic tendency; not a movement against the state, but one within it" (Stevenson & Burke, p. 282). This is a valuable insight. Although government initiatives may at times be empowering (itself a complex concept that will be examined shortly), the relationship between government institutions and community groups has disempowering qualities that many theorists relate to capitalist economies (Miliband, 1983; Offe, 1984).

Many health promoters acknowledge the disempowering qualities of government bureaucracies (often their employers) by contending that health promotion belongs to the whole community. Community groups do organize and act in the name of health promotion, however, they are more likely to do so around specific issues involving welfare rights, pollution, housing, safety, or employment concerns. The abstract concept of health promotion, like that of empowerment, is of more concern to professionals working for government agencies. To claim health promotion is a community phenomenon, especially when many health promotion initiatives remain focused on personal life-styles, could fulfill Stevenson and Burke's bleak prophecy of a bureaucratically conceived concept colonizing how people view their day-to-day lives: What is important is not your relationships, your work, your identity, your capacity; it is your cholesterol level.

Does health promotion's bureaucratic parentage mean that it surrenders any empowering potential to the co-opting "power-over" tendencies of government institutions? To the extent that health promotion becomes a marketing tool for government agencies and their agendas, the answer would be yes. But health promotion can also be regarded as a response to social movement groups and the challenges they make to government. Eyerman and Jamison (1991) discuss social movements as a form of cognitive praxis, in which social movement groups challenge dominant social beliefs and norms, generate new knowledge, and create new ways to look at old problems or relations. But vehicles must exist or be created through which this new social movement knowledge can be translated into broader social sectors, such as government institutions, if the knowledge is to influence how political and economic decisions are made.

The Ottawa Charter's concept of health promotion and community psychology's use of empowerment as an "exemplar of practice" (Rappaport, 1987) are such vehicles. Both terms in their elaborated definitions incorporate some of the critiques and new knowledge claims of the women's, environmental, gay/lesbian rights, and other social movements (Minkler, 1989). Both terms represent challenges to the narrowness and rigidity of the biomedical paradigm, the disempowering tendencies of professionals and the disabling qualities of bureaucracies and institutions. Health promotion is less a social movement in itself than a response to the new knowledge claims of social movement groups (1). Health promotion and empowerment exist as conceptual lenses through which professional (bureaucratic, within-the-state) practices can be revalued. The goal of this revaluing is a more empowering relationship between professionals and clients, between institutions and community groups. Although not sufficient in itself, such a relationship is a necessary strategy for healthy social change.

Health promotion and empowerment nonetheless exist between two perils: That of co-opting or neutralizing social struggle and conflict within the conservative ethos of institutions, and that of naively proclaiming the community as the solution to all sociopolitical and economic health problems. This tension, which arguably underpins all relations between government institutions and community groups, is embedded even within the concept of "empower" itself.

## KEY ELEMENTS OF THE EMPOWERING RELATIONSHIP

*Empower*, the central act in the new health promotion, is both a transitive verb, in which the subject acts upon an object, and an intransitive verb, in which the subject acts only upon itself. Used transitively, *empower* means bestowing power on others, an enabling act, sharing some of the power professionals might hold over others. But there is a danger in *empower*'s transitive meaning. Professionals, as the empowering agent, the subject of the relationship, remain the controlling actor, defining the terms of the interaction. Relatively disempowered individuals or groups remain the objects, the recipients of professional actions. Our language exerts considerable force in our world constructions (Seidman & Wagner, 1992). Continually stating "we need to empower this or that group" creates and reinforces a world of professional practice in which nonprofessional groups are incapable of their own powerful actions. This danger is illuminated by the intransitive meaning of *empower*: the act of gaining or assuming power (*Compact Edition of the OED*, 1971, p. 855). *Empower* used in this sense is reflexive; it takes no object. To some, this meaning of empowerment should stand as its litmus test. The only empowerment of any importance is the power seized by individuals or groups.

Even if we confine our use of *empower* to its intransitive meaning, there are different subjects: professionals and their clients. When professionals empower intransitively, they claim more power for themselves. If they do so with the intent to transform oppressive social structures, rather than to advance self-interests, this mutually empowers professionals and their clients. Many frontline health workers are relatively powerless in their organizations, and need to claim legitimacy for themselves in order to be effective in their work with less powerful individuals and groups. Schon (1983) warns that when such workers are not granted professional status, they have great "difficulty in establishing a reflective [empowering] contract with their clients" because they lack "enough voice in the situation to be able to do so" (p. 298). Much of the disabling power-over tendencies within professional practice may simply reflect a projection of professional disempowerment (Finne, 1982), or the self-evident truth: One must have power in order to share it.

When clients or community groups empower intransitively, the professional ensures that power can be taken. Professionals generally do have more power (status, legitimacy, access to or control over resources) than their clients. How is this power shared or given up in ways that do not patronize? How is power taken from those in empathy with relatively powerless individuals or groups in ways that do not become stuck in anger or resentment? These questions surround all social justice struggles that exist simultaneously at the interpersonal and social (intergroup) levels, for example, between women and men, indigenous and colonizing peoples, economic or status-defined social classes. Empower in these struggles is both transitive and intransitive; it exists only as a relational act of power taken and given in the same instance. The tension this invoked in professional practice became indentified as "power over" and "power with." Power over relies upon the reality of things—diseases, health behaviors, risk factors. These things are important, but they can lead to what McKinlay (1990) refers to as "terminal hardening of the categories," in which professionals get the answers they want to hear by virtue of the questions they ask. *Power with* looks to the reality of lived experiences in the language, images, and symbols that people use to give voice to them. *Power over* tolerates others' views. *Power with* respects others' views, trying to understand them within the context of the others' life. *Power over* tries to educate others to his terms, his ways of viewing the world. *Power with* tries to find some common ground between what she knows, and how she talks about it, and what communities know, and how they talk about it (2).

The act of naming one's experiences is essential to an experience of self-efficacy or empowerment. This does not mean that how one interprets one's experiences is true, or necessarily empowering. As Fay (1987) cautions, there is still the problem of false consciousness, of viewing one's life through the internalized and distorting conceptual lenses of those who hold power over one. The power of the word nonetheless draws attention to the professional need to respect how people identify their own health concerns an4 issues. If health workers fail to "start where people are" (Nyswander, 1956) they risk being irrelevant to the lives and conditions of many persons, further complicating and overwhelming peoples' lives by inserting into them more and more "urgent" problems that they must address and "buy into."

In an earlier work based on the workshops, I suggested that there are three broad clusterings of named health problems corresponding to diseases (e.g., cardiovascular disease, cancer, acquired immunodeficiency syndrome [AIDS], behaviors (e.g., smoking, diet, unsafe sex), and social conditions (e.g., poverty, unemployment, discrimination, pollution) (Labonte, 1989). Each of these clustered problems embeds a set of assumptions, comprising three reasonably discrete approaches to health: The medical, behavioral, and socioenvironmental approaches (Labonte, 1992, 1993b). These three approaches represent organizational biases; hospitals tend to work from a medical approach, state health agencies from a behavioral approach, and community groups from a socioenvironmental approach. These biases condition and constrain the ability of health workers to act effectively or legitimately within a different approach. They may create a situation in which the professional is unable to enter a dialogue with his community groups in search of some shared meaning; rather, he persists in actions that seek to educate these groups to the terms of the health agency.

An example of this tendency comes from a PATCH (or Planned Action Towards Community Health) program in the United States, developed by the Centers for Disease Control. A community opinion survey found that violence and drugs were major concerns. A behavioral risk factor survey identified heart disease. The community opinions were put on the back burner. Screening tests, life-style counseling, and referrals were offered, because those were the categories of the professionals to which the community must be educated (Bogan, 1992). Some Canadian PATCH programs have dropped the risk factor survey altogether (it is normally part of the PATCH protocol), believing that a commitment to reducing health inequalities must proceed with the knowledge that the most important act of power is naming one's experience, and having that naming heard and legitimized by others.

Although the behavioral or risk factor approach to health tends to take a power-over approach to health concerns of community groups, such programs can still be empowering, depending on how the health promoter views his task. For example: Two health promoters are developing heart health programs. One sees her clients solely in terms of cardiovascular outcomes. The other sees his clients in the richer terms of their family, community, and economic lives. Outwardly, the programs may appear to be similar, at least initially. But in the first case, heart health never transcends its encasement by cardiovascular disease. In the second case, heart health is simply one entry point into the more complex experiences of people that often include gendered, class-based, and cultural forms of oppression. In the first case, when people express concerns about these oppressions the health promoter is either deaf or shrugs that it is not heart health, not in her mandate. In the second case, the health promoter asks of himself: What can I and my health agency do to support these persons in these other endeavors? Asking and answering this question distinguishes an empowering from a disempowering health promotion practice. This distinction is most evocatively

FIGURE 18.1   **Model of Empowerment**

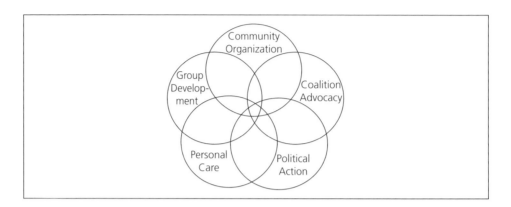

expressed in a challenge to professionals made by Lily Walker, an Australian aborigi-
nal woman: "If you are here to help me, then you are wasting your time. But if you
come because your liberation is bound up in mine, then let us begin" (Valvarde, 1991,
p. 4).

## THE EMPOWERMENT HOLOSPHERE

To illustrate this beginning, I will use a simple model of empowerment as a professional practice, developed during the workshops (Figure 18.1). The model identifies
the range of strategies that health professionals and health agencies need to employ if
they are to reduce or ameliorate inequitable social conditions. These strategies are
not the responsibility of any one health worker or discipline but, rather, are an organizational and interorganizational mandate. The individual professional's responsibility is to see that the whole process is engaged, and to find a place in its engagement.
Each of the model's "spheres" represents a different level of social organization and
relationship—interpersonal (personal empowerment), intragroup (small group development), intergroup (community organization), interorganizational (coalition building
and advocacy, political action). Heuristically, the model links in practice the individual, organizational, and community levels of empowerment discussed by Israel,
Checkoway, Schulz, and Zimmerman, 1994, and so overcomes some of the historic
limitations of professional actions. The model is discussed in detail elsewhere
(Labonte, 1992, 1993b; Labonte & Little, 1992); what follows is a summary of central practice concerns in each sphere. Although I have defined empowerment as a
relationship, and therefore professionals and the people or groups with whom they
work are both significant actors, the discussion that follows focuses on the professional half of the relationship.

## Personal Care

This sphere is one at which most front-line workers encounter individuals living in relatively powerless situations; it is the venue of direct service. McKnight (1987) argues that "resources empower; services do not." This witty play on the disabling tendencies of large "institutions nonetheless denigrates the community of caring professionals and reinforces a "we/they" polarity that creates and reinforces a false cleavage between professionals and community members, the former being bad, the latter being good. The irony of this cleavage lies in the formative mobilizing role often played by professionals and intellectuals who participate in social justice actions (Zald, 1988; Freeman, 1983; Eder, 1985). It also risks denying persons what they often require and request: Respectful services. One Canadian health center mistakenly drove a wedge between its clinical workers and its community workers, reversing the historic tables by extolling the importance of community development over medical care. The dissatisfied clinical team suffered rapid staff turnover, the poor neighborhood lost its continuity of care, and the health center lost some of its empowering credibility.

The two pillars that allow service delivery to be empowering are that they are offered in a supportive, noncontrolling way and that they are not the limit of the services and resources offered by the agency. This approach builds towards community organizing and coalition advocacy—the political elements of empowerment at the structural level remain explicit—while recognizing "that low income people have the right, here and now, to support in the face of difficulties…our credibility in working with disempowered groups rests to a large extent on whether or not these groups find community workers to be of practical usefulness" (Jackson, Mitchell, & Wright, 1988, p. 4). Some recent examples from Canadian public health practice include these:

1. Poor women in a state-run rooming house, who complain of giving blowjobs to use the bathroom, and a community health worker who believes them, who spends time with them, who advocates with them for better safety and more dignity in the house.

2. Nutritionists and health educators who visit elderly live-alones, maintaining their healthy diet by cooking with them, and sharing their meals.

3. Street people shut out by attitudes from the institutional services to which they are entitled, and public health nurses who take the personal care to where they live: in the hostels, in the 24-hour donut shops.

Unless professionals think simultaneously in both personal and structural ways, they risk losing sight of the simultaneous reality of both. If they focus only on the individual, and only on crisis management or service delivery, they risk privatizing by rendering personal the social and economic underpinnings to poverty and powerlessness. If they only focus on the structural issues, they risk ignoring the immediate pains and personal woundings of the powerless and people in crisis.

### Small Group Development

Community is often presented as the engine of health promotion, the vehicle of empowerment. It may be more accurate to say that the small group is that locus of change (3). The group is where we forge identities and create purpose. Only in interacting with others do people gain those healthful characteristics essential to empowerment: control, capacity, coherence, connectedness and critical thinking or conscientization (Wallerstein, 1992). Without the support of a group, many people will be unable to participate in more formalized (political, policy) venues of social change; they will remain the historically marginalized and uninvolved. Thus, continuing from the examples under the previous sphere:

1. A number of women roomers now meet weekly to share each other's burdens, to identify each other's strengths. The caring nurse has become the enabling facilitator.

2. A group of older shut-ins in high-rise isolation now pool their food and share their dining, brought together by a nutritionist who knew intuitively that eating even poor food in the warmth of others does more for health than digesting the finest quality nutrients in loneliness.

It often takes between one and two years before a group may form from the disconnected individuals, formation occurring when individuals self-identify as group members. When Minkler (1985) and her graduate students first began working with senior roomers in San Francisco's Tenderloin, it took a year of standing in the hotel lobby chatting with individual roomers, offering them counseling and an open ear, before the first group formed. Health workers in Ottawa, Canada, talk of how after a similar group of poor, older adults formed, they met for over a year sorting through their internal dynamics before they became interested in tackling such socioenvironmental problems as housing costs and community safety (Labonte, 1993a). This slow community-building process at the group level is not well understood by many program funders who often expect new groups to move into social action with demonstrable impacts within the first year. Although it is reasonable to demonstrate shifts in group dynamics over the first year or two of group development (for example, stronger group identity, role differentiation, agreement on issues, management of group functions, and organization) it is less reasonable to expect that newly formed groups should quickly turn their attentions to issues extrinsic to their own immediate interpersonal concerns.

There is also a tension that arises when groups begin to shift from an inward to an outward orientation. In the early years of a community garden project involving single mothers on social assistance, the group was split on the importance of the garden itself (Labonte, 1990). Some saw it as a metaphor, an organizing point for single mothers who, as their group strength grew, would be better able to do the "important" work of protest and lobbying for social assistance reform. Others saw the garden as the end in itself; empowerment existed in the simple acts of planting, tending, and harvesting tomatoes. Clearly, empowerment exists at both levels, and must be supported at both levels. Often small group developers or community organizers fail to recognize that these two levels—the personal or interpersonal and the sociopolitical—are not contradictory, but complementary. We need groups that nurture the soul, and groups that challenge the status quo.

## Community Organization

Community organization describes the process of organizing people around problems or issues that are larger than group members' own immediate concerns. Community organization implies choice on the part of professionals and their agencies to work with some community groups, and not with others. Although there is no true consensus within the health sector on which community groups warrant support, there is growing acceptance of an advocacy framework of action, explicitly recognizing that priority community groups are those whose income, educational, occupational, and general social class positioning place them low within the hierarchy of political and economic power (Labonte, 1993b; Watt & Rodmell, 1988; *City of Toronto*, 1991).

Although community organizing may strive for inclusivity in community-building, relatively powerless groups usually seek to correct their imbalance by limiting the power other groups have over them. These groups often create their group identity as a community in opposition to or conflict with those groups that are more powerful than themselves. This dynamic has been at the base of all Alinsky-style social action organizing efforts, the confrontational we/they approach to organizing that has been used successfully to create community groups from the seemingly intractable conditions of isolation and apathy (Ward, 1987). The healthful importance of conflict in social change processes is often overlooked in a health promotion/empowerment rhetoric of consensus, which frequently defines empowerment as a non-zero-sum commodity (Israel et al., 1994). In one respect, this is true; to the extent that consensual, caring social relations are nurtured, all will benefit, including those who currently occupy privileged hierarchical positions. This is intimated in research linking higher life expectancy rates with lower slopes in various measures of social hierarchy (Wilkinson, 1990). But coercive forms of one group's power over might only be restrained, in zero-sum fashion, by another group's ability to prevent it. This point is similar to the earlier argument that empowerment exists in power being simultaneously taken and given; power exists dialectically as an aspect of social relations, rather than as a commodity.

Community organizing often extends beyond mobilizing new groups to supporting existing groups on the issues important to group members. As relations between health agencies and community groups develop, health workers need to consider in what it is they are inviting community groups to participate, as the following story illustrates.

*A health educator for a city health department convened a committee on housing and health with activists from housing rights groups. These groups wanted safer, better heated and ventilated, and more affordable housing. The health educator agreed politically with their concerns. The housing and health committee met for a year, doc-umenting with studies and literature reviews that the activists' concerns were legiti-mate health issues. The report was presented to the health educator's manager, who agreed with the literature review but nayed most of the recommendations as "too radical." The report went back to the committee. The recommendations were rewrit-ten. The health educator's manager passed the report along, but his manager, although agreeing with the literature review, again nayed most of the watered down recommendations as "too radical." The report went back to the committee, which began to suffer the absenteeism of the housing group activists. The recommenda-tions were rewritten in the deft style of "public health parenthood" platitudes. (Everyone is against poverty; not everyone is against those economic structures that maintain the wealthy and create the poor.) The report made it all the way to City Council, where it was discussed for 90 seconds and unanimously passed. By this time the original committee was completely moribund, and the health educator was puz-zling over what had gone wrong.*

The mistake here was confusing participation in a bureaucratic process with par-ticipation in a social change process. The question the health educator should have been asking herself is "What activities are best suited to the end: Effecting political change in housing policy?" This requires a recognition that her organizational require-ments for change differ from those for community groups and, particularly, for activist leaders within those groups. This recognition would not deny her and her staff an important role in achieving the end, but would reconstruct it using a metaphor of a nutcracker, with the nut being the specific policy issue at hand (e.g., safe, healthy, affordable housing). Persons within the organization, in their role as legitimating pro-fessionals, provide the studies, creating a strong inner arm. Activist groups outside the organization provide the stories and, in their more powerful role as citizens, posit the more politicized demands, and at the appropriate political level (e.g., city council). Their concerns, buttressed by the concurrent internal validation made in the language of the organization, give decision-makers (politicians) less opportunity to refer the issue inwards for "more study," risking the conservatism illustrated by the story. The policy nut begins to crack.

The centrality of community to health promotion—the Ottawa Charter uses the term repeatedly and many commentators regard community as the venue for, if not the very definition of, the new health promotion practice (Green & Raeburn, 1988)—has both empowering and disempowering political and economic impacts, as Robertson and Minkler (1994) discuss at some length. Although community has diverse meanings and interpretations (Israel et al., 1994), the notion of community-as-locality (neighborhood) predominates in much community development, empower-ment, and health promotion literature. This construction of community may allow for programs unique to community groups and their perceived concerns (an empowering impact), but it can also, and in a politically reactionary way, mystify the reality that most economic and social policy is national and transnational in nature (a disempowering impact). Local decision-making can only be within narrow parameters at best, and is unlikely to include substantial control over economic resources. As Durning (1989) recently commented "Small may be beautiful, but it can also be insignificant" (p. 168). A similar point is made by Daly and Cobb (1989) in reference to environmental economics: Political decision-making must remain at the level at which economic decision making occurs, otherwise public policy, those decisions embodying community ethics, will devolve to private economic interests. Health workers must exercise particular caution that their support for community groups does not become an unintended buttress to political and public policy actions based upon economic theories that would see power continue to accumulate in fewer and fewer hands.

## Coalition Building and Advocacy

Coalition building and advocacy can overcome the political limitations of community organizing. Coalitions are groups of groups with a shared goal and some awareness that "united we stand, divided we fall"; advocacy means taking a position on an issue, and initiating actions in a deliberate attempt to influence private and public policy choices. The two are linked in the Holosphere model because advocacy usually involves coalitions.

There are three facets to advocacy in professional practice. First, professionals can aid community groups in their own advocacy by offering knowledge, analytical skills, information on how the political and bureaucratic structures function, and so on. Their support for advocacy is an extension of their support for community organizing. Second, health organizations can also support advocacy by creating policy documents and analyses that form the policy nutcracker's inner arm, thereby legitimizing the advocacy concerns of community groups with which they work. Institutions play a powerful role in shaping and defining what is important in social life (and consequently political discourse) through the implicit and explicit statements made by the types of services they offer, and the policies they create and make public. Third, professionals, individually or through their professional organizations, can increase the strength of their own political voices, taking positions on such policy issues as social welfare reform, housing needs or affordability, employment policies, environmental standards, or any other concerns that may be expressed by individual clients or community groups. An organized political voice of caring professionals may be crucial in moving us towards more just and sustainable forms of social organization: It is professionals who see the human costs of current economic and political practice, who have access to the knowledge and information on how the governing system works, and who have a degree of professional credibility in their statements. Empowerment for professionals, then, is both recognizing and claiming the power they already hold, not "over" others, but in relation to how governments and economic elites currently enact programs and policies.

In Ontario, public health has established itself as an important, legitimating voice in policy debates. When the Ontario Public Health Association (OPHA) argued a few years ago that welfare reforms were an essential investment in health that should be funded through freezes in hospital and physician expenditure increases, the Association helped to influence all party support for the reforms. As professional advocates, the OPHA met the institutions on their own terms. It gave them studies and debated in the language of policy, but the OPHA was not alone. The OPHA worked with coalitions of church groups, anti-poverty groups, unions, newly forged organizations of the poor themselves. There were peoples' stories behind the studies' statistics, and an incredible power that came in recognizing and honoring the differing but mutually supporting roles of community activists and professional advocates.

## Political Action

Political action represents an intensification of actions initiated under the rubric of coalition advocacy. Such action may be partisan or nonpartisan, local or national, participatory or representative in democratic form, legally enacted or civilly disobedient. The line between what comprises coalition advocacy and what constitutes political action is fuzzy; one important difference may lie in the role played by social movement organizations and groups and the degree to which health workers allow themselves to be scrutinized by these movements. This scrutiny often involves moments of conflict, as social movement organizations create their own political legitimacy and voice. But the healthy and often essential role that intergroup conflict plays in social change should not lead health workers to shun the necessity of uniting diverse, conflicting groups at some higher level of community. Pragmatically, the community born in conflict or struggle rarely survives the eventual peace "unless those involved create the institutional arrangements and noncrisis bonding experiences that carry them through the year-in-year-out tests of community functioning" (Gardner, 1991, p. 14).

Gray (1989) provides a comprehensive collaboration model for promoting those functions. There are several steps in effective collaborating, first and most important being problem-setting. Effective collaborating requires the efforts of persons Gray labels "midwives," the community developers of organizations-as-communities. These midwives (functionally distant from all of the stakeholders) work with the stakeholders before they come to the table, seeking to find the "superordinate goal" that Sherif (1966) years ago argued was the basis for initiating any reduction in intergroup conflict.

Using principles from collaboration theory, experiences based on case stories (Labonte, 1993b), and insights gleaned from attempts to forge relations between community health and social service centers and neighborhood volunteer centers in Quebec (Panet-Raymond, 1992), it is possible to propose some preliminary terms for effective (authentic) partnership. Although tenuously offered, these terms provide a starting point from which health agencies might ground an empowering health promotion in day-to-day practice:

1.  All partners have established their own power and legitimacy. This often requires a period of conflict, and some enduring strain between powerful and powerless groups, and a transfer of resources from the former to the latter.

2.  All partners have well-defined mission statements; they have a clear sense of their purpose and organizational goals.

3.  All partners respect each other's organizational autonomy by finding that visionary goal that is larger than any one of their independent goals.

4.  Community group partners are well rooted in the locality and have a constituency to which they are accountable.

5.  Institutional partners have a commitment to partnership approaches in work with community groups.

6.  Clear objectives and expectations of the partners are developed.

7.  Written agreements are made clarifying objectives, responsibilities, means, and norms; regular evaluation allows adjustments to these agreements.

8.  Community workers have clear mandates to support community group partners without attempting to get them to "buy into" the institutional partner's mandate and goal.

9.  All partners strive for and nurture the human qualities of open mindedness, patience, and respect.

## CONCLUSION

A few years ago, government plans to implement the welfare reform referred to earlier were stalled due to their costs, sparking the creation of a massive coalition of welfare advocates, organizations, professionals, church, and labor groups. A Toronto community health center joined in the fray. This center was a small neighborhood organization, providing primary health care, health education and promotion, community organizing, and other supporting services, all managed by an elected board of neighborhood residents. The neighborhood had a high ratio of single mothers on welfare. Many of these women come to the center for their medical services because the primary care team spent time with them, listening to their concerns about money, counseling them on their stresses and strains, hearing their loneliness, and applying the band-aids when they were needed.

But these services were not enough. The primary care teams knew that these women's health problems were less rooted in their bodies, and even in their health behaviors, than in the structured inadequacies of the welfare system. These teams, with the center's health educator, created small groups on health exploration for these women that offered a supportive learning experience, breaking through some of the isolation and learned helplessness engendered by poverty (Seligman, 1975). Some of the women, with the support of the health promoter, organized a community action group which, on its own and in coalitions with other organizations, lobbied for reform. The primary care teams also took case stories of these women's lives. These stories wove a tapestry with the studies collected by the health administrators in a powerful policy statement advocated by the board. Center staff, through their professional associations, lobbied senior government bodies, issued press releases, and joined with coalitions advocating reform. Board members met with politicians, met with media, addressed protesting rallies, made deputations before committees, and linked with social movement groups in their effort to locate the reforms within a larger social justice agenda. For a brief period of time much of the internal squabbling that often characterizes agencies and institutions disappeared in a focused endeavor, in which every staff person and citizen volunteer could see their role and its relation to other roles.

Although the Holosphere model of empowerment has proven a useful educational device in many public health settings, the health center story also implies a few of its difficulties.

1. Linkage across the spheres tends to occur in response to a particular crisis. It is hard to cross discipline and sectoral boundaries in "normal" service delivery situations.

2. A large internal investment of time is required if staff are to engage in the critical peer reflections necessary to move through their disciplinary boundaries.

3. The ability of different professions to support each other around the Holosphere may be constrained by status and financial inequities (power relations) between the professions themselves. For example, physicians are relatively free to expand their practice frames to small group, community organizing, or coalition politics, particularly when they work in salaried settings. Community workers or public health nurses do not have the reverse privilege of expanding their practice frames to personal service modalities monopolized by physicians.

4. The larger an institutional organization, the more difficult it becomes for the different hierarchical layers to maintain the informal contacts necessary for different staff to know when and how issues can be supported around the Holosphere.

Moreover, the Holosphere model presumes that professions and bureaucratic institutions are capable of transformation, meaning that their behaviors can change so that, on measure, they are less disabling than before. This presumption is akin to Wildavsky's dictum that "each policy solution is the beginning of the next problem, and success is when the next problem is smaller than the one for which it was a solution" (O'Higgins, 1992, p. 2).

This presumption, finally, is an act of faith. Faith, according to theologian and literary critic, Northrop Frye (1991), "starts with a vision of reality that is something other than history or logic . . . and on the basis of that vision begins to remake the world" (p. 18). What might prevent this faith from degenerating into rationalized self-interest is the extent to which professionals critically examine what has been both enabling and disabling about their practice styles and their organizations, and make the results of that examination public and accountable. I have argued that health promotion and empowerment function primarily as organizing concepts useful for this examination.

## ENDNOTES

1.  A social movement, whether formalized into a lobbying organization or existing as an informal support or consciousness-raising group, exists "out-there" in the associations of civil society, what John McKnight (1987) calls "social spaces" or the informal, unmanaged and associational sectors of society (Robertson & Minkler, 1994). This demarcation between state (government, bureaucracy) and social movement (civil society) is a tenet shared by both major social movement theory streams, resource mobilization theory and new social movement theory.

2.  I am alternating use of gendered pronouns in this article. Unless the context otherwise specifies, there is no gendered implication to my pronoun or adjective selection.

3.  *Small* only partly refers to size. Primarily, this functional social level of the Holosphere model refers to groups that look primarily inward, to the socioemotive needs of their members, that is, support groups. Normally, these groups are small in number, and many group theories hold that beyond a certain number (over twenty or so) the task/status structuration that arises leads intractably to more formalized relationships.

## REFERENCES

Bogan, G. III. (1992). Organizing an urban African American community for health promotion: Lessons from Chicago. *Journal of Health Education, 23*, 157–159.

*Compact edition of the Oxford English dictionary*. (1971). p. 855.

*City of Toronto: Advocacy for basic prerequisites for health* (policy paper). (1991). Toronto: Department of Public Health.

Daly, H., & Cobb, J. (1989). *For the common good*. Boston: Beacon Press.

Durning, A. (1989). Mobilizing at the grassroots. In L. Brown, A. Durning, C. Flavin, L. Heise, J. Jacobson, S. Postel et al. (Eds.), *State of the world 1989*. New York: Norton.

Eder, K. (1985). The "new social movements": Moral crusades, political pressure groups or social movements? *Social Research, 52*, 869–890.

Epp, J. (1986). *Achieving health for all: A framework for health promotion*. Ottawa: Health and Welfare Canada.

Eyerman, R., & Jamison, A. (1991). *Social movements: A cognitive analysis*. Philadelphia: University of Pennsylvania Press.

Fay, B. (1987). *Critical social science*. Ithaca, NY: Cornell University Press.

Finne, M. (1982). When non-victims derogate powerlessness in the helping professions. *Personality and Social Psychology Bulletin, 8,* 637–643.

Freeman, J. (1983). On the origins of social movements, and a model for analyzing the strategic options of social movement organizations. In J. Freeman (Ed.), *Social movements of the 60s and 70s.* New York: Longman.

Frye, N. (1991). *The double vision.* Toronto: University of Toronto Press.

Gardner, J. (1991). *Building communities.* Independent Sector Leadership Studies Program, Stanford University, Stanford, CA.

Gray, B. (1989). *Collaborating: Finding common ground for multiparty problems.* San Francisco: Jossey-Bass.

Green, L., & Raeburn, J. (1988). Health promotion. What is it? What will it become? *Health Promotion, 3,* 151–159.

Israel, B., Checkoway, B., Schulz, A., & Zimmerman, M. (1994). Health education and community empowerment: Conceptualizing and measuring perceptions of individual, organizational and community control. *Health Education Quarterly, 21,* 149-170.

Jackson, T., Mitchell, S., & Wright, M. (1988, April). *The community development continuum.* Second National Conference of the Australian Community Health Association.

Labonte, R. (1989). Community health promotion strategies. In C. Martin & D. McQueen (Eds.), *Readings for a new public health.* Edinburgh: Edinburgh University Press.

Labonte, R. (1990). Empowerment: Notes on community and professional dimensions. *Canadian Research on Social Policy, 26,* 64–75.

Labonte, R. (1992). Heart health inequalities in Canada: Models, theory and planning. *Health Promotion International, 7,* 119–128.

Labonte, R. (1993a). *Community health responses to health inequalities.* North York, Ontario: North York Community Health Promotion Research Unit.

Labonte, R. (1993b). *Health and empowerment: Practice frameworks.* Toronto: Centre for Health Promotion/Participation.

Labonte, R., & Little, S. (1992). *Determinants of health: Empowering strategies for nurses.* Vancouver, BC: Registered Nurses Association of British Columbia.

McKinlay, J. (1990). Comments at Health Promotion Research Conference. Toronto, Canada: University of Toronto.

McKnight, J. (1987). Comments at Prevention Congress III. Waterloo, Ontario.

Miliband, R. (1983). *The state in capitalist society.* London: Quartet Books.

Minkler, M. (1985). Building supportive ties among inner city elderly: The Tenderloin Senior Outreach Project. *Health Education Quarterly, 12,* 303–314.

Minkler, M. (1989). Health education, health promotion and the open society. *Health Education Quarterly, 16,* 17–30.

Nyswander, D. (1956). Education for health: Some principles and their application. *California's Health, 14,* 69–70.

Offe, C. (1984). *Contradictions of the welfare state.* Boston: MIT Press.

O'Higgins, M. (1992). Social policy in the global economy. In T. Hunsley (Ed.), *Social policy in the global economy.* Ontario: School of Policy Studies, Queens University, Ontario.

Panet-Raymond, J. (1992). Partnership: Myth or reality? *Community Development Journal, 27,* 156–165.

Rappaport, J. (1981). In praise of paradox: A social policy of empowerment over prevention. *American Journal of Community Psychology, 9,* 1–25.

Rappaport, J. (1987). Terms of empowerment/exemplars of prevention: Towards a theory for community psychology. *American Journal of Community Psychology, 15,* 121–148.

Robertson, A., & Minkler, M. (1994). The new health promotion movement: A critical examination. *Health Education Quarterly, 21*(3), 295–312.

Schon, D. (1983). *The reflective practitioner.* New York: Basic Books.

Seidman, S., & Wagner, D. (Eds.). (1992). *Postmodernism and social theory*. Oxford: Blackwell.

Seligman, M. (1975). *Helplessness: On depression, development and death*. San Francisco: W. H. Freeman.

Sherif, M. (1966). *Group conflict and cooperation*. London: Routledge, Kegan and Paul.

Stevenson, H. M., & Burke, M. (1991). Bureaucratic logic in new social movement clothing. *Health Promotion International, 6,* 281–290.

Valvarde, C. (1991). Critical theory in health education (mimeo). Montreal: Montreal DSC.

Wallerstein, N. (1992). Powerlessness, empowerment and health: Implications for health promotion programs. *American Journal of Health Promotion, 6,* 197–205.

Ward, J. (1987). Community development with marginal people: The role of conflict. *Community Development Journal, 22,* 18–21.

Watt, A., & Rodmell, S. (1988). Community involvement in health promotion: Progress or panacea? *Health Promotion, 2,* 359–368.

Wilkinson, R. (1990). Income distribution and mortality: A "natural" experiment. *Sociology of Health and Illness, 12,* 391–412.

World Health Organization. (1986). *Ottawa charter for health promotion*.

Zald, M. (1988). The trajectory of social movements in America. *Research in Social Movements, 19,* 19–41.

# PART

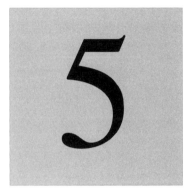

# FREEING/ FUNCTIONING IN HEALTH EDUCATION

*The freeing/functioning philosophy in health education offers an alternative approach and purpose. The focus of health education for a professional who espouses this philosophy would be a holistic and humanistic approach that acknowledges the whole person. Grounded in principles of humanistic psychology, the freeing/functioning philosophy promotes the development of the entire person. Early pioneers in the adoption of this philosophy by the health education profession include Russell (1975), Nolte (1976), and Greenberg (1978). This philosophy in health education is interested in how people function, totally, despite some practices not generally correlated with health.*

*Adoption of this philosophy would ensure that health education's commitment would be to human fulfillment, the focus would be positive, and the learner would be an active self-learner liberated to govern and make choices congruent with his or her own life. Within this philosophy people are free to make their own choices as long as the decisions do not adversely affect others.*

*Choosing freeing/functioning philosophy means concentrating on self-development with the focus on self-image, self-esteem, and self-worth. The premise of this philosophy is that people who have a positive, holistic perception of self are more likely to have and practice healthier lifestyles. Freeing/functioning philosophy focuses on encouraging clients and students to participate fully in life celebration and to be grateful for the opportunity to live and experience both life's joys and sorrows (Greenberg, 1978). This philosophy would argue that people who are unfulfilled and feel unworthy are more apt to practice negative lifestyle patterns. Teach people to love themselves first, and good health habits will follow. Advantages to this philosophy include a holistic approach to health education, honoring autonomy and democratic principles, and moving away from a piecemeal approach to health.*

## ARTICLES

The articles in Part 5 introduce readers to the principles of the freeing/functioning philosophy of health education. Greenberg (1978) introduces the notion of health education as freeing. He challenges health education professionals to move away from looking at only the behavioral minutiae of clients and instead trying to understand the whole person and the reasons behind health decisions being made. Greenberg urges health educators to stop overemphasizing the physical aspects of health to the detriment and neglect of others. Anderson & Ronson (2005) introduce the importance of following democratic principles in health promotion programs with special emphasis on autonomy. In the example they reported on, they found that health promotion should be a process in which people are encouraged to have control over their lives. By empowering the students, they found that the students were more apt to comply with health promotion principles when they felt listened to and respected. Hoyman (1971) guides the profession through a splendid description of human ecology as a route to personal fulfillment and a holistic means to health where examples within health education are explored. And finally, Hawks (2004) encourages health educators to take a holistic approach to the profession. He contends that with purpose, self-fulfillment, and meaning to life, good health practices follow. In order to find meaning in one's life, a commitment to autonomy and self-governance is paramount.

## CHALLENGE TO READER

As one reads through these articles to glean principles that you can apply in your professional practice, pay special attention to the purpose, the role of the teacher, the role of the learner, and the methods for implementation. How can you put these principles into practice as you interact with people in your everyday life?

# CHAPTER

## 19

# HEALTH EDUCATION AS FREEING

### JERROLD S. GREENBERG

I write this article out of a genuine concern for the direction in which I see health education moving, and out of the frustration of repeatedly being confronted with inconsistencies in the practices and philosophies of my colleagues. I propose that health education be considered a process in which the goal is to free people so that they may make health-related decisions based upon their needs and interests as long as these decisions do not adversely affect others. Though at first glance this definition of health education appears not much different from what others have offered, its application, as described here, certainly is. One implication of health education as a *freeing* process is the assumption that participants, voluntary or otherwise, are not initially free. One could consider the feelings of inferiority, hostility, and alienation; socioeconomic status; and emotional distress to be enslaving people so that they are not as free to choose health-related behaviors as they might otherwise be (see Suggested Readings). It is suggested here that health education should be directed at the elimination or diminishment of these enslaving factors so as to free the participants in the process.

Others have stated a philosophy similar to this, but when pressed to go further often become inconsistent. For instance, if the view of health education as a freeing process is supported, health educators must not be concerned with the particular behavior of their clients, but rather with the *process* used by their clients to arrive at that behavior. For example, if a client (student in school, adult in nursing home program, and so on) chooses to smoke cigarettes but has made that decision freely, the health educator has been successful.

This model is more democratic than the one many health educators have adopted. It does not entail programming clients to behave in predetermined ways that have been defined as "healthy," but rather attempts to eliminate or diminish the factors which influence the client's behavior so as to allow him or her to freely choose health-related behaviors consistent with his or her values, needs, etc. This model is a move away from the *1984* syndrome of operant conditioning and a push toward a more collaborative type of health education between educator and client.

Someone once said, "Give me a fish and I eat today, but teach me to fish and I can eat forever." Similarly, health education that teaches people the decision-making process will be more valuable than health education that tells people how to behave. In many instances, health scientists are not even sure which behaviors are healthy or unhealthy. For example, though there is sufficient evidence to conclude that serum cholesterol is related to coronary heart disease, the relationship between ingested cholesterol and serum cholesterol has not been agreed upon. Yet health educators teach people to lower ingested cholesterol, rather than present the debate surrounding this issue and let people decide for themselves whether or not reducing cholesterol makes sense to them. As Toffler (1971) and Pirsig (1974) have written, knowledge is expanding rapidly. The facts of today too often become the myths of tomorrow. The healthy behaviors that health educators program people to adopt today may become the unhealthy behaviors of tomorrow (swine flu inoculations?). Rather than training people to behave in pre-determined ways, let's teach them to analyze issues freely and decide for themselves how to behave.

Another aspect of this concept pertains to the relationship of mental, social, and spiritual health to physical health. Too often in determining which behaviors are "healthy," health educators emphasize the quantity of life to the detriment of the quality of life. Mortality and morbidity become the mainstays rather than happiness and comfort. Physical health is adopted as the objective often to the exclusion, or at least the deemphasis, of mental, social, and spiritual health. Greene (1971) writes of this issue:

> *A businessman might be fifteen pounds overweight for no apparent reason other than careless eating habits, an unawareness of the advantages of a trim physique, and ignorance of the basic principles of weight control. This should be classed as a remedial health defect and one important indicator of reduced health status. However, let us compare this case with the case of another businessman, equally overweight, who happens to be a well-informed and enthusiastic amateur gourmet. His library of cookbooks includes directions for preparing many of the most popular dishes of other cultures. He spends many interesting hours in offbeat markets shopping for hard-to-get food items. The meals he prepares constitute focal points of an interesting and satisfying social life. This man realizes he is overweight; he knows how to reduce and control his weight, and he may even suspect that his coronary may arrive a year or two ahead of schedule, but he does not care. His overweight*

*condition constitutes a health defect only in the absolute sense. When viewed in rela-*
*tion to his value system, it represents a logical concomitant to his particular pattern of*
*good health. (p. 114)*

In the health education model being proposed here, since the individual is responsible for choosing a health-related behavior, the value system is more likely to be a part of that decision than if someone else made the decision for the individual.

The objectives of this new health education are concerned with enslaving factors. Some of these factors are described below. Some objectives pertain to the development of skills, others to the acquisition of knowledge, and still others to understanding derived through introspection. The goal is to help the client either eliminate these factors from influencing behavior, diminish their effect, or have them surface so the client can freely and knowingly allow them to influence behavior.

1. Poor self-esteem is associated with many health-related behaviors and should be improved. People who don't think well of themselves cannot be expected to have confidence in their own decisions and can be expected to be unduly influenced by others.

2. Alienation consists of social isolation, normlessness, and powerlessness. Social isolation is a lack of significant others in which one can confide. Normlessness is a lack of rules, regulations, and standards that one can choose to live by. Powerlessness is a feeling of not being in control of one's own destiny. Alienation, like self-esteem, is related to many decisions. People cannot freely make decisions if, for instance, they have high powerlessness since they would not believe those decisions were important to their lives.

3. Most people are influenced by others in some way and health educators should be able to show others the effect of peer group pressure in their lives. The needs derived from peer status, such as friendship, respect, etc., should be discussed and their importance analyzed by each client. The realization of the influence of peer group pressure and status in decisions made by each participant will lead to a more conscious influence. That is, it is hoped that awareness will lead to the ability to spot the pressure when it occurs and then to decide, consciously, to allow or not allow it to affect behavior.

4. Values clarification activities have gone far to help people develop values that make sense to them and to act more consistently with these values. Since a lack of understanding of one's value system could be expected to result in confused or inconsistent behavior health educators should concern themselves with this topic.

5. Health knowledge is necessary, though not a sufficient factor, to make decisions which are most appropriate for oneself.

6.  Health skills must be teamed. One is not free to choose to brush and floss one's teeth, for example, unless one has learned the skills.

7.  Internal locus of control is the belief that events can be influenced fey oneself. External locus of control is the belief that events are beyond one's control. Those who don't believe a "healthy" behavior can influence their health cannot be expected to adopt that behavior. Health educators should help people realize they can influence their own health by developing an internal health locus of control within their clients.

Some other enslaving factors are lack of problem solving skills; lack of decision-making skills; lack of assertiveness; lack of communication skills; and fear of physicians, death, dying, and pain.

I propose that the objectives of health education not be decreasing the incidence of smoking, drug abuse, or any other health-related behavior. Rather, the objectives should be to improve self-esteem, decrease alienation, help students realize the effects of peer group pressure, learn health knowledge and skills and so on. In other words, free people to make their own decisions about health-related behaviors. It's more democratic, makes more sense in terms of ever-changing facts, and interestingly enough, can probably be expected to result in clients adopting "healthy" behavior to a greater extent than they do now.

## EVALUATION OF RESEARCH

The implications of this new health education for evaluation of health education programs are profound. Presently we pre and posttest program participants in terms of their health related behaviors (such as questionnaires regarding use of drugs) with the hope that less unhealthy and more healthy behavior will occur at the program's end than beginning. There should be less venereal disease (or earlier detection), less alcohol abuse, less cigarette smoking, better nutritional value, more exercising, etc. Under the new health education, health-related behaviors would not be measured. Instead, self-esteem scales, alienation scales, locus of control scales health knowledge and skills tests, etc. would be administered before and after. Improvement on these enslaving factors would indicate the effectiveness of the health education program. Improvement would also indicate that program participants were freer to decide on a personal set of health behaviors. As an additional outcome, though not a specific objective of the program, the health educator might look at the decisions these freer people made about their health. Further research could include the following:

■   The development of more valid and reliable measures of enslaving factors.

■   The relationship between the degree of the enslaving factors and health-related behavior; for instance, do freer people behave in ways traditionally described as healthy (social, mental, and spiritual, as well as physical) to a greater extent than those less free?

- The development and testing of instructional strategies designed to eliminate or diminish enslaving factors.

- The development of effective means to "sell" this new health education to various groups: parents, students, legislators, administrators, etc.

*Health education* as used in this article refers to primary prevention. The applicability of this model to other aspects of health education has not been considered.

## REFERENCES

Greene, W. (1971). The search for a meaningful definition of health. In D. A. Read (Ed.), *New directions in health education: Some contemporary issues for the emerging age*. New York: Macmillan.

Pirsig, R. M. (1974). *Zen and the art of motorcycle maintenance*. New York: Bantam Books.

Toffler, A. (1971). *Future shock*. New York: Bantam Books.

## SUGGESTED READINGS

Cahman, W. J. (1968). The stigma of obesity. *Sociological Quarterly, 9*, 283–299.

Calhoun, J. F., & Zimering, S. (1976). Is there an alcoholic personality? *Journal of Drug Education, 6*(2).

Greenberg, J. S. (1972, Fall–Winter). A theory of health education. *New York State Journal of Health, Physical Education, and Recreation, 25*(1), 50–52.

Greenberg, J. S. (1978). *Student-centered health instruction*. Reading, MA: Addison-Wesley.

Jacobs, M. A., et al. (1966). Orality, impulsivity, and cigarette smoking in men: Further findings in support of a theory. *Journal of Nervous and Mental Disease, 143*, 207–219.

Jones, M. (1968). Personality correlates and antecedents of drinking patterns in adult males. *Journal of Consulting and Clinical Psychology, 32*, 10.

Warner, R. (1971, October). Alienation and drug abuse: Synonymous? *National Association for Secondary School Principals Bulletin*, 59.

# CHAPTER

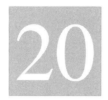

# DEMOCRACY: THE FIRST PRINCIPLE OF HEALTH PROMOTING SCHOOLS

ANDY ANDERSON

BARBARA RONSON

In Canada, the premiers of each province and territory recently forged a Ten-Year Plan to Strengthen Health Care. Within that plan, they committed to "working across sectors through initiatives such as Healthy Schools. This is excellent news. Leaders in the art and science of "health promotion" have long been advocating the need to go beyond the health care sector and build better partnerships with other sectors as one means of improving the health of populations and communities. "Healthy Cities" and "Healthy Schools" movements around the world are examples of efforts to improve health in its full sense—including physical, mental, social and spiritual components— through such collaboration. They have taught us, moreover, that partnerships need to be built at the highest as well as the grass roots levels.

Countries around the world have found that when their ministers of education and health work in genuine partnership for the well-being of their citizens, reflecting and modeling partnerships at the local level, unprecedented progress can be made. Furthermore, Healthy Schools require roots in key principles such as democracy, equity, empowerment and active learning. Unfortunately, too little of the dialogue concerning Healthy Schools draws on this learning today. We hear mostly of issues such as vending machines in schools and time for supervised physical activity. While attention to such issues can be important starting places, little sustained improvement will result if these deep learnings from the Health Promoting School movement are ignored.

In this paper, democracy, the first principle of the European Network of Health Promoting Schools, will be examined in depth to illustrate how the Healthy Schools initiatives in Canada can go beyond a narrow focus on physical health of students and become a leading force for school reform in its broadest sense. Democracy will be examined on a civic level as presented by Alexis de Tocqueville and Robert Putnam; and on a school and classroom level as presented in the more recent work of Glickman, Fenstermacher, Palmer, and Giroux. The work of Don Nutbeam and Katherine Weare on Health Promoting Schools will help to illustrate how democracy links to healthy citizens and schools. An organizational guide for Healthy Schools will be offered and examples of what healthy schools might look like will be presented. It is hoped that this paper will help to broaden the dialogue on Healthy Schools to take best advantage of the opportunities we now have to create lasting improvements in our schools. Our discussion of democracy is part of our ongoing research efforts to understand how health promotion might (a) appeal to wider audiences, (b) inform school operations such as governance, instructional practice, school climate and service delivery, and (c) contribute to the theory and practice of school improvement, specifically as a way to make schools smarter, stronger, and safer.

## AN OVERVIEW OF THE HEALTH-PROMOTING SCHOOLS MOVEMENT

One of the most highly regarded and successful international educational endeavors is the concept of the Health Promoting School. The WHO (1996) defines a health promoting school (HPS) as "a school that is constantly strengthening its capacity as a healthy setting for living, learning, and working." In partnership with a range of human service providers, health promoting schools aim to provide the conditions that optimize opportunities for both students and teachers to learn. Underlying the concept of health promotion is the notion that to achieve good health persons must have some measure of control over the decisions and conditions they encounter over time and across circumstances. Decisions are the result of an interpretative process both in understanding what the needs are and what can and should to be done about them. Drawing on information, experience, goals, anticipated consequences, and ideally morals, we can make reasoned, responsible choices. At the heart of these choices are the feelings (values, motives, care) we have about the situation. Whether we are enthusiastic, troubled, outraged by a certain situation, or not, will have a bearing on our interpretation, reaction, and choice of action.

Dispassionate views of human functioning have been around for centuries. Vesalius (*De Humani Coporis Fabrica*, 1543) and Harvey (*Exercitatio de Motu Cordis*, 1628) helped foster the emerging metaphor of the body as a machine, emphasizing the lever-like action of muscles and joints and the analogy between circulation and pumps, valves and conduits. Newton's *Principia* (1687), by describing the simple mechanical laws governing the universe, further entrenched the desire to understand all natural phenomenon, including health and disease in mechanical terms. Thus, theories of health and disease during the Renaissance followed other scientific movements of the era. Health and disease were explained either in terms of general mathematical or physical principles, in keeping with Copernicus, Kepler, Galileo, and Newton, or in accordance with chemical principles, as described by Boyle, Willis, and Mayow. Bodily functions were explained in terms of their chemical (iatrochemical) or mathematical (iatrophysical or iatromathematical) principles.

These efforts to understand bodily functioning and the mechanisms of disease continue today. The result of this work is a comprehensive knowledge that has led to the development of antibiotics, drugs, vaccines, and other procedures used to treat and prevent various illnesses. As we move into the twenty-first century, the focus of this research is becoming more microscopic with endeavors such as the Human Genome Project. Upon completion of this project, our understanding of the composition and functions of the human body will increase dramatically. This knowledge will result in a different approach to the prevention and treatment of disease.

Perhaps the greatest advance in health policy achieved as a result of scientific conceptions of health is the implementation of universal health care in many countries. The philosophy behind this service is that the health of the population will improve if all of its members have access to medical services rooted in scientific understanding.

Contemporary versions of health which cast humans as constructivists and creationists, having determination over their well-being, focus on building within people their capacity to "make a life" by enhancing their ability to learn—cope, adapt, and make sense of their environments and relationships. Subsequently, health promotion is defined as "the process of enabling people to increase control over and to improve their health. To reach a state of complete physical, mental, and social wellbeing, an individual or group must be able to identify and to realize aspirations, to satisfy needs, and to change and to cope with the environment" (WHO *Ottawa charter*, 1986).

The European Network of Health Promoting Schools, supported jointly by the World Health Organization, the Council of Europe, and the European Union, consists of approximately five hundred schools from forty-one countries reaching 8,000–10,000 teachers and 500,000 students. In Canada and the United States, the conceptual roots of health promotion in school settings date back to the 1980s where there was a strong call for continuous Comprehensive School Health Education (CSHE) from kindergarten to school leaving. Proponents of CSHE argued that health habits and knowledge acquired early in life could impact lifelong health status. Health education portrayed simply as a course of study was not considered effective. Rather, the curriculum should be part of schoolwide and community efforts to promote healthy living. The curriculum for health education should address, therefore, a wide array of topics, every year, that developmentally built the skills and habits of mind needed to cope with divergent needs and evolving circumstances related to health and well-being. Health education, like other subjects offered in school, should prepare young people to be lifelong, autonomous, and responsible learners and as such represent an important area of study related to human development.

Later, Comprehensive Health Programs sought to include health services and school environments—hallways, playgrounds, cafeterias—that were considered equally important for children's and youths' health. Perhaps the classic example of incongruence between health education and school environments has been the tension between nutrition education aimed at promoting healthy food choices and the sale of junk food in vending machines and school fund-raising campaigns. Unless the "school" is committed to healthy eating the effects of the health education program are undermined.

In the United States, the *Journal of School Health* (1987) dedicated a special issue to comprehensive school health programs featuring an article by Allensworth and Kolbe, which proposed eight components of a comprehensive program:

- Health education

- Physical education

- Health services

- Nutrition services

- Counseling, psychological, and social services

- Healthy school environment

- Health promotion for staff

- Parent/community involvement

Clearly, the responsibility for health promotion has been broadened and enriched to involve a wide spectrum of services and supports. With strong support from the Centers for Disease Control and Prevention, this model, like the Canadian model has endured. In 1995 the word *coordinated* replaced *comprehensive* because people tended to confuse comprehensive school health programs with comprehensive school Health Education (instruction) and felt that the term *comprehensive* might discourage an overburdened education system from implementing the model.

## The Term "Coordinated School Health" Now Predominates in the United States

At the heart of each school health promotion model are a number of principles which serve as a moral compass for decisions about the purpose, structure, and engagement of people within organizations, institutions, and programs of study. These principles are seen not only as central to campaigns for the health promotion in schools but also as fundamental rights and entitlements for children and youth leading to the formation of a just and civil society. Ten principles listed as fundamental to the WHO Health Promoting Schools framework are democracy, equity, empowerment, teacher development, collaboration, community development, curriculum, sustainability, school environment, and measuring success. Like the Coordinated School Health Model, these education principles recognize schools as a key setting for health promotion because it is capable of providing universal access to knowledge, skills, services and supports, building within individuals and communities their capacity for change agentry and growth. Further, health promotion "works" when it is presented in a way that is consistent with the goals and mandates of the organization and presented systematically. School experiences managed in relation to these principles are posed as a way to broaden and intensify students' involvement in what Habermas (1990) has termed the *lifeworld* of schools: cultural traditions, ceremonial rituals, participation in clubs, and teacher-student relationships; and the *systemsworld* of the school: programs of study, school governance. Authentic involvement in school life can build feelings of affiliation and connectedness. Enriched student participation builds trust and a greater awareness of students' needs, interests, talents, values and goals as well as mutual understanding between teachers and students. When students feel like they are listened to, respected, and have a voice, they are more likely to contribute to and comply with school mandates. In other words, following health promotion principles such as democracy should be thought of as a way to make schools stronger.

The health promoting school is also celebrated as a way to forge stronger links between the community—local culture, context, customs—and approaches to health promotion. In this way, health promotion builds on resources unique to each school community. Community characteristics are viewed as assets to be developed not problems to be overcome. Lerner and Benson's *Developmental Assets and Asset-Building Communities* (2003) provides a review of programs and research that make a convincing argument for the notion of growth change in relation to community resources—strengths, imagination, hopes. Increasingly, community service groups such as the Lion's International are taking up this challenge through programs such as the Lion's Quest program which is used in thousands of schools across America and Canada. Accordingly, principles of health promotion activate community involvement which enables schools to get smarter about the specific needs and opportunities that exist within communities.

School environments that work to respect the right everyone has to enjoy school attendance, share ideas and insights openly, challenge the status quo, and question existing practices and power relationships foster rich opportunities for critical and alternative thinking. Under these conditions, we propose, schools are safer (Anderson, 2003).

In this paper we examine the first principle of a health promoting school: democracy. Initially, we consider democracy relative to the educational opportunities presented in school, in general. We thread into this dialogue the implications these ideas and beliefs about democracy hold for the HPS as an integral part of overall efforts to improve schools for "public" good, that is, the betterment of society, responsible citizenry, care for self and others. Finally, we present ideas about how democratic thinking might impact programs of study in health education to promote healthy living, social responsibility, and active citizenry.

Conceptually, we examine democracy as

- a stance or disposition toward learning, for example, openness to ideas, respect for alternative views and realities, acknowledgement of learning as a social process linked to time, place, and context;

- a way of being in the classroom, community, or world, for example, actively pursuing meaning from multiple texts, protecting and promoting opportunities for everyone to learn by creating environments that are inviting and safe;

- a way of belonging, for example, relating learning to citizenry, contribution to the betterment of society, relating knowing and doing to community participation—communities of scholarship, communities of care;

- an organizational model, for example, how people, programs, policy and partners interrelate and work together in relation to common values and principles such as equity and empowerment.

## UNDERSTANDING DEMOCRACY FROM A SOCIAL PERSPECTIVE

The Greeks tell us that the early meaning of the word *democracy* was "strength of the people." Most people today think of democracy in terms of its dictionary definition:

> *government by the people, rule of the majority, government in which the supreme power is vested in the people and exercised by them directly or indirectly through a system of representation, usually a political unit that has a democratic government [with] absence of hereditary or arbitrary class distinction. (Webster's New Collegiate Dictionary)*

Alexis de Tocqueville suggests democracy was meant to provide greater and more equitable access to the informational and intellectual resources that enable everyone to participate in the affairs and decisions that affect our lives. In his sociological study *Democracy in America*, first published in 1835, he describes how greater equality in America was evident through the independence of the judiciary, freedom of the press, the rule of law, and also through the habits, opinions, manners and morals, families, and religion of the people. One of the most recent well-known writers on this subject is Robert Putnam, director of the Harvard Center for International Affairs. Putnam's seminal work, *Making Democracy Work: Civic Traditions in Modern Italy* (1993), puts forward the idea that prosperity is related more to democratic traditions and civic engagement than to the acquisition of material goods. His conclusions are in agreement, he says, with hundreds of empirical studies in a wide range of disciplines that have shown that higher civic engagement and social connectedness produce better schools, faster economic development, lower crime as well as more effective government. Researchers in such fields as education, urban poverty, unemployment, the control of crime, drug abuse, and health have discovered that successful project outcomes are more likely in civically engaged communities. Civic societies have denser networks of social connectedness and there is general agreement on basic values, consensus is valued, and the power structure is more democratic and less hierarchical or authoritarian (Wilkinson, 1996).

In Putnam's later work, "Bowling Alone" (1995), he painstakingly documents the decline in "associational memberships," community engagement and "social capital" in the United States. He says, for example:

*The voting rate has declined by nearly a quarter between the 1960s and 1990. Church association has decreased from 48% in the late 50s to 41% in the early seventies and has remained steady or further declined since then. The number of people reporting attendance at a public meeting on town or school affairs in the previous year decreased from 22% in a survey to 13% in 1993. The number of those in the non-agricultural workforce who belonged to a union declined from 32.5% in 1953 to 15.8% in 1992. 12 million people belonged to Parent Teacher Associations in 1964 compared to 5 million in 1982 and approximately 7 million now. Membership in civic and fraternal organizations has come down since the mid-sixties, along with the general level of volunteerism in such organizations. As well, the number of people who socialize with neighbors more than once a year has declined from 72% in to 61% in 1993.*

Though there may be some countertrends, such as an increase in participation in "support groups," the paid workforce and cause-related organizations, the overall tendency towards increased isolation and splintering of families and groups is difficult to dispute. Putnam calculates that at all educational (and hence social) levels of North American society, and counting all sorts of group memberships, the average number of associational memberships has fallen by about a fourth over the last quarter century.

Kellner (1990) in *Television and the Crisis of Democracy* laments:

*The commercial system of television sells television advertising to corporations and political candidates who can afford to purchase highly expensive airtime, thus ensuring control of the economic and political system by the wealthy and powerful. It is precisely this system of corporate-controlled and television mediated elections that has "turned-off' the electorate, giving the United States the lowest rate of participation in major elections among major capitalist democracies. And it is the paucity of information provided by commercial television that renders the electorate highly uninformed and thus incapable of intelligently participating in the political process. (p. 180)*

Kellner pleads for a critical theory of television which "conceptualizes both sides of the existing society and culture—namely the forces of domination and those that prefigure and struggle for a better society." Increases in the formation of street gangs are often considered the result of alienation, displacement and loneliness experienced by young people. The need for affiliation and affection provided by gang membership can often undercut concerns about personal health.

In a democracy that is flourishing we would probably experience less central control and greater community and neighborhood involvement in the decisions and actions taken to provide what the community values in health, education and community life. Arrangements would be in place that would enable people to take care of each other, support efforts to grow, and deal directly with the obstacles and threats to peace and good order. For example, in communities with high social cohesion people feel that the community is looking out for their best interests, they believe their children are safe in the streets and playground areas, and in troubled times the community will rally to support them. Feelings of belonging extend beyond families and neighborhoods to include business and industry, faith communities, and municipal agencies. Clearly, these adages would represent a sense of community: We're all in this together. Nothing about us without us. It takes a whole village to raise a (whole) child.

### Democracy from an Educational Perspective—What Giroux Has to Say

In Henry Giroux's *Stealing Innocence* (2000) and later in *The Abandoned Generation: Democracy Beyond the Culture of Fear* (2003) critical arguments are presented about democracy in education which can be traced to constructivists' beliefs about learning. Learning is a sense-making process. Accordingly, individuals consciously strive for meaning, to make sense of their environment in terms of past experience and their present state in an attempt to create order, resolve incongruities, and reconcile external realities with prior experience.

Giroux emphasizes that knowledge is mainly acquired through social processes wherein culture, context, and community are logically and philosophically active. He concludes politics and pedagogy are subsequently inseparable. Hence Giroux pushes for an approach to education that engages students in not only critical analysis of the context but of the implications this knowledge has for how we think, behave and participate in our life experiences. Content is not neutral; rather it is located in a social-political and cultural milieu. Giroux makes it clear that for full participation in a democratic society, students must be prepared to examine knowledge in relation to the "knower," how ideas are never without interpretation tempered by the knowledge, beliefs, and experiences of the examiner. Consider, for example, health in relation to knowledge, beliefs, and experiences of the person. The idea of health then becomes more than just views about health that center largely on disease avoidance, prevention, and treatment. Views about health that focus on what is happening in a person's life—such as level of income, relationships with close and intimate others, participation in social and civic life, employment stability, to name a few—are seen as determinants of health which impact the capacity one has to live to the fullest.

The links between democracy and education, Giroux argues, are rooted in the notion that learning is a journey toward self-knowledge, self-mastery, thus liberation. Accordingly, education is not a matter of handing out "encyclopedic knowledge" but of developing and disciplining awareness which the learner already possesses. To educate means to bring out but also intensify and enlarge one's perception of the larger social order versus simply gathering information. He complains that assessment and standardized testing, for example, aimed at mastery of discrete skills and bodies of knowledge have little to do with teaching students to develop critical thinking skills, socio-cultural maps, and an awareness of the powers that enable individuals to locate themselves in the world and to effectively intervene and shape it.

Giroux portrays the classroom as a place where students think critically about the world around them but also offer a sanctuary and forum where they can address their fears, anger and concerns about events such as 9/11 and how it affected their lives. He pushes for discourse within academic study which discusses the meaning of democratic values, the relationship between learning and civic engagement and the connection between schooling and public "good" versus private interests. The learning of skills, disciplinary knowledge, rigor are not valuable in and of themselves. One of the principal aims of education, therefore, is to develop a critical awareness of the values and ideologies that shape the form of received knowledge. This aim suggests a constant probing and criticism of received knowledge as part of civic and social engagement in community affairs.

Accordingly, school work must be linked to larger purposes such as creating more equitable and just public spheres within and outside educational institutions—exercising rights and entitlements—as a part of active citizenry. Giroux draws on the work of Freire, who argues that it is through the sort of critical and moral engagement with subject matter that educators build a sense of hope, not despair and disappointment. He encourages progressive educators and their students to stand at the edge of society, to think beyond existing configurations of power in order to imagine the unthinkable in terms of how they live with dignity, justice, and freedom (p. 146). Within acts of "moral imagination" students are posing problems that begin with "What if" and "Why not." This approach to pedagogy in general is based on the idea that there is more hope in the world when teachers and students can question what is often taken for granted in their text books, classrooms, and larger social order versus memorization of predigested information.

The key point here is that learning is seen as essentially a social process. Knowledge because of its relative nature is dependent upon communication among learners, teachers, and others. In order to be effective, therefore, health promoters must find their inspiration in not only understandings of health but of the fundamental purposes of school and beliefs about learning.

## What Fenstermacher Says

In the educational literature, democracy is more often discussed in terms of learning environments where students are encouraged to contribute their understandings and reasonings about the subject matter as part of a process of making sense of the concepts and ideas in relation to students' lives and real world problems. The goal, therefore, of democratic education is for students to participate actively in the construction of knowledge rather than simply consume it. As an educational principle, democracy should run deeply throughout the school informing organizational culture, personal and interpersonal associations, and the pursuit of knowledge from the classroom level up to the highest levels of decision-making.

Fenstermacher (1999) refers to democracy as "a way of living wherein each individual holds an entitlement to envision an ideal future for him or herself and is ensured sufficient freedom to pursue that vision." In a democratic classroom the content students learn should in some way connect to or resonate in the lives they are living. Fenstermacher encourages involvement in the many disciplines of human knowledge and understanding "so that children become acquainted with these in ways that not only permit their understanding of them, but also lay the groundwork for the eventual contribution to these disciplines." Student involvement, namely, the experience of connecting and contributing to an understanding of the subject matter and then applying and relating it to real world problems, is democratic education. Specifically, learners who are actively engaged in the learning process are more likely to understand the material, that is, know why, know how, and know when the material relates to situations and problems that affect their lives.

Content becomes knowledge as a result of individuals in some way putting that information to "good" use, that is, applied responsibly to real world problems. Information has educational value relative to the impact it can possibly have on our quality of life. We might, therefore, want to consider how educators help students transform information into knowledge through a process of putting what we know and value to "good use," that is, making a positive difference in people's lives. Knowing in a democracy should have implications. Knowing that thousands of people will die of HIV/AIDS unless medical supplies are available must be accompanied by consideration of the social, political, and economic forces that interact to allow this situation to occur. What does it take to provide medical services to countries financially unable to buy expensive medical supplies? Why is the delivery of soft drinks to these desperate areas of the world more efficient than the delivery of essential medical supplies?

## What Glickman Says

Democratic learning is "a set of purposeful activities always building toward increasing student activity, choice, participation, connection, and contribution. It always aims for students individually and collectively to take on greater responsibility for their own learning" (Glickman, 1999). In practice, democratic learning involves

- students actively working with real world problems, ideas, materials, and people as they learn skills and content;

- students having escalating degrees of choices, both as individuals and as groups, within the parameters provided by the teacher;

- students being responsible to their peers, teachers, parents, and school community to ensure that educational time is being used purposefully and productively;

- students sharing their learning with one another, with teachers, and with parents and other community members, that is, "function as a community of learners";

- students deciding how to make their teaming a contribution to their community;

- students assuming responsibility for finding places where they can apply and further their learning, that is, attend to process, how knowledge is obtained, whose knowledge counts;

- students working and learning from one another individually and in groups at a pace that challenges all (Glickman, 1999).

## What Palmer Says

What sort of curriculum and instruction would enable students to learn democratically? Palmer describes a curriculum that has as its subject matter practical public problems and citizen action (Palmer, 1998). These matters of civic importance and the process by which they are carefully examined should be the subject of classroom study. Discussions are studied for their content but also for who is speaking and who is not. Whose ideas count? Who gets air time? Who doesn't? Whose voice is missing? Palmer, like Giroux tells us that there is a need for democratic discussion that examines not only what is said, but who is saying it and, whose voice is left out.

## What Nutbeam Says

Democratic approaches to the study of subject matter aligns with what Nutbeam (2000) has described in health education as "critical literacy." The health literate citizen is concerned not only about knowledge and interpersonal relationships but social justice, equity, and involvement—Whose interests are being served? Who dominates? Who is silent? How do determinants of health interact with decisions for health? For example, why are the smoking rates double among First Nation adolescents? Why are people in upper income households half as likely to require hospital care as people living in low income households? Why are white women most likely to become anorexic? How do speech patterns and clothing present subtle barriers to participation in certain activities?

## What We Say

Engagement, participation, expression, equality, justice, responsibility, individual rights to liberty and freedom—these all represent democratic collaboration well done, not only in school but in all areas of life. Teachers must ask themselves, What would teaching and learning for democracy look like? What would students achieve and demonstrate in classrooms if democracy were practiced as the most powerful pedagogy of learning for all students? Our attempt to answer this question follows:

- Students are involved in setting some of the formats, structures, and rules of learning.

- Textbook material and worksheets are emphasized less while reference materials, electronic media, technology, and hands-on activities are relied on more.

- Students are sometimes contracted for work to be done with a final demonstration, subject to peer, parent, and community review.

- Students tutor other students and contribute to schoolwide projects.

- Students are provided with opportunities to work in the field.

- Homogenous groupings, including age groupings, are minimized.

Education for democratic learning means involving students in varied and alternative discussions about the subject matter, presenting opportunities to see the subject matter from their perspective, the perspective of others, different places of understanding, different cultures, different times in history, different locations and positions of power or lack of outlooks. The example we present later proposes the question, What might be the implications of changing our eating habits to include the recommended daily consumption of fresh fruits and vegetables outlined by National Food Guides? Imagine the number of different points of view/concerns expressed about this proposition. Imagine what students can learn about the politics of promoting policy for public good.

## What Weare Says

In her paper "The Health Promoting School—An Overview of the Concept, Principles and Strategies and the Evidence for Their Effectiveness," Katherine Weare writes that democracy needs a balance between participation, warm relationships, clarity and autonomy (1998).

"Participation" and the closely aligned concept of empowerment underlie the famous definition of *health promotion* by the Ottawa Charter as "the process of enabling people to increase control over, and to improve, their own health." Empowerment, she explains further, aims to be genuinely democratic by ensuring that the action or process is done with, rather than to, people. There is overwhelming evidence, she writes, that the level of democratic participation in schools is a key factor in producing high levels of both performance and satisfaction in teachers and pupils. Therefore a key strategy for a health promoting school is to ensure that its organization, management structures and ethos are empowering and encourage participation. Her description is apt (Weare, 1998):

*Empowerment and participation take many interlinked and mutually supportive forms: They include consultation of staff and students, a democratic, "bottom up" approach to decision making, and open communication. The role of the head teacher in an empowering school is as facilitator rather than a despot, the leader of a team of staff rather than the apex of a rigid hierarchy, a team that genuinely collaborates with pupils and parents in the running of the school, is responsive to their needs and wants, and attempts to create a sense of common ownership of the school's processes, policies and decisions. Such schools see themselves as accountable to parents, to pupils, to local education authorities, and to the local community. Pupils' parliaments, parents' councils, and school planning groups that include members of the local community are just some of the ways in which empowering and democratic intentions can become reality.*

The importance of "warm relationships" to learning is also well documented, she says. Poor relationships between pupils and staff and between teachers and their colleagues is one of the most commonly cited causes of staff stress, while high levels of support reduce the likelihood of staff "burnout." Better achievement of outcomes, both cognitive and affective, are found in classrooms with "higher levels of cohesiveness" and "less social friction." Competencies that underpin our ability to make good relationships include the capacity for empathy, genuineness, and respect.

The third element for effective schools she defines is "clarity," which is related to the word *transparency*, a term frequently referred to in the health promoting school literature. Clarity involves structure and boundaries, having people know what is expected of them and what they can expect of others, understanding what their role is, and what the norms, values, and rules of the organization are. Students can form better relationships, have higher attainments, enjoy learning, and attend better when there is clear leadership by teachers and they are certain of what they are doing. Teachers also perform better when goals are clear. They become better motivated and more effective in their job performance. Clear, timely feedback to pupils and teachers about their performance is also important.

The fourth element she describes is "autonomy" which she defines as "self-determination and control of one's own work and life, thinking for oneself and being critical and independent, while able to take full responsibility for one's own actions." This, she says, is essential if pupils are to be prepared to become full citizens in the democracies of the free world. Students need to learn to think for themselves and to work independently as their age, stage, and personality allows.

Democracy in schools requires each of the four elements in the right proportion. She explains that too much emphasis on warm and supportive relationships, participation and individual autonomy without clarity can lead to a laissez-faire environment in which people have an unrealistic sense of their own personal importance, everyone competes, no one knows what the rules and boundaries are, and little is achieved or learned. But an emphasis on clarity alone leads to an authoritarian, inflexible, over-regimented and autocratic environment, in which people may know the rules but may not care about following them, and can feel unvalued and alienated. The third way that achieves the right balance between these extremes has been described as "democratic." It is one in which people feel cared for, part of the organization and able to act with a degree of personal control, but know too that there are clear boundaries, that they are but one among many, and their needs have to be set alongside everyone else's (Weare, 1998).

## PROGRAM, POLICY, PARTNERSHIPS, PEOPLE

In this section we outline an organizational guide for health promotion in school communities with democracy in mind. Underlying this proposed guide are key concepts related to democracy and health promotion presented earlier:

■ the process should involve those directly involved or concerned about the health issue, especially students,

■ the process by which decisions are made and actions are carried out should be egalitarian,

■ throughout the process, participants should be encouraged to examine the change process itself, the factors that interact to stimulate change, stages of change, and obstacles to change,

■ the process should clearly reflect the notion that health is more than a course of study—it is a way of thinking about and interacting with others to produce sustainable improvements that reflect local needs and citizenry.

Four elements comprise the guide: program, policy, partnerships, and people. To demonstrate the confluence of curricular, pedagogical, and political dialogue that teachers and students might address in the study of health promotion as an in-depth exploration of the way various bodies of knowledge inform decision making, we propose students address a real-world contemporary issue. Around this question, educators and students are invited to bring to bear creative, divergent, and innovative thinking: What are the implications of converting our dietary habits in North America to include fresh fruit and vegetable consumption as per recommendations by National Food Guides (*Canada's Food Guide* recommends that about 5–10 servings of our daily food consumption should be made up of fresh fruits and vegetables; current consumption patterns indicate Canadians consume about one-half the recommended amounts—www.dieticians.ca).

### Program

A program of study must be in place, suitably, resourced, and timetabled to ensure students have regular and sufficient class time to participate in a planned sequence of study including topics that are suitable and relevant to the age group involved and are presented by a qualified and effective educator. Effective teachers ensure all students have a chance to explore the topic from a wide range of views, to enter into debates, discussions, and dialogue about the material, to explore alternative realities related to the topic and to consider the reasoning behind opposing perspectives. In-class study is an opportunity to present how knowledge is created, reasoned, fathomed in a democratic society—the effects of culture, climate, and economics. Under these conditions students begin to realize that knowledge resides in the individual studying it. Truth is not absolute, existing in some independent form, rather its existence is embodied in the lives, minds, behaviors of those who experience it—cognitively, affectively, metacognitively. In-class study is an opportunity to participate in a community of scholarship activities: posing questions, looking deeply and broadly at the underlying factors, looking at propositions from the perspective of other disciplines, questioning authority and status quo, probing for meaning, asking critically important questions such as who's interests are being served? Who's voice is not present in this discussion?

A health promotion inspired curriculum would be alert to opportunities to put content knowledge and skills to good use, that is, relate knowing to doing the "right" thing. For example, a class might use their addition skills to calculate the weight of their daily garbage and then graph the results over a period of several days. The success of a classroom campaign to reuse, recycle, reduce their waste will become evident in the numbers and charts that portray the results of their concerted actions to be environmentally responsible.

Senior classes might begin a unit of study by brainstorming the possible outcomes of a nation converting to a diet rich in fresh fruit and vegetables. Determine why fruits and vegetables are such an important part of a healthy diet—what's in them that's good for us! Encourage students to use their communication skills to gather information about this proposal from the perspective of beef, pork, and chicken farmers, restaurant owners, fast food chains, and advertisers. Challenge students to work in small groups to consider the economic prospects and pitfalls associated with a major change such as this. Another group might consider the environmental benefits of reducing the production of beef. Students might interview agricultural experts and visit a Web site such as www.ecohealth.org to obtain information about the importance of conservation-minded land use. Students interested in examining this issue from a business perspective might interview the manager of a fast food chain restaurant to find out how menu changes would impact profits, the businesses image and marketing strategies. Medical researchers would also have important insights to add to this discussion in terms of health benefits such as reductions in some forms of cancer, weight management, and heart disease, as well as the health care savings that would accrue from diets that emphasize fresh fruits and vegetables.

The opportunity to debate the issue gives students a chance to put forward ideas in a reasoned, logical, persuasive manner. The sides of the debate can also be presented in the form of marketing campaigns and journalistic reports published in school newsletters. Letters to legislators give students a chance to construct their arguments and present them as conscientious members of society.

## Policy

Policy underpins the overall school environment, the school culture or ethos that permeates the life and times at school. Policy statements (formal and informal) are often a way to look for the degree to which schools nurture the democratic values, for example, rights to access, expression of ideas discussed in their classrooms. Students need to understand that policies are statements of beliefs and values. A class, a family, or an individual can create policies and then try to live by them. An increasing number of people have a no-smoking policy in their home, their vehicles, and their workplace. Considering our question re food consumption habits, examine school and district policies related to food consumption in schools, vending machines and cafeteria menus. Define policy. Who forms policy? Under what conditions does policy become a reality? Consider the implications of a policy that would affect what can be sold in the cafeteria and vending machines, consumed by students and teachers during lunch breaks or sold for fundraising. Try to write a policy that could be defended and presented to the school administration that would encourage fresh fruit and vegetable consumption. Track student, teacher, parent, school nurse, health educator, and administrative responses to policy proposals to see how power straggles emerge.

## Partnership

Access to community resources is a critical and integral part of school organization and student health. Health promoting schools seek to coordinate and optimize access to community services: immunization, vision/hearing tests, family and youth counseling, protective services, health services, career services, mentoring programs. Consider the resources available through public health, food and agriculture, and environmental groups to help students sort through the various issues related to this dietary proposition.

## People

At the centre of efforts to promote health is the development of a certain kind of person rather than a person who knows certain things. In schools where democracy is evident, resources and relationships are mobilized in such a way that the development of young people—socially, morally, spiritually, physically, intellectually—is paramount. This commitment is aimed at an overall institutional capacity to prepare young people for participation in a just and civil society.

Students are perhaps the most underutilized resource in school reform, yet have the most to gain or lose in the process. Health promotion that listens to the voice of students is the first step. The voice and involvement of students is essential to school improvement: to increase their motivation and educational productivity; for the valuable feedback they can give about their learning; because it is their learning; because they can be powerful partners in school improvement as co-researchers; because their involvement in responsible debate about their education should reflect the level of responsibility that many have in their lives outside school; and because school must work with and reflect the students'world (Pickering, 1997).

Students must consider their participation in the exploration of this dietary change question as part of a process aimed at preparing them to work through an issue with information that is biased, hence the need to develop knowledge, skills, and attitudes such as

- *critical thinking skills*: the ability to assess viewpoints and information in an open-minded and critical way and to be able to change one's opinions, challenge one's own assumptions and make better judgments as a result

- *an understanding of sustainable development*: recognition that the earth's resources are finite, precious, and unequally used

- *co-operation skills*: the ability to share and work with others effectively, to analyze conflicts objectively and to find solutions acceptable to all sides

- *ability to argue effectively*: to find out information and to present an informed persuasive argument based on reason

- *belief that people can make a difference*: individuals can act to improve situations and a desire to participate and take action

- *respect for diversity*: everyone is different but equal and we can learn from each other

## CHALLENGES

Health promotion should be studied as a way to link theory and practice, knowing and doing what's right. The Greeks tell us the early meaning of the word *democracy* was "strength of the people." Health promotion initiatives should help students find their talents, put their imaginations and insights to good use, and enable them to be part of ongoing efforts to make the world a better place for everyone. Health promotion could be thought of as a way to work together to understand ourselves, our ambitions, and to turn our aspirations into realities.

In one community, the school is near a minimum security prison where families come for periods of time and then return to their communities. Turnover is the highest of any school in the province. The school, however, ensures each child who attends this school will take with them a scrapbook containing pieces of their work, a story about the school, pictures of the child involved in activities at the school, and a personal note from the teacher about the time they spent together. In another school children make friendship bracelets they take to the senior citizens in a nearby home for the elderly. And in yet another community, students give their labor to people and organizations in the community in return for monetary donations which are then used to buy supplies and services to send to people in the Caribbean who are victims of recent hurricanes.

These activities are the heart of democracy.

## CONCLUSION

Democracy as the first principle of a health promoting school can be viewed as a moral compass used to navigate the struggles of school management and curricular reform. Thinking about health promotion in schools as part of a democratic process challenges educators to consider the importance of

- student involvement in the way schools operate and improve,

- classroom study that addresses real-life issues,

- creating school environments that are open to discussion and debate about human events to help prepare young people for involvement in community and civic affairs, and

- the school as a setting for experiencing the attributes of a democratic society.

Learning about democracy through health promotion initiatives is proposed in this paper as an important way for students to put their knowledge, skills, beliefs and convictions to good use, to feel like they are a part of their school's ethos and progress, and to enjoy the freedom to be deterministic and expressive about the meanings they are making relative to course content, world events, and personal experience. Education with democracy in mind should ultimately heighten students' awareness of the relationships between knowing and being, the links between behavior and beliefs, the importance of character development (care for others, honesty, trust, responsibility, sacrifice) honed through scholastic endeavors, and the value of participation in communities of learning and service in schools, neighborhoods and beyond.

## REFERENCES

Allensworth, D. D., & Kolbe, L. J. (1987). The comprehensive school health program: Exploring an expanded concept. *Journal of School Health, 57,* 409–412.

Anderson, A. (2003). Using comprehensive approaches to school health to make schools stronger, smarter, safer. *Physical and Health Education Journal, 68*(4), 14–20.

*Canada's food guide.* (2007.) Ottawa, Ontario: Office of Nutrition Policy and Promotion, Health Canada. Retrieved from http://www.hc-sc.gc.ca/fn-an/food-guide-aliment/index-eng.php

de Tocqueville, A. (1835). *Democracy in America.* Retrieved from http://booksjniHOT.org/gb.tocqueville.html

Fenstermacher G. (1999). Agenda for education in a democracy. In *Leadership for educational renewal: Developing a cadre of leaders.* San Francisco, CA: Jossey-Bass.

Freire, P., & Macedo, D. (1987). *Literacy: Reading the word and the world.* South Hadley, MA: Bergin & Garvey.

Giroux, H. (2000). *Stealing innocence: Youth, corporate power, and the politics of culture.* New York: St. Martin's.

Giroux, H. (2003). *The abandoned generation: Democracy beyond the culture of fear.* New York: Palgrave Macmillan.

Glickman, C. D. (1999). *Revolutionizing America's schools.* San Francisco, CA: Jossey-Bass.

Habermas, J. (1990). *Moral consciousness and communicative action.* (Trans. C. Lenhardt & S. W. Nicholson). Cambridge, MA: MIT Press.

*The health promoting school—An investment in education, health, and democracy.* (1997). Conference report, Thessaloniki-Halkidiki, Greece, May 1–5.

Kellner, D. (1990). *Television and the crisis of democracy.* Boulder, CO : Westview Press.

King, A. J. C., Boyce, W., & King, M. A. (1999). *Trends in the health of Canada's youth.* Ottawa: Health Canada. Lerner, R. M., & Benson, P. L. (2003). *Developmental assets and asset-building communities: Implications for research, policy, and practice.* New York: Kluwer Academic/Plenum.

Nutbeam, D. (2000). Health literacy as a public health goal: A challenge for contemporary health education and communication strategies into the 21st century. *Health Promotion International, 15,* 259–267.

Palmer, P. (1998). *The courage to teach.* San Francisco: Jossey Bass.

Pickering, J. (1997). Involving pupils. *School Improvement Network Research Matters* (No. 6). London: Institute of Education.

Putnam, R. D. (1993). *Making democracy work: Civic traditions in modern Italy.* Princeton, NJ: Princeton University Press.

Putnam, R. D. (1995). Bowling alone: America's declining social capital. *Journal of Democracy* 6(1), 65–67.

Raphael, D. (2004). *Social determinants of health: Canadian perspective.* Toronto: Canadian Scholars Press.

Steinhauer, P. J. D. (1996). Toward improved developmental outcomes for Ontario children and youth. *Ontario Medical Review, 44.*

*Toward a healthy future: Second report on the health of Canadians.* (1999). Federal, Provincial and Territorial Advisory Committee on Population Health.

Weare, K. (1998). The health promoting school: An overview of concepts, principles and strategies and the evidence for their effectiveness. In European Network of Health Promoting Schools, *First workshop on practice of evaluation of the Health Promoting School* (pp. 9–18). Retrieved from http://www.schoolsforhealth.eu/upload/pubs/FirstWorkshoponpracticeofevaluationoftheHPS.pdf

World Health Organization. (1986). *Ottawa charter for health promotion.* Retrieved fromhttp://www.who.int/hpr/NPH/docs/ottawa_charter_hp.pdf

World Health Organization. (1996). *Promoting health through schools—The World Health Organization's Global School Health Initiative.* Geneva: World Health Organization.

# CHAPTER

21

# HUMAN ECOLOGY
# AND HEALTH EDUCATION

### HOWARD S. HOYMAN

The twentieth century has confronted us with some crucial questions: Does man have a future? Will there be a year 2000 for us and our children? Can man survive and prevail in the "asphalt jungle" of our cities? Can man escape from the crippling and lethal dangers of our technotronic world? Or are we clever "naked apes" destined to go the way of the dinosaurs in an ecological booby trap of our own making? Will there be no human voices echoing down the corridors of time (Shepard & McKinley, 1969; Love & Love, 1970; Odum et al., 1970)?

Each generation of man and each person has a rendezvous with destiny. The new ecological Jeremiahs, aided by Sartre and Camus, have confronted us with the supreme "challenge and response" situation of our time: the realization that human life is absurd and in danger of being snuffed out like a candle cannot be an end for man but only a beginning (Ehrlich & Ehrlich, 1970; Environment section staff, 1970).

## MAN'S ECOLOGICAL COEXISTENCE

Modern ecology is a comparatively new scientific field—with taproots in the past—whose time has come in the twentieth century. Human ecology has emerged out of our modern existential human predicament and the ecological crisis now facing us. It

*Note:* This article is intended to be read for its pholosophical perspective. Originally published in 1971, it may contain factual material or examples that are dated.

encompasses mankind evolving and adapting—for better or for worse—as the dominant species on earth (Dobzhansky, 1962; Dubos, 1965). Modern man's health and life depend upon how well he can adapt to and manipulate his environment to meet selection pressures and goals, and there is a premium on how fast he can do it. Environmental changes—many of them manmade—are occurring so rapidly that man can now be born in one age and live and die in another. Man has demonstrated amazing adaptive potentialities and the ability to change his environment to suit his own ends. But his greatest strength may turn out to be his Achilles heel, for there are limits to man's adaptive potentialities and limits to the life-support systems of our finite Spaceship Earth.

Fortunately, scientific discoveries such as the theory of evolution, plus our ecological crisis, have finally led us to rediscover our environment and to reconsider our place in nature and the dynamic web of life (biosphere). We are now learning the hard way that man cannot live by and for himself alone, because man's destiny is linked with nature. If we continue to devastate the earth, ruthlessly plunder natural resources, kill off other forms of life, and decimate our fellow man, we have signed our own death warrant.

Coined about one hundred years ago and unknown ten years ago except to a few scientists, *ecology* is now a household word and headline news in the mass media (Farb et al., 1963). What is it? Ecology is the study of the interrelationships of living things with each other and with their environment. General ecology includes plant, animal, and human ecology. Ecologists study the interactions between individual organisms and populations and their environment (autecology), and between populations and species and their environment (synecology).

Living things do not live alone (Bates, 1960). The plants, animals, and microorganisms, and humans that live in a *biotic community* are all interconnected by an intricate dynamic web of relationships. Living things—including man—live in what biologists and ecologists call *ecosystems*. The ecosystem concept emphasizes the functional relationship among organisms and between organisms and their physical environment. Ecosystems include both a place and a way of life, and the more complex, the more stable they are. Food webs are an example of those complex functional relationships, by means of which energy flows and chemical elements essential to life and health move through an ecosystem. The concept of ecosystem-interrelated organisms, populations, biotic community, and environment is a complex and dynamic set of flows, factors, forces, exchanges, and feedback regulations. Human ecosystems are exceedingly complex and dynamic because they include the sociocultural as well as the physical and biotic dimensions of environment. Man has both a nature and a history, and he lives—coexists—both in the biosphere and noosphere (Teilhard de Chardin, 1959). Biologists and geologists study biotic communities and ecosystems because all living things—including man—are inseparable from each other and their environment.

An understanding of ecosystems and the ecology of public health is very important for health educators. On the negative side, the concept of ecosystem is related to our concepts of disease, disability, aging and death; and on the positive side, to our concepts of the epigenetic human life cycle—with its critical stages, healthy growth and development, and our quest for self-identity and self-fulfillment (Erikson, 1963, chapter 7).

An understanding of the flow of energy and the cycling of essential materials in ecosystems is a prerequisite to our growing awareness of the potential destruction—by man's own shortsighted activities—of the ecosystems and food webs upon which the survival and health of mankind finally depend. A dramatic example is the concentration of toxic substances such as DDT and methyl-mercury in food webs involving man. We are finally coming to see that the population explosion, plundering of natural resources—some of them nonrenewable—and environmental pollution have placed our ecosystems and man himself in jeopardy (Cloud et al., 1969). It is a sign of the times when housewives and school children discuss eutrophication.

## ECOLOGICAL MODELS

Human ecology is based on a *unitive* view of man, as a self-regulating, self-actualizing organism. It is concerned with the whole man, as an open-system, in his reciprocal dynamic transactions with his total environment—physical, biotic, and sociocultural. Human ecology is concerned with the unique individual as well as with populations and "statistical man," with his personality as well as his tissues and organs, and with his spiritual outlook on life and need for personal fulfillment, as well as with his biologic needs for survival.

Public health is one of the major sectors of human ecology (Colloquium on Man's Health and His Environment, 1970). Human ecology is not a new approach to the study of health, disease, aging and death. However, the increased interest in and growing emphasis on human ecology and epidemiology in relation, to public health and medical theory and practice is timely and exceedingly important. The emerging epidemiologic, multiple-causation approach, within the broad framework of human ecology; is certainly a step in the right direction. The results so far indicate that the "causal webs" of human health, disease, aging, longevity, and death are all interlinked dynamic processes in the organism-personality, and are far more complex than appears on the surface (Hoyman, 1962). A man's level of health and disease, his rate of aging, and his length of life are all dynamic ecological resultants—as well as major operative factors. Figure 21.1 is a crude model of the ecology of health and disease (Hoyman, 1965).

### Ecology of Health

Fortunately, we do not have to start from scratch in developing an ecological health model. Health educators have long stressed the need to view health as a dynamic process, involving the whole person and his *unique* life style, in his total environment. We have described and defined health in terms of the actualization and fulfillment of man's *desirable* adaptive and creative potentialities. For instance: *Health is personal fitness for survival and self-renewal, creative psychosocial adjustment, and self-fulfillment.*

Health is a multidimensional unity. It has dimensions such as physical fitness, mental health, psychosocial well-being, and ethical and spiritual outlook (Hoyman, 1956). Health is determined by the reciprocal, ecological interaction of genetic, environmental,

## FIGURE 21.1 An Ecologic Model of Health and Disease. Example of favorable and unfavorable dynamic, interacting hereditary, environmental, and personal ecologic factors and conditions that are determinants of the levels of health and disease on a continuum

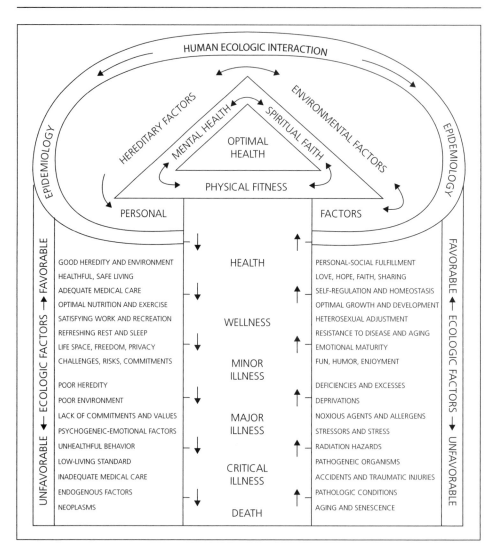

*Source*: H. S. Hoyman. (1971). Human ecology and health education II. *Journal of School Health, 41*(10), p. 540. (Adapted in part from *Our Modern Concept of Health*, by H. S. Hoyman. Courtesy of the American School Health Association.)

and individual factors, some of primary and others of secondary or lesser importance. The *ecological causal web of health* is all finally centered, at the human level, in the life cycle and developing self in its quest for identity and fulfillment. Viewed from this vantage point, health is much more than the absence of disease, disability, pain, and decay; it encompasses physical fitness, social well-being, personality development, and a zest for full, fruitful, creative living.

Health then is more than wellness. Our postulate is that a well person can become healthier. Man's health potential ranges from zero health (death) to optimum health, on a health-disease continuum. An *ecological elevator effect* is depicted in Figure 21.1, based upon the postulate that *favorable* ecological factors tend to push one up into the zones of wellness and health, and *unfavorable* ecological factors tend to push one down, into the zones of disease and death.

Healthful living involves a paradox. Aim directly at health and one is sure to miss the target. We must risk health to gain it. Health is expendable in genuine living; it cannot be hoarded and "saved for a rainy day." The miracle of human, health is a many-splendored thing. It is rooted in man's flesh, grows and develops in his heart and mind, and flowers in his ethical and spiritual life.

Health is a moving, evolving target. Our model of health changes with the times. The science-fiction dream of perfect health is a mirage, for as Rene Dubos (1959) has pointed out, new times bring new health hazards and problems and new diseases.

## Ecology of Disease

In health education, we have focused more on specific diseases than on models and theories of disease—and this approach has serious limitations.

The complexity of human disease is indicated by the somewhat conflicting and bewildering array of theories of disease that have been advanced. Some major examples are the demoniac theory, divine theory, humoral theory, animal magnetism theory, miasma theory, Christian Science theory, naturopathic theory, subluxation theory, germ theory, psychosomatic theory, stress theory, psychoanalytic theory, and the ecologic-epidemiologic theory of disease. As yet we are far from having any fully and widely accepted *unified* theory of disease, but we seem to be aiming at that as an eventual goal. What the future holds remains to be seen. But the ecologic-epidemiologic approach to disease etiology and cures and to prevention, and control, does seem to provide a sufficiently broad theoretical framework within which to work.

What is disease? No definitive answer can be given. As we now view it, disease is a dynamic process involving any disease, disorder, dysfunction, or any pathological condition of the body, mind, or personality. Strictly speaking, the whole person is always ill or diseased. The range of disease is from critical illness to the milder disorders that occur even in persons with optimum health. Disease is caused by multiple interacting variables and co-factor agents, not usually by single factors acting alone—although Liebig's "law of the minimum" must be taken into account (1). Predisposing, precipitating (triggering), and perpetuating factors—genetic, environmental and individual—are all involved. Instead of single factor, linear cause-and-effect etiology, the newer the concept of an *ecological casual web of disease* seems closer to the truth—as crudely illustrated in Figure 21.1.

Epidemiologists (medical detectives) tackle the problem of the causation, and prevention and control, of communicable and noncommunicable diseases in population groups, within a broad ecological framework, relative to the agent-host-environment complex. Tuberculosis is a classic example of the way ecological variables may be involved in the causation, and prevention and control, of a communicable disease, with the TB germ as the *necessary*, but not the *sufficient*, cause in the infection equation (Engel, 1962). And coronary heart disease (CHD) is a dramatic example of the way ecological variables may be involved in noncommunicable disease causation and prevention and control. Although the etiology of CHD is not known, apparently genetic, environmental, and individual factors are involved, as related to risk factors such as obesity, diet, blood cholesterol and triglyceride levels, cigarette smoking, lack of physical exercise, high blood pressure, emotional stress, personality type, and age and sex. The compound probability for the coronary prone person is much higher if two or more of these risk factors are present.

Human, disease is a universal phenomenon. At this juncture, the goal of eradication of all human disease is a utopian dream. The very processes and goals of living involve disease, and new times bring new killers and disablers. A comparison of the major killers in 1900 vs. 1970 in the affluent developed countries (DCs) underscores this key fact. For example, in the United States today [1971] about two out of three people who die are killed by heart disease, cancer, or stroke—far different major killers than in 1900.

## Ecology of Longevity

Will science eventually conquer aging and death? Will man's life expectancy at birth be 100 years by the year 2000? Will scientists soon discover some X factor that will increase man's potential life span to anywhere from 150 to 1,000 years?

Man has not yet discovered the Fountain of Youth, although he is still searching (McGrady, 1968). We know very little about the enigma of human aging and death from so-called natural causes. We have a plethora of aging theories (e.g., biological clock theory, wear and tear theory, cumulative poisoning theory, evolutionary theory). But we have few hard facts to back them up. Man's potential life span—the maximum number of years man can live even under the most favorable circumstances—apparently has not changed for at least the past 10,000 years. Human aging and death take no holidays; they are universal phenomena. Death lurks ahead in the shadows for each one of us. Self-awareness brought death awareness, as Dobzhansky (1967) has pointed out. And death awareness profoundly affects our views about life and health, as Tolstoy brings home to us so dramatically in his fascinating story "The Death of Ivan Ilyich."

What is modern man's longevity potential? The *maximum* human life span falls in the 110–115 year range, as judged by the authenticated records of the longest-lived people. However, the average potential life span is lower, of course, than the maximum, and the potential life span of individuals varies so that some persons are potentially longer or shorter lived than others. There is much science fiction, but little "hard" evidence to support the claims that man will soon live from 150 to 1,000 years.

Our great world need today is to increase man's *health span*, not his life span. Who wants to survive as a human vegetable? An ounce of prevention is still worth a pound of cure, and it costs far less. The real tragedy is to die without having really lived, be it at 50 or 150.

Man's average life expectancy at birth has increased markedly in the DCs during the past one hundred years, and it is now about 70 years—due mainly to the gains in infancy and childhood. But barring a major scientific breakthrough in death control, we may expect much smaller gains in life expectancy in the DCs by, say, the year 2000.

In our current concern over personal and environmental factors, we must not overlook the great importance of heredity. The whole set of genes a person inherits from his parents is called the "genotype." Health, disease, aging, and longevity are phenotypical phenomena, determined by the ecological interactions of the genotype with the total environment. Nature and nurture work together in joint sovereignty. From the standpoint of health, disease, senescence, and longevity, some individuals have good and others poor hereditary endowment. Some gene mutations are lethal, causing serious diseases or fetal deaths; others are sublethal, killing off or weakening most of the carriers; and still others are subvital, impairing health in various ways (Scheinfeld, 1965).

## HEALTH EDUCATION IMPLICATIONS AND OPPORTUNITIES

In health education "health" is the goal and "education" is the process. Oberteuffer (1964) has spelled out incisively the vital, reciprocal ties between health and education. Equally important, he has called for bold, imaginative planning and action in developing modern health education in our schools and communities. So what are some of the implications and opportunities of an ecological approach to health and health education?

### 1. Integrated Community-School Programs

Students live in communities. We need to develop more integrated community-school health education programs in the 1970s (Hoyman, 1966). Boys and girls need a more consistent, pattern in the health education they learn at home, at school, and in the community—especially now that we are faced with a wider generation gap. The ecological complexity of personal, family, and community health problems necessitates a community wide approach to study, planning, and action—involving all school age and adult groups. Many public-health problems—such as environmental pollution—

are of such magnitude and so complex that action on a wide front is indispensable for their resolution. And in the long run success or failure will depend upon a participating and committed health-educated public. For example, the Russians claim good results for their integrated "one package" public health plan—including school and adult health education—with the development of community health centers and public health lecture series in the USSR (Hoyman, 1963).

## 2. Improved Health Science Curricula

A national health and safety curriculum for Grades K–12 will not meet the needs of all students, schools, and communities, in a pluralistic, pragmatic democratic society such as Canada or the United States, based upon an experimental lifestyle. However, perhaps certain principles should be followed in all the health science curricula. For example, the health science curricula should be (1) organized for grades K–12 inclusive to provide for vertical and horizontal articulation related to personal-social health interests, needs, and problems; (2) planned as a *flexible* scope and sequence framework, with basic concepts as organizing central themes, as well as major health instruction areas; (3) developed so as to help insure a *spiral* learning progression from elementary to advanced levels, aimed at improving knowledge and skills, changing attitudes and beliefs, developing sound health practices, and organized to avoid boring, unplanned repetition of topics; (4) organized to utilize modern health education methods and materials; and (5) planned to include evaluation as an integral part of the curriculum as related to student participation and achievement, as well as to appraisal of the health-science curriculum itself.

A schematic health science curriculum organized to provide a *spiral* learning progression, with both depth and breadth, in the following fourteen major areas of health instruction, has been outlined elsewhere: (1) human ecology and health, disease, longevity; (2) human ecology and growth, development, maturation, aging;(3) healthful living and physical fitness;(4) nutrition and personal fitness; (5) alcohol, tobacco, and drugs; (6) prevention and control of disease; (7) community and environmental health; (8) consumer health education; (9) rise of modern scientific medicine; (10) safety education; (11) first aid and home nursing; (12) personality development and mental health; (13) family life and sex education; (14) health careers (Hoyman, 1965, pp. 115–121).

We need to sink deeper taproots in health education by grounding it in the ecology of health, disease, aging, and longevity and in the whole epigenetic human life cycle with its various stages from conception to death. All major health instruction areas and health units should be taught from an ecological viewpoint. Three major areas of scope are listed below to illustrate this assumption:

1. *Human ecology and health, disease, longevity.* Man as a whole open-organism-environment-system, capable of adaptive behavior for survival and personal fulfillment; an ecologic view of health, disease, aging, longevity, and death; the personal health triangle: physical fitness, mental health, and spiritual faith; hereditary, environmental (including sociocultural factors) and personal factors

affecting levels of health and disease; the health and disease spectrum; epidemiology of health and disease; the agent-host-environment complex and multiple versus single factor etiology; life span and life expectancy differences and interrelationships; modern man's health and longevity potential; human ecology and health in the space age.

2. *Human ecology and growth, development, maturation, aging.* Structure and function of the human. body, including the male and female reproductive systems; human heredity and human reproduction; highlights of the physical, psychological, and sociocultural characteristics of life cycle stages from birth and infancy to old age and death; physical growth and development; growth charts—values and limitations; male and female body types; individual differences in puberty and in adolescent growth changes, including secondary sexual characteristics and psychosexual development; major theories of aging and longevity; age and sex differences in morbidity, mortality, and longevity; relationship of growth, development, aging, and homeostasis to health, disease, and longevity.

3. *Community and environmental health.* Public health goals, services, principles, and organization; legal aspects of public health as an official governmental agency; full-time official public health departments—local, regional and state; economic aspects of public health; national and international public health organizations; cooperative relationships such as those with school health programs and occupational hygiene programs: selected elements of vital statistics and demography and the population explosion; major current public health problems and points of attack; voluntary, commercial and professional health agencies; public health personnel and career opportunities in public health and the health sciences; environmental health and safety: (1) water purification (2) sanitary sewage disposal, (3) garbage and refuse disposal, (4) insect and rodent control, (5) food sanitation, (6) housing, lighting, heating and ventilation, (7) air pollution, (8) radiation health hazards, (9) pesticides and herbicides, (10) sociocultural factors such as urbanization, industrialization, secularization, and health and safety, (11) protection from accident hazards; rise of the modern public health movement; public health as a one-world ecological problem in the space age; the ecological crisis and environmental pollution and quality control

In developing health curricula, we should avoid a crisis-oriented, piecemeal approach. Critical health problems—such as drug abuse, cigarette smoking, and sex education—should be included as an integral part of comprehensive health education for grades K–12. Some examples of health curricula of this type are Oregon's Four-Cycle Health Curriculum, started in 1945, which was the first spiral-cycle health curriculum developed for grades 1–12 in the United States (Hoyman, 1945); the School Health Education Study's *Health Education: A Conceptual Approach to Curriculum Design* (1967), which is by far the best example of a concept approach in the United States; Hoyman's Health Science Spiral Curriculum, for grades 1–12, which was the first curriculum in the United States based upon ecological models of health, disease, and longevity and upon an ecological approach to health education (Hoyman, 1965); and the recently completed New York State Health Curriculum for grades K–12, based upon the New York Health Education Law, which has been designed, in part, from an ecologic-epidemiologic viewpoint in all five major strands of the curriculum: physical health, sociological health problems, mental health, environmental and community health, and education for survival (New York State Curriculum Materials, 1970 & 1971). These curricula are all steps in the right direction because they enable us to keep the student, the subject, and society all in focus. But it would be fatal for us to treat them as sacred cows, because if we do, they are apt to become frozen instead of fresh. They all need critical evaluation and continuing revision if we are to move ahead in health curriculum development.

The concept approach to curriculum design is *one* sound way to structure health education as a functional field of knowledge, in relation to health and modern life. Man makes his concepts, and then his concepts make man. Some examples of unifying ecological health education concepts are the following:

1.  Health is a dynamic ecologic process, involving the whole person in his total environment—physical, biotic, and sociocultural—as he lives and moves through the stages of his lifecycle from conception to death, guided by his personality and lifestyle and expressed in his motives, goals, ideals, and values.

2.  Health is a multidimensional unity, with dimensions such as physical fitness, social well-being, mental health, and ethical and spiritual outlook—all entwined in man's struggle for survival and fulfillment.

3.  Human health, disease, aging, and longevity are all interlinked dynamic emergents from the ecological causal web of genetic, environmental, and individual factors—and are not usually caused by single X or XYZ factors operative alone. Some of the ongoing changes are reversible, others irreversible.

4.  Human life involves an ecological elevator effect: *favorable* ecological factors tend to push man up into the zones of wellness and health; *unfavorable* ecological factors tend to push him down into the zones of disease, disability, and death.

5.  Human disease and death control, without effective birth and population control, has led to the world population explosion with its potential threat to man's survival as a species and to his life at a more fully human level.

6.  Man is the dominant, but endangered, species on Spaceship Earth; and his personal-social fulfillment, if not his survival, are threatened by the interrelated ecological effects of the population explosion, environmental pollution, and the plundering of natural resources—some of them nonrenewable.

7. Public health and the ecological crisis are interlinked one-world problems that confront us with an urgent need for a health-educated public, as well as for improved comprehensive public health and medical care planning, services, and research.

## 3. Functional Health Teaching and Learning

Inert health facts and isolated, memorized health concepts keep no better than fish—they both start to smell within one day. We need to link up health concepts and facts with current problems, issues, options, and choices. Students are not interested in "cadaver hygiene." Nor are they motivated by things supposed to be "good for their health." They view health as a means to an exciting, adventurous life, not as an end in itself. They want to tackle real health problems and issues head-on. They are activists and they want to live concepts and principles, not just talk about them. They like to participate in independent study, problem solving, classroom dialogue, and open-forum discussions, based upon realistic learning experiences.

Take the population problem as an example. The big issue is one of controlled versus uncontrolled population growth and density distribution. Some options—expressed as annual percent increase and population doubling time—that could be critically discussed follow: zero population growth; 0.5 percent, doubling time 140 years; 1.0 percent, doubling time 70 years; 2.0 percent, doubling time 35 years; 3.0 percent, doubling time 24 years; uncontrolled population growth—except for natural controls. How do these options relate to personal, family, and community health?

Another example is the problem of physical fitness in a sedentary society. The basic issue is a sedentary versus a physically active life. Examples of options are no regular exercise or physical work; light exercise and physical work; moderate exercise and physical work; and heavy exercise and physical work (Hanson, 1970). How do these options relate to health, disease, and longevity throughout the human life cycle?

A third example is the problem of cigarette smoking. The basic issue is to smoke or not to smoke—and if so, how much? Examples of options are nonsmoker, light smoker, moderate smoker, heavy smoker, and ex-smoker. How do these options relate to health, disease, and length of life?

A final example is the problem of sexual behavior. One basic issue is premarital coitus versus premarital abstinence. Examples of options are the four major sexual standards in America: premarital sexual abstinence for both sexes; the double standard, with greater sexual freedom for the male; premarital sexual permissiveness with love and affection, for both sexes; and premarital sexual permissiveness without love and affection, for both sexes (Reiss, 1960; Hoyman, 1969; Hoyman, 1971). How do these options relate to human sexuality and conduct?

Some additional examples of gut issues in human ecology and health education follow:

1.  Ecology of drug use vs. drug abuse

2.  Prevention and control vs. eradication of disease

3.  Wellness vs. optimum health

4.  Zero population growth vs. a 0.5 percent annual increase

5.  Ecology of food production and distribution vs. obesity and famine

6.  Multiple vs. single factor theories of diseases causation

7.  People impact vs. Spaceship Earth

8.  Population growth vs. population density distribution

9.  Human survival vs. human fulfillment

10. Death control vs. birth control vs. population control

11. Population control vs. genocide and ethnocide

12. Length of life vs. quality of living

13. Renewable vs. nonrenewable natural resource

14. Environmental quality vs. cost control and the GNP

15. Environmental pollution vs. a democratic solution

16. Euthanasia vs. "human vegetables"

17. Man mastering nature vs. man mastering himself

18. Family planning vs. population control

19. Abortion vs. contraception—babies by choice instead of by chance

20. Ecological optimism vs. the new Jeremiahs and Paul Reveres

21. Science vs. values

## 4. More Realistic Teacher Preparation

The preparation of prospective health teachers is top-heavy with theory. The last thing a graduating health teacher encounters is a student. To a mission-oriented teacher the confrontation often comes with a brutal shock. Health teachers need much more practical work in their preparation, such as nurses get in good nursing schools and training hospitals. Apprenticeship experiences should be started in the freshman and sophomore years. Juniors should be required to take a field work course in community health education. School observations plus realistic microteaching should lead up to student teaching—preferably off campus. I feel that a full year of student teaching is highly desirable with some experience in urban schools and ghetto areas.

Prospective health teachers are often long on methods and short on content. Focusing on methods to the neglect of content is another case of "throwing out the baby with the bath water." They need a better understanding of the ecology of health, disease, aging and longevity; and the health and safety hazards of the various critical stages in the epigenetic human life cycle. They need a better understanding of contemporary health problems, issues, and options. They need more course work in human ecology and the behavioral sciences and in health education courses organized and taught from an ecological viewpoint.

## 5. Improved Research Needed

We need more sophisticated research related to the theory and practice of health and safety education (Veenker, 1963). A first step is to develop research laboratories in colleges and universities offering doctoral programs in health education. For example, during the past decade, we have developed a Health Education Laboratory and a Safety and Driver Education Laboratory in the Department of Health and Safety Education at the University of Illinois. These research laboratories are used by graduate students and faculty members (Creswell, 1970). There is also an acute need for more interdisciplinary team research in dealing with complex health education problems that cut across several fields, such as drug abuse, anti-smoking education, alcohol education, VD prevention and control, and accident prevention. Fortunately there is much more grant money available now to fund well-designed research studies in health and safety education than was the case ten years ago, when we started the research laboratories. Another "straw in the wind" is the establishment of the Research Council of the ASHA and the research reports and publications of the National Society of Public Health Educators.

## HUMAN SURVIVAL IS NOT ENOUGH

In sum, we need a vastly improved ecological working model of man in nature, in society, and in the world. One that takes into account man's body, mind, spirit and milieu. A model that faces up to man's hopes and fears and loves and hates, to his rational-irrational nature, and to his potentialities for both good and evil (Barrett, 1958; Sperry, 1964). One that is grounded in the dignity of man, as guided by worthy motives, goals, ideals, and values. A model of man evolving and adapting that goes beyond animal survival, as the dominant species on earth. One in which there is room for emergent novelty and creativeness, and in which, hopefully, man can aim at self-transcendence and self-fulfillment at a more fully human level. We must beware of reductionist and the "nothing but" fallacy—man is nothing but an animal or a robot. As we face up to the ecological crisis now confronting us, we need a model of a man that includes all of human nature, for as the noted psychoanalyst Erik H. Erikson has recently pointed out, "there is a core to each man which transcends his psychosocial identity." As part of our task we need to critically reexamine the dangerous half-truth that there are no bad people, only bad environments.

As we look ahead, let's thank God that we have some Paul Reveres sounding the ecological crisis alarm. We need to be jolted out of our arrogant complacency, before it is too late. In the human heart, hope triumphs over experience. And I keep hoping that we may now be on the verge of man's coming of age in an Ecological Renaissance. If so, our human survival and fulfillment will depend upon our learning to live in harmony with nature, with other people, and with ourselves. We must learn to cultivate and cherish the simple joys and delights of daily life. We must learn to seek aesthetic, sensual, ethical, and spiritual as well as materialistic—values and goals. For as Emerson put it, over one hundred years ago, things are in the saddle and ride mankind.

Public health is riding the ecological hobbyhorse into the future. We health educators must think, plan and act now in terms of an ecological approach—or get left behind. So far, health educators have been strangely silent about the vital ties between human ecology and health education—a luxury that we can no longer afford (Russell, 1969).

Public health is people, and it is a one-world problem. On a global scale, there are millions upon millions of little children and adults who are sick, hungry, some starving, some cold, uneducated, with little or no hope for a better life; many dying prematurely. And according to some modern prophets, we humans are now facing potential extinction as a species on earth.

We must use all of our world and public health resources—services, education, research—to help stem this tidal wave of human waste and suffering and loss of hope. In this great mission, health education must play a much greater public health role in the future than it has in the past. In health education, our greatest resource is our firm conviction that we can work cooperatively with others—children and adults, in school and out—to help shape and improve the future of mankind. Let this conviction wither away in our hearts and minds, and health education will soon "die on the vine."

In conclusion, I believe that our ecological problems *can* be solved. Whether they *will* be solved remains to be seen. The blue chips are down and the name of the game is human survival and fulfillment. Our modern spiritual drama has an awe-inspiring Old Testament grandeur, with its Heaven and Hell and prophetic sense of impending salvation or doom for man on earth—shot down by the Four Horsemen: famine, pestilence, war, and death.

We must stop our ruthless war with nature. We must change our strategy and tactics and aim at population control—without deterioration of the human gene pool; reduction of environmental pollution; and wiser use of natural resources. We do need economic growth an expanding GNP, and scientific and technologic development—*but not at any cost*. Hopefully, the science and art of human ecology, applied to global public health, may help us to cure our arrogant narcissism so we can live in harmony with nature and free ourselves from our spiritual nihilism and alienation in the modem world (Belgum, 1967). We must start now with man and the world as they are today and work in the spirit of Luther's dictum that "God carves the rotten wood and rides the lame horse."

## ENDNOTE

1.  Justus von Liebig established a scientific principle, over one hundred years ago, that became known as the "law of the minimum": essentially the growth of a population or the life of an individual organism will be limited by whatever essential factor(s) is in shortest supply. The Ehrlichs (1970, p. 51) discuss space, heat, available energy, nonrenewable resources, food and water, and air as examples of some of the potentially limiting factors for human individuals and populations.

## REFERENCES

Barrett, W. (1958). *Irrational man*. Garden City, NY: Doubleday.

Bates, M. (1960). *The Forest and the sea: A look at the economy of nature and the ecology of man*. New York: Random House.

Belgum, D. (Ed.). (1967). *Religion and medicine: Essays on meaning, values, and health*. Ames, IA: Iowa State University Press.

Cloud, P., et al. (1969). *Resources and man: A study and recommendations*. San Francisco: W. H. Freeman.

Colloquium on Man's Health and His Environment (presentations). (1970, January). *Archives of Environmental Health, 29*(1), 72–140.

Creswell, W. H. et al. (1970). *Youth smoking behavior characteristics and their education implications*. Champaign, IL: University of Illinois Press.

Dobzhansky, T. (1962). *Mankind evolving: The evolution of the human species*. New Haven, CT: Yale University Press.

Dobzhansky, T. (1967). *The biology of ultimate concern*. New York: New American Library.

Dubos, R. (1959). *Mirage of health*. New York: Harper.

Dubos, R. (1965). *Man adapting*. New Haven, CT: Yale University Press.

Ehrlich, P. R., & Ehrlich, A. H. (1970). *Population, resources, environment: Issues in human ecology*. San Francisco: W. H. Freeman.

Engel, G. L. (1962). *Psychological development in health and disease*. Philadelphia: Saunders, pp. 244–249.

Environment section staff. (1970, February). Fighting to save the earth from man. *Time, 95*(5), 56–63.

Erikson, E. The quest for identity. (1970, December 21). *Newsweek* (special report), *76*(25), 89. Quoted by permission of *Newsweek*.

Erikson, E. H. (1963). *Childhood and society*. New York: Norton.

Farb, P., and the editors of *Life*. (1963). *Ecology*. New York: Time (Life Nature Series).

Hanson, D. (1970). *Health related fitness*. Belmont, CA: Wadsworth.

Hoyman, H. S. (1945). *Health guide units for Oregon teachers (Grades 7–12)*. E. C. Brown Trust, University of Oregon Medical School for the Oregon State Department of Education.

Hoyman, H. S. (1956). The spiritual dimension of man's health in today's world. *Journal of School Health, 36*(2), 52–63.

Hoyman, H. S. (1962, September). Our modern concept of health. *Journal of School Health, 32*(7), 253–264.

Hoyman, H. S. (1963, February). Impressions of health education in the USSR. *Journal of School Health, 33*(2), 49–61.

Hoyman, H. S. (1965, March). An ecologic view of health and health education. *Journal of School Health, 35*(3),110–123.

Hoyman, H. S. (1966, June). Bottlenecks in health education. *American Journal of Public Health, 56*(6), 957–961.

Hoyman, H. S. (1969, September). Our most explosive sex education issue: Birth control. *Journal of School Health, 39*(7), 458–469.

Hoyman, H. S. (1971, April). Sweden's experiment in human sexuality and sex education. *Journal of School Health*.

Love, G. A., & Love, R. M. (Eds.). (1970). *Ecological crisis: Readings for survival*. New York: Harcourt Brace Jovanovich.

McGrady, P. M. (1968). *The youth doctors*. New York: Coward-McCann.

New York State curriculum materials in health and safety education for the elementary and secondary schools. (1970 & 1971).

Oberteuffer, D. (1964, March). Vital ties between health and education. *NEA Journal*.

Odum, E. P., DeMott, B., & the editors of *The Progressive*. (1970). *The crisis of survival*. Glenview, IL: Scott, Foresman.

Reiss, I. L. (1960). *Premarital sexual standards in America*. Glencoe, IL: Free Press.

Russell, R. D. (1969). Toward a functional understanding of ecology for health education. *Journal of School Health, 39*(7), 702–708.

Scheinfeld, A. (1965). *Your heredity and environment* (rev. ed.). Philadelphia: Lippincott.

School Health Education Study. (1967). *Health education: A conceptual approach to curriculum design* (Grades K–12). St. Paul, MN: 3M Education Press.

Shepard, P., & McKinley, D. (Eds.). (1969). *The subversive science: Essays: Toward an ecology of man*. Boston: Houghton Mifflin.

Sperry, R. W. (1964). Mind, brain, and humanist values. In J. R. Platt (Ed.), *New views of the nature of man* (Ch. 4). Chicago: University of Chicago Press.

Teilhard de Chardin, P. (1959). *The phenomenon of man*. New York: Harper.

Veenker, C. H. (Ed.). (1963). *Synthesis of research in selected areas of health instruction*. Washington, DC: School Health Education Study.

# SPIRITUAL WELLNESS, HOLISTIC HEALTH, AND THE PRACTICE OF HEALTH EDUCATION

STEVEN HAWKS

Seeking to climb stairs in the dark, on a staircase with missing or unequal treads, is a recipe for bruised shins and thwarted ascension. Just so, it is the argument of this article that the attainment of health education objectives is being hampered by a lack of appreciation for the functional role of spiritual wellness—a tread that is currently misaligned in the stairway of effective health education. This position is clarified by reviewing the definitions and goals of health education, considering philosophical inconsistencies in current practice, and outlining a foundational role for spiritual health education, that, if actualized, may improve the likelihood of successful outcomes.

## THE UNREACHABLE GOAL OF HEALTH EDUCATION

It is the general goal of health education to improve the health knowledge and attitudes of individuals and thereby inspire personal behaviors that lead to optimal health and wellness, or high levels of functioning in all of the various dimensions of health (Butler, 2001). Underlying this goal are several assumptions or beliefs about the nature of health. First, *health* is typically defined in our literature as being multidimensional, the realization of which requires a degree of depth and balance among such diverse elements as physical health, emotional health, intellectual health, social health, and spiritual health (Cottrell, Girvan, & McKenzie, 2002). Further, these dimensions are considered to be dynamic inasmuch as the status of one dimension often influences the condition of another (Butler, 2001). Finally, it is argued that health is functional because most people value it primarily for its usefulness in the pursuit of higher aims, rather than merely as an end in itself (Read, 1997).

And yet the profession of health education seems philosophically inconsistent in its methodology, in that efforts at health promotion often ignore all three of the concepts presented in the preceding definition. First, the multidimensional nature of health is effectively discounted; most published health education objectives include only physical health variables as primary outcome measures (for example, *Healthy People 2010*). Outside of educational settings that offer courses on personal health, it is difficult to identify more than a few health education interventions that target, say, intellectual health, social health, or spiritual health as principal dimensions of interest with specific outcome objectives. Why bother to comment on the multidimensional nature of health if in most settings we overlook all dimensions save one?

If the multidimensional nature of health is disregarded, then its dynamic nature can hardly be appreciated or capitalized on. Although it is well documented, for example, that emotional well-being exerts a profound influence on cardiovascular health, we do not often consider emotional health variables as outcome goals for cardiovascular prevention programs (Williams et al., 1999). Similarly, social support is a significant factor in understanding a multitude of health outcomes, including various types of cancer, cardiovascular disease, immune function (Callaghan & Morrissey, 1993; Uchino, Cacioppo, & Kiecolt-Glaser, 1996), women's health (Hurdle, 2001), and positive health practices (McNicholas, 2002). And spiritual well-being influences such diverse outcomes as recovery from addiction (Pardini, Plante, Sherman, & Stump, 2000), teen sexual activity (Holder et al., 2000), depression (Nelson, Rosenfeld, Breitbart, & Galietta, 2002), eating disorders (Hawks, Goudy, & Gast, 2003), breast cancer (Feher & Maly, 1999), long survival with AIDS (Ironson et al., 2002), and a number of health behaviors (Waite, Hawks, & Gast, 1999). Yet, with few exceptions (for example, Weaver & Cotrell, 1996; White & Dorman, 2001), health educators seldom attempt to measure or influence social health or spirituality in health education interventions. Without an appreciation of multidimensionality, we are unable to investigate the dynamic nature of these health dimensions in terms of how they interrelate with and impact one another (Karren, Hafen, Smith, & Frandsen, 2002).

Instead physical health is generally promoted by health educators as a sufficient end in itself, with no consideration for some larger purpose that might justify its need in the first place. The functional nature of health, its basic role of serving higher human interests, is thus lost in a fervor of physical health promotion, which implies that good physical health is apparently the greatest achievement possible. In contrast, it seems likely that most individuals become interested in improving health behaviors only when they see a vital connection between enhanced health status and the realization of a self-defined, higher purpose in life (Hawks, 1994; Hawks, Hull, Thalman, & Richins, 1995).

Consider the overweight, middle-aged, divorced gentleman, hopelessly entangled in a dead-end career, who spends inordinate amounts of time on the couch in front of the TV—eating chips, smoking cigarettes, drinking beer, and feeling sorry about his lonely and meaningless existence. In fact, he believes that his TV, stimulants, and snacks are the only things that make his otherwise unbearable life somewhat tolerable. How will this good man respond to the modern health educator who—without stopping to consider the various dimensions of health involved (for example, social, emotional, spiritual, intellectual) and without contemplating the general lack of purpose in this person's life—enthusiastically promotes dietary restraint, nicotine patches, and treadmills as the path to good physical health? Our client will likely roll his eyes with boredom, dismiss the notion of "health" altogether, and reach for another smoke.

And thus by failing to equitably consider and promote all dimensions of health, and without appreciating the true motivation that must underlie successful health behavior change—active engagement in a self-defined higher purpose—the realization of health education goals is substantially hindered. Indeed, as currently promoted, the primary goal of health education (substantial health behavior change at the population level) may be largely unreachable.

## INCONSISTENCIES IN THEORY AND PRACTICE

Our preoccupation with physical health is not hard to understand given the foundational influence of the seventeenth century Cartesian duality that firmly separated mind and body (Gorham, 1994; Tomaselli, 1984). The subsequent development of physical medicine, and the later emergence of public health and health education professions that primarily target the prevention of physical illness, was perhaps inevitable (Rubin & Wessely, 2001; Switankowsky, 2000). The national health objectives for most developed nations (for example, *Healthy People 2010*), and thus their public health funding mechanisms, continue to revolve almost exclusively around the prevention and treatment of physical illness (U.S. Department of Health and Human Services [USDHHS], 2000). Acceptance of this paradigm on the part of our profession implies the belief that if we simply take care of physical health, the apparently lesser dimensions will fall into place of their own accord. Or, if necessary, the clergy, psychologists, and social workers can tend to the emotional, social, spiritual, and intellectual maladies of humanity.

Such a one-dimensional, fractured approach is inconsistent with our philosophical allegiance to holistic health promotion (Switankowsky, 2000). We now have firm evidence that the mind and body, far from being separate, are intimately interwoven—and that there truly are many dimensions of health that interact with each other

(Karren et al., 2002). Therefore, it is less effective, if not negligent, to promote physical health without simultaneously addressing the other dimensions of health in a truly integrative model (Grace, 1998).

As it now stands our practice is inconsistent with our philosophy, and our effectiveness may be limited as a result. If things continue as they are, then ethically we must take a step backward and redefine health as consisting of a single static dimension that represents an end in itself (physical health). Alternatively, we might relabel our profession as that of physical health educator with a disclaimer that the complexity of multidimensional health cannot be promoted by a single discipline (at least, not by ours). Then again, we might rise to the occasion by fully embracing our current definition of health, initiating research agendas that help us understand the interconnectedness of all dimensions of health, and devising theory-based educational programs that might advance them evenhandedly.

## BARRIERS TO PROMOTING MULTIDIMENSIONAL WELLNESS

There are several barriers that hinder progress toward a health education practice that genuinely promotes a dynamic, multidimensional wellness from a functional perspective. Perhaps the most daunting barrier is the inertia of a vast public health system that has settled around the focal point of physical health as the ultimate outcome objective. Physical health is tangible, understandable, measurable, and objective—and it is therefore easy to target. Given this reality, national physical health objectives that drive funding and other resource allocation mechanisms place inescapable pressure on health educators to pursue agendas that are consistent with those objectives (USDHHS, 2000).

A second barrier is the ambiguity of dealing with dimensions of health that have not achieved a consensus definition, are intangible, and are seemingly immeasurable. One introductory health education text, for example, presents a standard overview of the five dimensions of health but concludes that the meaning of spiritual health must "be left to the individual reader" (Cottrell et al., 2002, p. 7). As opposed to this hopeless ambiguity, each dimension of health must be acceptably defined, operationalized, and have a means of valid, reliable measurement, so that it can become a legitimate outcome goal for health education programming. This has yet to happen for many of the core dimensions of health. Most aspects of the physical dimension, by contrast, have already achieved this status (such as blood pressure, blood lipid profiles, morbidity and mortality rates, body mass index), thereby contributing to the preponderance of research and practice that focuses on the physical dimension.

Finally, the trepidation of stepping into such politically charged arenas as the promotion of spirituality leaves the profession hesitant in acting on its own definition of health. One school health educator complained to the author that use of the word *condom* in a public secondary school classroom posed far fewer ramifications than use of the word *spirituality*. Even though it seems clear that spirituality can be promoted without violating the separation of church and state (Weaver & Cotrell, 1996), discomfort with this dimension remains even higher than other controversial arenas such as sexuality education.

## OVERCOMING BARRIERS

Several steps have to be taken to bring the practice of health education into harmony with its philosophical foundations. The first step is to pursue organized efforts, possibly within the context of professional associations, to clearly define the various dimensions of health in a way that builds consensus. Numerous scholarly articles have been written about the nature of spiritual health (Banks, 1980; Bensley, 1991a, 1991b; Chapman, 1986; Hawks et al., 1995; Seaward, 1995), but a lack of professional consensus forces readers of introductory texts to come to their own conclusions as to what it really represents and whether it is important. The recent process used to bring about consensus in relation to a professional code of ethics might represent a useful pattern for defining each health dimension (Cottrell et al., 2002). Likewise, previous efforts by jointly established committees to achieve consensus in health education standards and terminology might offer another plausible approach (Joint Committee on Health Education Standards, 1995; Joint Committee on Health Education Terminology, 1991).

The second step, also pursuable through the avenue of organized efforts by professional associations, is to place pressure on the crafters of national health objectives to develop public health objectives that represent a dynamic, multidimensional view of health. They should be encouraged further to design a stronger mechanism for increased local control over resource allocation that might include intervention and evaluation priorities that target nonphysical dimensions of health. Although the value of *Healthy People 2010* cannot be overestimated in terms of its ability to focus multilevel efforts on urgent problems (Cottrell et al., 2002), the process that leads to national objectives can be criticized as being too top-down in its orientation and too focused on the physical dimension of health.

Finally, there is a real need for individual health education researchers who are willing to commit time and energy to designing, implementing, and evaluating the impact of programs that target various nonphysical dimensions of health. Ideally, such a research agenda would lead to valid, reliable measures of these dimensions that include both quantitative and qualitative instruments and methodologies (Hawks et al., 1995). In 1990 J. R. Bloom challenged medical care researchers to develop a body of knowledge in relation to social support and health (Bloom, 1990). Within a few years dozens of research reports were published that clearly documented several mechanisms by which social support might be influencing health (Uchino et al., 1996).

As a result the health care community is working diligently to incorporate social support into treatment protocols (Hurdle, 2001; Luskin et al., 1998). Based on more recent research efforts there is growing interest in incorporating spiritual support into patient care strategies (Castledine, 2003; Graber & Johnson, 2001; Kearns, 2002;

Lemmer, 2002; Schweitzer, Norberg, & Larson, 2002). The same research and practice efforts that are taking place in patient care settings should also be taking place in health education and health promotion settings (Hawks et al., 1995).

## A DYNAMIC, MULTIDIMENSIONAL, FUNCTIONAL MODEL FOR HOLISTIC HEALTH

One step toward the harmonization of practice and theory in health education is the refinement of theories and models that represent a dynamic, multidimensional, functional characterization of health, and that can guide future approaches to health education. As previously suggested in the literature, the linchpin in such a philosophical model may be spiritual health (Meeks, 1977; Waite et al., 1999; Young, 1984). As defined by one author, spiritual health involves high levels of commitment to a well-defined worldview (Hawks, 1994). The worldview provides personal clarity in understanding the purpose of life and one's place in it. The worldview further offers a value system and an ethical path for fulfilling the higher purpose that life affords. The importance of relationships, the nature of a higher power or larger reality, and a sense of personal worth are also encompassed within the spiritual worldview. Even in modern secular societies it may be the strength of the spiritual worldview that provides grounding, direction, personal peace, coping skills, and the hope of fulfillment (Brown, 2003).

In a dynamic functional model of holistic health (Figure 22.1), spiritual health represents purpose and higher meaning in life along with the value system that

**FIGURE 22.1**   **A Dynamic, Functional, Multidimensional Model of Holistic Health**

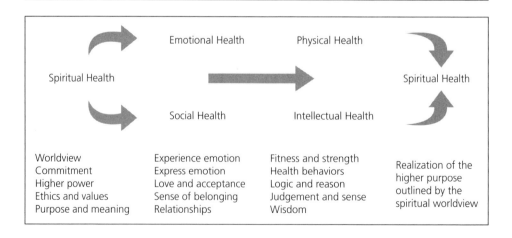

defines proper actions and the nature of relationships. As such, good spiritual health fulfills foundational needs and provides the impetus for achieving positive emotional and social health. Emotional health is generally defined as the ability to experience and express the full range of human emotions in appropriate ways, whereas social health involves the quality of our relationships, satisfaction in our social roles, our sense of belonging, and feelings of love and acceptance (Hawks, 1994). As shown in the model, and as demonstrated in the literature, high levels of spiritual, emotional, and social health can positively impact physical and intellectual health outcomes, including a heightened enthusiasm for practicing positive health behaviors—the real goal of health education (Hammermeister & Peterson, 2001; Uchino et al., 1996; Waite et al., 1999; Williams et al., 1999). To the degree attained, physical and intellectual health become the tools for realizing the higher purpose that is encompassed within the spiritual worldview and the cycle continues. Once inspired by the possibility of spiritual fulfillment, the couch-bound gentleman described previously may be more eager to consult with the health educator as to the best methods for giving up addictive substances, increasing exercise, and managing his diet.

For the limited instances in which such a comprehensive approach has been taken, mostly in the medical field, the level of success has been exceptional. By including program strategies that target spiritual and emotional development as the prerequisites to health behavior change, atherosclerosis has been reversed (Ornish et al., 1998) and medically unmanageable pain has been mitigated (Kabat-Zinn, Lipworth, & Burney, 1985). The implications for *illness* prevention and health education are intriguing, but remain largely unexplored (Hawks et al., 1995).

As dictated by our modern definition of health, this model is truly multidimensional, dynamic, and functional. But implementation of this paradigm will be far more challenging than the current strategy of focusing on new strategies to creatively dispense physical health information to an unmotivated population. Although inexpensive, at least in comparison with medical treatments, the multidimensional approaches alluded to in the previous paragraph are nevertheless very time- and energy-intensive. Programs last many weeks, or even months, and the level of involvement for both educators and participants is high. Although a single dose of a small pill might be preferred by the client, an intensive, comprehensive approach that addresses all dimensions of health is capable of providing lasting, life-altering solutions that can be achieved in no other way (Kabat-Zinn et al., 1985; Ornish et al., 1998).

The growing levels of alienation, apathy, and unhealthy lifestyles that are apparent in many modern societies are perhaps a reflection of diminished spiritual and emotional well-being (Cowley, 2002). It thus behooves health educators to better understand the dynamic and influential nature of spiritual health (an acknowledged yet largely ambiguous dimension in our definition of health) and devise appropriate ways to promote it along with social, intellectual, and emotional health.

## CONCLUSION

The profession of health education, if so inclined, is in a position to more fully encourage and support a holistic health and wellness transition in the populations it serves. This requires efforts at both the individual and the national level. First, there must be a push within the profession to clearly define and operationalize concepts associated with the various dimensions of health. Second, there must be an effort to incorporate nonphysical outcomes into national and local health objectives. This must also include national and local resource allocation mechanisms that encourage health education researchers to design, implement, and evaluate programs that target the full spectrum of health dimensions. Finally, it requires that as individual researchers and practitioners we become better versed in the various dimensions of health by conducting appropriate program design, implementation, and evaluation agendas that further refine models and theories and guide more effective practices. Along the way we must be willing to run contrary to popular notions against meddling with such things as spirituality and step into uncharted territory in terms of the knowledge and educational strategies that must become the new tools of health education (Hawks et al., 1995).

Other helping professions, including medicine, nursing, social work, psychology, and health counseling are already incorporating spiritual, emotional, and social protocols into their treatments, practices, and professional preparation programs (Dudley & Helfgott, 1990; Gelo, 1995; Kearns, 2002; Matthews et al., 1998; Tart & Deikman, 1991). Commitment to such a course by the profession of health education will perhaps represent the beginnings of a process that will allow us to become a leader in promoting the type of health in which we profess to believe, and thereby enable us to realize more effectively the ultimate goals of health education. Each step up the stairway that leads to the realization of health education objectives will gradually become a sure one.

## REFERENCES

Banks, R. (1980). Health and the spiritual dimension: Relationships and implications for professional preparation programs. *Journal of School Health, 50*, 195–202.

Bensley, R. J. (1991a). Defining spiritual health: A review of the literature. *Journal of Health Education, 22*, 287–290.

Bensley, R. J. (1991b). Spiritual health as a component of worksite health promotion/wellness programming: A review of the literature. *Journal of Health Education, 22*, 352–353, 394.

Bloom, J. R. (1990). The relationship of social support and health. *Social Science & Medicine, 30*, 635–637.

Brown, C. (2003). Low morale and burnout: Is the solution to teach a values-based spiritual approach? *Complementary Therapies in Nursing & Midwifery, 9*(2), 57–61.

Butler, J. (2001). *Principles of health education and health promotion* (3rd ed.). Belmont, CA: Wadsworth.

Callaghan, P., & Morrissey, J. (1993). Social support and health: A review. *Journal of Advanced Nursing, 18*, 203–210.

Castledine, G. (2003). Developing a spiritual approach to health care. *British Journal of Nursing, 12*, 451.

Chapman, L. (1986). Spiritual health: A component missing from health promotion. *American Journal of Health Promotion, 4*(1), 18–24, 31.

Cottrell, R. R., Girvan, J. T., & McKenzie, J. R. (2002). *Principles and foundations of health promotion and education* (2nd ed.). San Francisco: Benjamin Cummings.

Cowley, G. (2002, September 16). The science of happiness. *Newsweek*, 46–49.

Dudley, J. R., & Helfgott, C. (1990). Exploring a place for spirituality in the social work curriculum. *Journal of Social Work Education, 26*, 287–294.

Feher, S., & Maly, R. C. (1999). Coping with breast cancer in later life: The role of religious faith. *Psychooncology, 8*, 408–416.

Gelo, F. (1995). Spirituality: A vital component in health counseling. *Journal of American College Health, 44*, 38–40.

Gorham, G. (1994). Mind-body dualism and the Harvey-Descartes controversy. *Journal of the History of Ideas, 55*, 211–234.

Graber, D. R., & Johnson, J. A. (2001). Spirituality and healthcare organizations. *Journal of Healthcare Management, 46*(1), 39–50

Grace, V. M. (1998). Mind/body dualism in medicine: The case of chronic pelvic pain without organic pathology: A critical review of the literature. *International Journal of Health Services, 28*(1), 127–151.

Hammermeister, J. L., & Peterson, M. (2001). Does spirituality make a difference? Psychosocial and health-related characteristics of spiritual well-being. *American Journal of Health Education, 32*, 293–297.

Hawks, S. R. (1994). Spiritual health: Definition and theory. *Wellness Perspectives, 10*(4), 3–13.

Hawks, S. R., Goudy, M. B., & Gast, J. A. (2003). Emotional eating and spiritual well-being: A possible connection? *American Journal of Health Education, 34*, 30–33.

Hawks, S. R., Hull, L., Thalman, R., & Richins, P. (1995). Review of spiritual health: Definition, role, and intervention strategies in health promotion. *American Journal of Health Promotion, 9*, 371–378.

Holder, D. W., DuRant, R. H., Harris, T. L., Daniel, J. H., Obeidallah, D., & Goodman, E. (2000). The association between adolescent spirituality and voluntary sexual activity. *Journal of Adolescent Health, 26*, 295–302.

Hurdle, D. E. (2001). Social support: A critical factor in women's health and health promotion. *Health and Social Work, 26*(2), 72–79.

Ironson, G., Solomon, G. R., Balbin, E. G., O'Cleirigh, C., George, A., Kumar, M., et al. (2002). The Ironson-Woods spirituality/religiousness index is associated with long survival, health behaviors, less distress, and low cortisol in people with HIV/AIDS. *Annals of Behavioral Medicine, 24*(1), 34–48.

Joint Committee on Health Education Standards. (1995). *National health education standards: Achieving health literacy*. Atlanta, GA: American Cancer Society.

Joint Committee on Health Education Terminology. (1991). Report of the 1990 Joint Committee on Health Education Terminology. *Journal of Health Education, 22*, 173–184.

Kabat-Zinn, J., Lipworth, L., & Burney, R. (1985). The clinical use of mindfulness meditation for the self-regulation of chronic pain. *Journal of Behavioral Medicine, 8*, 163–190.

Karren, K., Hafen, B., Smith, R., & Frandsen, K. (2002). *Mind/body health: The effects of attitudes, emotions, and relationships* (2nd ed.). San Francisco: Benjamin Cummings.

Kearns, M. L. (2002). Managing the spiritual needs of patients. Simple steps to enhance well-being. *Advance for Nurse Practitioners, 10*(3), 101–104.

Lemmer, C. (2002). Teaching the spiritual dimension of nursing care: A survey of U.S. baccalaureate nursing programs. *Journal of Nursing Education, 41*, 482–490.

Luskin, F. M., Newell, K. A., Griffith, M., Holmes, M., Telles, S., Marvasti, F. F. et al. (1998). A review of mind-body therapies in the treatment of cardiovascular disease. Part 1: Implications for the elderly. *Alternative Therapies in Health and Medicine, 4*(3), 46–61.

Matthews, D. A., McCullough, M. E., Larson, D. B., Koenig, H. B., Sywers, J. P., & Milano, M. G. (1998). Religious commitment and health status: A review of the research and implications for family medicine. *Archives of Family Medicine, 7*, 118–124.

McNicholas, S. L. (2002). Social support and positive health practices. *Western Journal of Nursing Research, 24*, 772–787.

Meeks, L. (1977). The role of spiritual health in achieving high level wellness. *Health Values, 2*, 222–224.

Nelson, C. J., Rosenfeld, B., Breitbart, W., & Galietta, M. (2002). Spirituality, religion, and depression in the terminally ill. *Psycho-somatics, 43*, 213–220.

Ornish, D., Scherwitz, L. W., Billings, J. H., Brown, S. E., Gould, K. L., Merrit, T. A., et al. (1998). Intensive lifestyle changes for reversal of coronary heart disease. *Journal of the American Medical Association, 280*, 2001–2007.

Pardini, D. A., Plante, T. G., Sherman, A., & Stump, J. E. (2000). Religious faith and spirituality in substance abuse recovery: Determining the mental health benefits. *Journal of Substance Abuse Treatment, 19*, 347–354.

Read, D. A. (1997). *Health education: A cognitive-behavioral approach.* Boston: Jones and Bartlett.

Rubin, G. J., & Wessely, S. (2001). Dealing with dualism. *Advances in Mind Body Medicine, 17*, 256–259; discussion 270–276.

Schweitzer, R., Norberg, M., & Larson, L. (2002), The parish nurse coordinator: A bridge to spiritual health care leadership for the future. *Journal of Holistic Nursing, 20*, 212–231.

Seaward, B. L. (1995). Reflections on human spirituality for the worksite. *American Journal of Health Promotion, 9*, 165–168.

Switankowsky, I. (2000). Dualism and its importance for medicine. *Theoretical Medicine and Bioethics, 21*, 567–580.

Tart, C. T., & Deikman, A. J. (1991). Mindfulness, spiritual seeking, and psychotherapy. *Journal of Transpersonal Psychology, 23*(1), 29–52.

Tomaselli, S. (1984). The first person: Descartes, Locke and mind-body dualism. *History of Science, 22* (pt. 2), 185–205.

Uchino, B. N., Cacioppo, J. T., & Kiecolt-Glaser, J. K. (1996). The relationship between social support and physiological processes: A review with emphasis on underlying mechanisms and implications for health. *Psychological Bulletin, 119*, 488–531.

U.S. Department of Health and Human Services (USDHHS). (2000). *Healthy people 2010.* Washington, DC: Author.

Waite, P., Hawks, S., & Gast, J. (1999). The correlation between spiritual well-being and health behaviors. *American Journal of Health Promotion, 13*, 159–162.

Weaver, R. I., & Cotrell, H. (1996). A non-religious spirituality that causes students to clarify their values and to respond with passion. *Education, 112*, 426–435.

White, M., & Dorman, S. M. (2001). Receiving social support online: Implications for health education. *Health Education Research, 16*, 693–707.

Williams, R., Kiecolt-Glaser, J., Legato, M. I., Ornish, D., Powell, L. H., Syme, S. L. et al. (1999). The impact of emotions on cardiovascular health. *Journal of Gender Specific Medicine, 2*(5), 52–58.

Young, E. (1984). Spiritual health—An essential element in optimum health. *Journal of American College Health, 32*, 273–276.

# PART

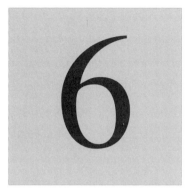

# SOCIAL CHANGE IN HEALTH EDUCATION

*The purpose of social change philosophy in health education is to advocate for environmental, economic, and political conditions that make healthy choices possible. Social change philosophy asserts that focusing on individual's responsibility for health is ineffective and distracts from the environmental and economic factors that have larger effects on the health of a nation. According to social change philosophy, individual emphasis on health fails to acknowledge inequalities in society which effectively determine the health of individuals.*

*Health education programs designed to support this philosophy would be based on social morality and justice in order to influence social determinants of health and illness. In social change philosophy, the practitioner would work toward a more equitable health care system, place greater emphasis on policy changes, and be an advocate of health as a human right. The primary purpose of social change philosophy is to legislate certain changes in order to benefit society as a whole. A macro-level approach to health education does not damn individuals for poor health choices but instead looks to change the context in which their choices are made. Changing the context and environment would allow individuals to make better lifestyle choices. Advantages to the adoption of this philosophy for the health education profession include the recognition of social variables that influence individual health. Social policies are advocated according to the criterion of bringing the greatest amount of good to the greatest number of people. Health topics addressed through social-change-based health education programs include community health advocacy, empowerment, quality of school health education programs, federal government support for health education, health care cost containment, universal health care coverage, and economic and social improvement.*

## ARTICLES

Using health education as a tool to bring about social change is not a new concept. Grounded in the social movements in the 1960s and 1970s, health education has taken a fresh look at what social change means in the contemporary world. Robertson and Minkler (1994) provide a critical examination of what they refer to as the "new health promotion movement." This exploration features an "introduction to new ideas, new language, and new concepts about what constitutes health and how health promotion efforts should be configured to achieve health." Leviton (2002) discusses health education as a means to bring global peace, the ultimate in restructuring social change. Coulter, Allbrecht, Guliotz, Figg, and Mahan (1999) put forth the argument that health education professionals have an obligation to embrace social change as a way to assure that the health of the public is protected and improved. O'Rourke (2002) explores moving beyond defining health as medical care, addresses the task of making health care affordable, and offers alternative funding scenarios for a viable health care system. Auld and Dixon-Terry (1999) review historical social movements that legislated successful interventions for health promotion and education. They encourage the health education to use these principles to advocate for advancement of the profession. Allegrante, Morisky, and Sharif (1999) encouraged the discipline to use advocacy to remove disparities in health care. Applying social change principles to "stimulate community political action and economic and environmental changes" can afford individuals opportunities to make good health decisions. As one searches for the underlying causes of illness, one finds that many social inequities are contributing factors.

And finally, Pinzon-Perez (2003) examines the interconnectedness of health care systems globally. She reiterates that the purpose of health education is to take an active stand against disparities in health care, advocate for essential human rights (better housing, better sanitation, good employment opportunities) and provide guidance in environmental protection measures.

## CHALLENGE TO THE READER

The articles in Part 6 will allow the reader to gain an understanding of the social change philosophy for health education, and the role of the health education practitioner within this approach. Here, the role of the health educator is to work within the political arena demanding and legislating changes that create the greatest amount of good. Eliminating health disparities is the main focus. The client is not the individual but society at large. A social change health educator is a good networker working at the macro level to create social justice. What are the concepts and principles you can glean from these readings? How can this knowledge be applied to the practice of health education?

# CHAPTER

23

# NEW HEALTH PROMOTION MOVEMENT: A CRITICAL EXAMINATION

ANN ROBERTSON

MEREDITH MINKLER

In 1986, Marshall Becker wrote a paper entitled "The Tyranny of Health Promotion," in which he critiqued the individual lifestyle approach to health promotion and cautioned against its tendency to equate "being ill" with "being guilty" and to substitute "personal health goals for more important, humane societal goals" (p. 20). Since the publication of that paper, we have witnessed a revolution in the field of health promotion. Guided to a large extent by position papers disseminated by the World Health Organization (WHO) Europe Health Promotion Office (1984), and furthered by the Ottawa Charter (1986b), the Epp Report in Canada (Health & Welfare Canada, 1986), the Healthy Cities project (Duhl), and others (Hancock, 1986; Labonte, 1986; Milio, 1981), this new health promotion movement has resulted in a fundamental shift in the ways in which many health professionals think, talk, and write about health, the determinants of health, and the strategies for achieving health. Both the philosophical core and one of the central strategies of the new health promotion is articulated in the concept of empowerment. The intent of this paper is to critically examine the concept of empowerment and its relationship to the notions of health and community participation.

Also known as "community health promotion," the new health promotion movement has given birth to a new group of experts with new knowledge bases, new language, and new skills. Like many social movements, it has come to represent the emergence of a new domain of knowledge and discourse (Foucault, 1977). The new health promotion movement has emerged largely by challenging the truth claims—the building blocks of any knowledge domain—of more traditional health education and health promotion approaches. Some of the prominent features of this new health promotion movement include the following:

1. Broadening the definition of health and its determinants to include the social and economic context within which health—or, more precisely, non-health—is produced

2. Going beyond the earlier emphasis on individual lifestyle strategies to achieve health to broader social and political strategies

3. Embracing the concept of empowerment—individual and collective—as a key health promotion strategy

4. Advocating the participation of the community in identifying health problems and strategies for addressing those problems

Although some practitioners of the earlier, more traditional approach to health promotion had attempted to employ one or more of these features, the new health promotion movement goes considerably further to consolidate them into a coherent, clearly articulated theory and approach to practice.

The new health promotion movement is to be applauded for having moved the field beyond the narrow confines of the earlier individual lifestyle approach. Nevertheless, in the spirit of Becker's paper (1986), we argue that critical self-reflection with respect to the terms and concepts used to articulate this new health promotion is needed, if we are to avoid simply substituting one tyranny for another. We suggest that, for the revolution in health promotion to be more than a revolution in professional discourse, critical examination of the new knowledge domain represented by the new health promotion is needed.

The paper is offered as a contribution to the continuing development and refinement of theory, research, and practice related to the concept of empowerment. To that end, we shall explore, in turn, the multidimensional and contested nature of health, empowerment, and community participation. We begin with a brief general discussion of what we mean, in the context of this paper, by multidimensional and contested.

## CONTESTED DOMAINS

The new health promotion movement is punctuated by words like *empowerment* and *community participation*. But what do these words mean and do they mean the same to all who use them? To invoke these words is to invoke powerful symbolic concepts.

This paper will explore the various meanings that surround these terms as well as the very notion of health. By getting underneath the meaning of the words and concepts used to frame community health promotion, this paper also seeks to unpack some of the underlying ideological conflicts and accompanying turf battles that have arisen in the wake of the new directions that health promotion has taken.

A fundamental ideological conflict exists about the goal of health promotion: Should the goal be improved health status (individual and collective)—health as an end? Or should the goal be social justice (Beauchamp, 1976)—health as a means? Emerging from that conflict are other related ideological conflicts, including micro-level (individual) change versus macro-level (structural) change; individual lifestyle strategies versus community-based approaches; and professional ownership versus public ownership.

We will demonstrate that much of what is contested in relation to concepts like empowerment and community participation, and their operationalization in health promotion practice, can be understood as boundary issues. What is contested frequently depends on whether we take a macro or a micro view of the meaning of health and the ways to achieve it. Because this macro/micro perspective is a critical lens through which we will examine in more detail these contested domains, it is important to say something briefly about this analytical framework.

Although it is true that the larger structural (economic, political, cultural, organizational) forces (the macro level) in any society shape the everyday lives of individuals (the micro level), it is also true that the everyday practices of individuals shape those same larger structural forces. This position tempers the notion of sociological determinism with the notion of human agency. To illustrate in the health arena: On the one hand, many epidemiological studies demonstrate the often profound role of poverty and other social, economic, and political factors in influencing individual health status (Ehrenreich & English, 1990; Haan, Kaplan, & Camacho, 1987; Marmot, Rose, Shipley, & Hamilton, 1978; Miller, 1990; Ratcliffe, 1978; Syme & Berkman, 1976; Syme, 1986). On the other hand, individuals have been able to reshape the social context within which they live, and thus affect their health.

For example, although the multibillion-dollar cigarette industry promotes tobacco subsidies, the right to advertise through the mass media, and other government policies that in turn encourage and support smoking on the individual levels the individuals who mobilize their colleagues to achieve a smoke-free workplace, or who lead a fight to curtail cigarette advertising targeted at people of color in poor neighborhoods, may also be contributing to broader institutional and/or policy level change. Similarly, disability rights groups, such as the Independent Living Movement, have enabled persons with disabilities to reframe as social pathology what previously had been framed as individual pathology. That is, disability was reconceptualized as resulting from a social environment that disregarded the existence of people with disabilities by making it difficult, if not impossible, for them to participate in public life. The solution was, in part, to reform the social and physical environments by making public spaces accessible to persons with disabilities (Driedger, 1989). In C. Wright Mills' terms

(1959), disability rights advocates succeeded in recasting their personal troubles as public issues.

Much analytical and operational power is lost by setting up the ideological dichotomy of the macro level versus the micro level referred to above. A much more constructive approach is to frame these two spheres as being in a dialectical relationship with each other: Each informs, produces, and reproduces the other, mediated by the mid-level sphere of social organizations (Bellah, 1991; Glendon, 1991; Moody, 1988). Such organizations, often referred to as "mediating structures" (Berger & Neuhaus, 1977), typically include churches, neighborhood organizations, schools, service organizations, and other such voluntary organizations and groups, as well as the networks which link them.

We suggest that to understand the new health promotion movement—indeed, for the community health promotion movement to move beyond the present internecine turf battles—the three spheres of health, empowerment, and community participation must be disentangled and critically examined, both separately and in relation to each other. Within the new health promotion there is much overlap between these spheres, both conceptually and in practice. However, in the interests of making explicit some of the ideological issues underlying the new health promotion, we shall examine each of these spheres in turn.

## RECONCEPTUALIZING HEALTH

One of the major contributions of the new health promotion movement has been to broaden the conceptualization of health to include an understanding of the social, political, and economic determinants of health. In this spirit, WHO (1986a) now defines health as

> the extent to which an individual or group is able, on the one hand, to realize aspirations and satisfy needs; and, on the other hand, to change or cope with the environment. Health is, therefore, seen as a resource for everyday life, not the objective of living; it is a positive concept emphasizing social and personal resources, as well as physical capacities. (p. 73)

In this macro or socialized version of health, health is seen as instrumental, a means rather than an end. Health is what one must have to accomplish other things in one's life. Although in general this broader concept of health captures more accurately the complex dimensions of health, at the same time it makes interventions to achieve health more difficult not only to define but to implement.

More narrow medicalized or micro conceptualizations of health tend to identify people with their illness, lack of health, or disability, lapsing at times into blaming the victim. Indeed, we have seen evidence of this in the case of acquired immunodeficiency syndrome (AIDS), where people who are diagnosed with AIDS, and even those diagnosed as human immunodeficiency virus (HIV) positive, have become stigmatized as the agents of disease in the classical epidemiological triangle of host, agent, and environment. Similarly, current injury prevention programs, which feature people with disabilities in their visual ad campaigns accompanied by slogans like "Don't let this happen to you," make an identification of the person with the disability. As Wang (1992) has pointed out.

> if the public health perspective rightly contends that *becoming* disabled is an unacceptable risk in our society, it paradoxically often fails to acknowledge the stigmatizing notion that *being* disabled is an unacceptable status in our society (p. 1093; emphasis in original).

A socialized conceptualization of health, like that of WHO, makes a separation between people and their health status. On the one hand this provides a refreshing alternative to the above noted tendency to stigmatize and marginalize persons with a disease or disability by identifying them with their disease or disability. On the other hand, however, the separation between individuals and their health may itself be problematic to the extent that it ignores or minimizes the everyday reality that constitutes that person's life. Regardless of the social context of their condition, people with diseases or disabilities do have pain, discomfort, and difficulties in managing their everyday lives.

The lifestyle approach to health promotion was criticized for turning health into a commodity, something to be bought and sold in the marketplace, which now included not simply the physician's office or the hospital but also the health food store, exercise club, or stress management program. Ironically, however, it could be argued that by redefining health more broadly as a resource—like wealth or education—which is variously distributed among people, we may risk further commodifying the notion of health. Health becomes even more than before something that resides outside of oneself, determined now by the entire social context, and conferred by a new set of experts with new knowledge bases and new skills. As a result, people may feel even less control over their health than before.

Becker's (1986) caution against health becoming "the paramount value of our society" in the lifestyle approach to health promotion also deserves to be carefully examined where the new health promotion is concerned. For in broadening the concept of health to embrace the whole of life, advocates of a socialized version of health may inadvertently make of health a moral value. Health risks becoming "health-ism," that is, a monolithic concept that attempts to explain everything and, thereby, ends up explaining nothing. If health becomes the analytical lens through which all social issues are seen, it may dilute and obfuscate not only health-related efforts but other social and political efforts as well.

Much of this difficulty with the definition of health can be resolved if we realize that health has both a micro-level individual dimension and a macro-level structural dimension. In her discussion of the political implications of different theories of disease causality, Sylvia Tesh (1988) is critical of the "web of casuality" theory because it "hides its politics" (p. 70). On the other hand, she goes on to say:

> The multicasual theory lacks guidelines for policy makers whereas the structural view lacks guidelines for individuals. We often need, it seems, personal policies that are

*different from public ones. We need to know what interim, individual actions we can*
*rely on until public policies are in place. (p. 81; emphasis in original)*

Thus, we must incorporate, not only into the discourse of the new health promotion movement but also into its practice, this notion of both micro and macro conceptualizations of health. As an example of how we might do that, we now turn to an examination of another fundamental concept of the new health promotion movement over which there is considerable ideological conflict: the concept of empowerment.

## EMPOWERMENT REVISITED

It is now well documented that health is significantly affected by the extent to which one feels control or mastery over one's life, in other words, by the amount of power or powerlessness one feels (see Wallerstein [1992] for an excellent review of this literature). For this reason, the new health promotion movement places an emphasis on empowerment as a primary health promotion strategy. With its roots in community psychology (Rapport, 1985), feminist theory (Gutierrez, 1990), liberation theology (Freire, 1973, 1988), and social activism (Alinsky, 1972), *empowerment* can be defined very broadly as "a process of increasing personal, interpersonal, or political power"(Gutierrez, 1990).

At the core of the notion of empowerment is the concept of power, defined as the ability to control the factors that determine one's life. Conceived of in this way, power is an attribute of individuals and communities. In Pinderhughes' (1983) words:

*power and powerlessness operate systemically, transecting both macrosystem and*
*microsystem processes. The existence or nonexistence of power on one level of*
*human functioning (e.g., interactional) affects is affected by its existence or nonexis-*
*tence on other levels of functioning—for example, intrapsychic, familial, community-*
*ethnic-cultural, and societal. (p. 332)*

The larger political aspect of power is emphasized by Gutierrez (1990), who writes: "Empowerment theory is based on a conflict model that assumes that a society consists of separate groups possessing different levels of power and control over resources" (p. 150). In other words, power is a nonmaterial resource differentially distributed in society.

If power is the ability to predict, control, and participate in one's environment, then empowerment is the process by which individuals and communities are enabled to take such power and act effectively in transforming their lives and their environment (Miller, 1985). With the concept of empowerment, the new health promotion movement, borrowing from earlier feminist conceptualizations of power (French, 1986), attempts to reframe power not as "power over" but rather as "power to" (O'Neill, 1990) or as "power with" (Labonte, 1992). This, in turn, suggests the notion of partnerships between professionals and individuals or communities rather than the more traditional hierarchical provider/client relationship. Yet as Siler-Wells (1989) has pointed out, "behind the euphemistic phrases of community participation and empowerment lay the uncomfortable realities of power, control and ownership" (p. 43).

As a consequence of these realities, the move towards partnerships and other more egalitarian arrangements, although certainly a positive step, may nevertheless ignore the very real structural distinctions that exist between professionals and individuals or communities. Professionals often are more educated, have more access to sources of information, and use a different language to discuss health issues than either the individuals or the communities for whom or for which they work. In addition, the health professional's very location in service agencies or health bureaucracies—what Gruber and Trickett (1987) call their "institutional embeddedness" (p. 358)—confers a certain power on them. This is primarily what Simon (1990) has called the power "to set boundaries around the domain of issues that will be considered germane" (p. 32); in other words, the power to decide the health agenda.

The operationalization of the notion of empowerment may thus be inherently problematic. Many health promotion practitioners have become familiar with the idea of empowerment and see their professional role now as being someone who empowers or gives power to individuals and communities. In this conceptualization of empowerment, there is no break up of the old provider/client power arrangement, for there exists a priori a power differential between the empowerer and the empoweree. As Rappaport (1985) has argued, empowerment occurs not when power is given, but when power is taken by individuals and communities to enable themselves to set and achieve their own agendas.

What is it, then, that health promotion practitioners are to do in the light of this conceptualization of empowerment? According to Rappaport (1985), "What those who have [power] and want to share it can do is to provide *the conditions and the language and beliefs* that make it possible to be taken by those who are in need of it" (p. 18; emphasis added). In other words, empowerment occurs in a climate that first of all fosters it ideologically. In a similar vein, Labonte (1990a) has argued that the role of health promotion professionals concerned with empowerment is

> to nurture this process and remove obstacles, the first being our own need to define health problems for the community [since] the power of defining health belongs to those experiencing it. (p. 87)

What this means is that, in the spirit of community organizer Saul Alinsky (1972) and adult educator Paulo Freire (1973), health promotion practitioners who truly facilitate empowerment do so by assisting individuals and communities in articulating both their health problems and the solutions to address those problems. By providing access to information, supporting indigenous community leadership, and assisting the community in overcoming bureaucratic obstacles to action, such practitioners may contribute to a process whereby communities increase their own problem-solving abilities—what Cottrell (1983) has termed *community competence*. Indeed, as Rappaport (1985) and community activists like John McKnight (1987, 1992b) have argued, empowerment ideology is based on the notion of the already existing capabilities and competencies of individuals and groups. In Rappaport's words:

*There are at least two requirements of an empowerment ideology. On the one hand, it demands that we look to many diverse local settings where people are already handling their own problems in living. On the other hand, it demands that we find ways to take what we learn and make it more, rather than less, likely that others not now handling their own problems in living, or shut out from current solutions, gain control over their lives. (1985, p. 18; emphasis added)*

By incorporating concepts of power and empowerment into its analysis and repertoire of strategies, the new health promotion movement has helped to move the field beyond the victim blaming rhetoric that often has accompanied the lifestyle approach. At the same time, however, the new health promotion has tended to cast the notion of empowerment as meaning that nothing short of collective political action counts as a legitimate health promotion strategy. In so doing, it has tended to ignore or disregard the multidimensionality of power—the earlier discussed essential interdependence between individual empowerment and empowerment at a more political level. As Shor and Freire (1987) point out:

*While individual empowerment, the feeling of being changed, is not enough concerning the transformation of the whole society, it is absolutely necessary for the process of social transformation. The critical development of [people] is absolutely fundamental for the radical transformation of society…but it is not enough by itself. (p. 6)*

Labonte (1989, 1990b) and Jackson, Mitchell, and Wright (1989) have discussed in detail this notion of the multidimensionality of empowerment in terms of an empowerment continuum. Empowerment can occur at many levels from personal empowerment through community organization to political action. What this continuum implies is that for an individual to join a smoking cessation program and succeed in quitting smoking may be as empowering for that individual as a community taking action to prohibit cigarette advertising on its local billboards may be for the community.

What the empowerment continuum also means is that not all health promotion practitioners necessarily have to work at all points on the empowerment continuum for their work to be constituted as empowering. To politicize health and health promotion strategies, as the new health promotion movement tends to do, does not mean that only political action now constitutes health promotion; it means framing health problems and their solutions in their social, political, and economic context. One's practice can be at the individual level—nutrition education classes for teenage mothers, for example—and be empowering.

The importance of recognizing and acknowledging the empowering potential of effective health promotion practice, including direct services on the individual level, is underscored further when we recall the potential misuse of the notion of empowerment to cut back or delegitimate the provision of such services. In the United States, for example, some conservative policy makers and organizations have combined the notion of empowerment with the political ideology of personal responsibility to suggest that people, individually and through such mediating structures as their churches and voluntary associations, must do for themselves rather than rely on the direct services of health and social service professionals to assist them in meeting their needs (Berger & Neuhaus, 1977; Pilisuk & Minkler, 1986). Although couched in the language of freeing people by decreasing their dependence on larger societal institutions, this kind of thinking has been used to justify the withdrawal of needed health and social services in times of fiscal conservatism (Binney & Estes, 1988; Estes, 1984; Schwartz, 1990).

Direct services can be empowering to individuals and to communities. A maternal and child health clinic in a low income neighborhood, for example, not only empowers individual women and children by ensuring their optimal health—especially if we think of health as a resource for daily living—it also has the potential to create solidarity and community among the women who use the services of the clinic. The important criterion in terms of empowerment is how the direct services are delivered: Are the women considered as supplicants to or beneficiaries of the service, or are they regarded as being entitled to good perinatal health because they are members of the community? Empowerment ideology would dictate the latter.

Much has been written on the importance of health and social services to, what is essentially, capacity building. In health education and health promotion circles, capacity building is conceived of as the nurturing of and building upon the strengths, resources, and problem-solving abilities already present in individuals and communities (Cottrell, 1983; McKnight, 1987). Community-based support services for family caregivers of the elderly, for example, may be essential to allowing and enabling family members to continue to function effectively. Unless such support services are provided, family support systems may break down, leading to adverse health outcomes as well as feelings of powerlessness among both the recipients of care and the providers of this informal support (Gallagher, 1989). Thus, not only may services provided to individuals and communities be empowering—depending on the ideology of their provision, as noted above—but services may be essential to maintaining the supportive capacity of families, networks, and communities (Pilisuk & Minkler, 1986).

This brings us to an examination of another piece of the new health promotion movement over which there is much ideological confusion and conflict: the notion of community participation.

## RHETORIC AND REALITY OF COMMUNITY PARTICIPATION

Together with the concept of empowerment, it is the notion of community participation that the new health promotion movement invokes as its defining feature, as what sets it apart from more traditional individualized approaches to health promotion. Community participation—sometimes the term *public participation* is used—represents the legitimizing concept of the new health promotion movement in terms of both analysis and intervention. But, probably more than any of the other contested domains examined in this discussion, the concept of community participation may be the most chameleon like. The reason for this is the many ways in which community and partici-pation are defined.

There have been numerous attempts to clarify the concept of community (see McMillan and Chavis [1986] for an excellent overview). According to Rifkin, Muller, and Bichmann (1988), *community* can be defined as concretely as "a group of people living in the same defined area sharing the same basic values and organization," or as abstractly as "a group of people sharing the same basic interests" (p. 933). The former definition is a static geographically based version of community whereas the latter, a more fluid version stressing relationships, admits that "the interests change from time to time with the consequence that the actual members of the 'community' change from time to time" (p. 933).

In the face of these competing definitions of community, McKnight (1987) rightly asks: "How will people know when they are in community?" (p. 57). He answers by arguing that communities are characterized by four features:

1. An emphasis on capacity as opposed to the deficiency approach of professionals

2. An informality, which often gives the appearance to professionals of communi-ties as "disordered, messy, and inefficient" (p. 58)

3. Community stories that "allow people to reach back into their common history and their individual experience for knowledge about truth and direction for the future," and which are often ignored and even threatened by professionals who want communities to "count up things rather than communicate" (p. 58)

4. The incorporation of celebration, tragedy, and fallibility into the life of the community

Inherent in the above characterization of community is a sense of connectedness, a sense that McKnight elaborates further when he goes on to describe community as

*the* social space *used by family, friends, neighbors, neighborhood associations, clubs, civic groups, local enterprises, churches, ethnic associations, temples, local unions, local government, and local media. In addition to being called the community, this social environment is also described as the informal sector, the unmanaged environ-ment, and the associational sector. (p. 56; emphasis added)*

These social spaces that McKnight names constitutes the mediating structures that intervene between the domain of the everyday life of individuals (the micro level) and the larger social/political/economic context within which these lives are lived out (the macro level). It could be argued that it is at the level of these mediating structures— that is, at the level of community—where the dialectical relationship between micro and macro forces discussed earlier happens, where they meet, produce, and reproduce each other. One aspect of the notion of capacity building, referred to earlier, is strength-ening individual membership in mediating structures—a micro level strategy that may be itself health enhancing (Leighton & Stone, 1974; Thomas, 1985). At the macro level, another aspect of capacity building is strengthening the ability of these mediating structures to participate in political and economic decisions, thereby enhancing the health of communities (McKnight, 1990).

Thus, the emphasis on community in the new health promotion movement is explicitly political. Glendon (1991) calls communities "the seedbeds of civic virtue" (p. 109). McKnight (1987) says that communities, as "the forum within which citizenship can be expressed," are "the vital center of democracy" (p. 57). The cornerstone of this political aspect of community is the notion of participation.

In embracing community participation, the new health promotion movement has pushed the field beyond the twin pillars of earlier, more traditional health promotion efforts: individual responsibility and professionally based interventions. However, there are still many unresolved issues surrounding the notion of community participation, both as a theory and as a practice, including: What does it mean for communities to participate in health promotion strategies to achieve health? How will we know when participation is occurring? Are there some forms of participation that are better than others?

Coming out of the social planning movement of the late 1960s, Sherry Arnstein (1969) developed a ladder of participation, adapted in Figure 23.1, by which the degree of participation could be measured. At the bottom of the ladder are manipulation and

## FIGURE 23.1    Ladder of Participation

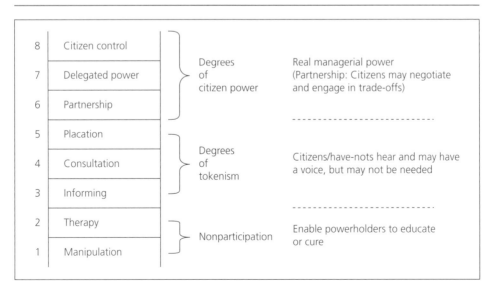

*Source:* Adapted from S. Arnstein, A ladder of citizen participation, *Journal of American Institute Planners,* July 1969.

tokenistic forms of participation. It could be argued that much of current health promotion practice, although using the rhetoric of community participation, in fact operates at these levels when professionals attempt to get people in the community to take ownership of a professionally defined health agenda. This occurs when professionals have decided to focus on particular health issues in a community—low birthweight or heart health, for example. Community participation in these instances often consists of the professionals convincing the community to take responsibility for and to carry out activities to address these issues, without the members of the community ever having decided whether these are the issues of interest to them. As Labonte (1990b) has pointed out, such an approach raises "the specter of using community resources primarily as free or cheaper forms of service delivery in which community participation is tokenistic, at best, and co-opted at worst" (p. 7).

Full community participation occurs when communities participate in equal partnership with health professionals in setting the health agenda—in defining their health problems and developing the solutions to address those problems. For that reason, Rifkin et al. (1988) offer the following definition of *community participation*:

> Community participation is a social process whereby specific groups with shared needs living in a defined geographic area actively pursue identification of their needs, take decisions and establish mechanisms to meet these needs. (p. 993)

If we accept the above definition of community participation, the role of professionals must be carefully reexamined. In the new health promotion movement, the role of the professional is recast from that of an expert who defines the community's needs and provides the solutions through professionally oriented strategies to that of a consultant to the community; someone who, in the Alinsky (1972) tradition, facilitates the mobilization of the community by providing technical and informational support. Rather than service provider and client, the community and the professionals are equal partners in setting the health agenda for the community. Within this view, the capacity of communities is facilitated by health education and health promotion efforts that strengthen the ability of those social units that we have called mediating structures—families, networks, neighborhoods—to identify and meet the needs of its members (McKnight, 1990; Eng, Hatch, & Callan, 1985). Such capacity building further may involve facilitating processes whereby disparate groups within a given community are enabled to interact more closely and effectively, ideally achieving some joint community problem-solving as a consequence of their collaboration (Brown, 1987).

Although we consider the shift in emphasis from a preeminent role for professionals to the need for a central role for communities to be a welcome change in the field of health promotion, we must also consider the question, Has the tyranny of the professional been replaced by me tyranny of community? As Hoffman (1989) has suggested, there may be a tendency in the community health promotion movement either to simplify or to romanticize the notion of community, "not only its unity and desire for service, but its degree of support for political action" (p. 197).

Communities are not homogeneous. In any geographical community there may be several diverse communities of interest. Rather than generating consensus, a community focus may, in fact, generate conflict and confrontation (Reynolds & Norman, 1988). Such "dis-sensus" has been witnessed in the United States, for example, where efforts have been made to mobilize low income communities around experimental needle exchange programs designed to reduce the spread of AIDS among intravenous drug users. With parts of the community heavily invested in needle exchange as a literal matter of life and death, and others arguing that such programs not only break the law but also condone and encourage drug use, efforts to achieve community cooperation and consensus on needle exchange programs have been fraught with difficulty.

Besides the local community, moreover, there are other stakeholders related to health promotion that constitute communities or "publics." The fact of these multiple stakeholders increases still further the likelihood of conflict over perceived health needs and resources, and hence over the formulation of health promotion policies and strategies. Among these other publics, which must be considered in public or community participation, are recipients of service; middle and upper income groups, the main supporters of public health as taxpayers; medical and other health providers; the media, which shape the perception of community issues; public policy makers; and public health workers (Minkler, 1990).

The dangers in casting communities as homogeneous entities and ignoring these diverse constituencies is that, as Farrant (1991) observes, there is "little encouragement to systematically analyze power relations within and between communities" (p. 431). As long as policy makers determine resource allocation, as long as the media play such a large role in shaping public attitudes and consumer choices, as long as business, industry, and the upper income groups have a loud voice in what happens and does not happen in the policy arena, these other publics must be a critical focal point for health promotion efforts. For example, health education and health promotion professionals are in a critical position to show these other publics that community coalitions comprised primarily of professionals and, at best, a handful of community residents with the time and energy—and, more importantly, a sense of personal power and efficacy—to devote to such work are unlikely to reflect the needs and interests of the most vulnerable and disenfranchised members of the community.

For these reasons, the notion of community participation implies a more politicized role for professionals vis-à-vis the community (Labonte, 1990b, McKnight, 1992). However, this may be problematic for both professionals and the community. In her analysis of the community activist movement in health and social planning of the 1960s, Lily Hoffman (1989) found that when community groups were politically radical, they often sought to use activist professionals and their services to gain power for their own ends. For their part, communities claimed that the adoption of political roles on the part of professionals deprived them of power, and that professionals who were politically radical were often found to be professionally conservative both with regard to defining the contents of services and in sharing expertise and control.

The new health promotion places a great emphasis on communities identifying their own needs and strategies to meet those needs. In general, this represents a welcome shift in health promotion practice. However, an unintended consequence of embracing the notion of community participation is that communities may assess social problems and propose solutions that reflect racism, sexism, ageism, or other problematic and divisive approaches. One only has to look at the anti-gay rights groups in Colorado and Oregon, for example, that recently sought to amend human rights legislation by removing the prohibition to discriminate against gays and lesbians in housing, employment, and other areas to see such troubling community mobilization at work. Indeed, in the study referred to above, Hoffman (1989) found that professionals were often disillusioned with the political and social conservatism of communities. The flip side of communities being co-opted by professional agendas is the potential for professionals to be used by communities to accomplish certain exclusionary agendas, such as the isolation of persons with AIDS, for example (Kirp, 1989). This may raise ethical and moral issues for health promotion practitioners when the agenda of the community conflicts with the larger agenda of equity and social justice.

Finally, health promotion practitioners must be ever vigilant that community participation, like the notion of empowerment, is not used as part of the rhetoric to justify budget cuts in professional and direct services. Using the rhetoric of community participation, medical providers may retreat from responsibility to improve health care institutions, and public officials may retreat from responsibility to regulate providers. As true partners with the community, health promotion practitioners may find themselves advocating for more direct individual services, more medical care facilities, and more health care providers. Brown's case study (1983–1984) of the role of health educators and other health professionals who worked alongside community members to fight the proposed closure of several county hospitals in California during the early 1980s provides an excellent example of such advocacy. Far from disempowering communities, moreover, this effort succeeded both in helping prevent several of the proposed closures, and in demonstrating to low income community members the efficacy of collective action.

## CONCLUSION

In the interests of not substituting one tyranny for another, the intent of this paper was to examine critically the new health promotion movement. To that end, we have discussed in detail the theoretical and practice implications of the concepts that form the building blocks of the new health promotion—namely, the reconceptualization of health, the concept of empowerment, and community participation.

We have argued that much of what continues to be contested in terms of concepts like empowerment and community participation, as well as the very notion of health, results from their multidimensionality. Broader socialized definitions of health, although taking into account, the social, political, and economic factors that affect health— thereby expanding the scope of what constitutes health promotion—may place the realization of health further out of the reach of many people by increasing its potential for commodification and obfuscation. As we have argued, the adoption by the new health promotion movement of a unidimensional notion of empowerment may obscure the interdependence of individual empowerment and collective empowerment. Finally, the rush to embrace community participation may lead to an over-idealized view of community solidarity and, in addition, may inadvertently subvert needed professionally based, direct services.

In health education and health promotion, empowerment provides the link between health and community participation both conceptually and in practice. Health, broadly defined as a resource for everyday life, is a desired outcome of empowerment strategies at both the individual and community levels. Similarly, high-level community participation, which increases capacity on the individual and community levels, is both an effective empowerment strategy and an outcome of empowerment.

We do not argue for a single framework to embrace notions of health, empowerment, and community participation. Rather, our intent was to make explicit the multiplicity of meanings surrounding these concepts, thereby revealing their inherent contestedness. Indeed, we suggest that to ignore the extent to which these concepts continue to be contested is to underestimate their power for analysis and practice. We suggest that the field of health education and health promotion is advanced by bringing these issues into open discussion.

One of the issues not addressed in this paper, and which needs to be addressed in future analyses, is the whole area of research. How are we to evaluate the effectiveness of the new health promotion movement? As McLeroy, Steckler, Goodman, and Bordine (1992) note with respect to health education, "whether labeled as capacity building, empowerment, or other terms, what is missing from our literature are methods for measuring changes in problem solving ability at various levels of analysis" (p. 2). In a similar vein, health practitioners who advocate the new health promotion cannot continue to implement these strategies simply because they sound good. Rather, practitioners must be able to demonstrate that the approaches advocated indeed do achieve more health and social benefits for more people than previous approaches. Otherwise, how will we know if anything has changed with respect to health promotion other than the language we use to talk and write about it?

Finally, proponents of the new health promotion must continue to scrutinize themselves, their theory, and their practice. Medicalized versions of health and individual lifestyle health promotion efforts represent stable knowledge domains with their own language, theories, and experts who possess specific skills. The new health promotion movement emerged as a new knowledge domain by challenging these existing domains and has created its own language and theories and experts. For the new health promotion not to become itself another imperialistic ideology, we must heed the warning of John McKnight (1992b) when he writes, "the possibility of health in a modern society depends upon our ability to free the idea of health from its subordination to managed, commodified and curricularized activities" (p. 3). As health professionals committed to the promotion of health, we must be vigilant that the new health promotion is not just a revolution in professional discourse, not just another tyranny.

## REFERENCES

Alinsky, S. (1972). *Rules for radicals*. New York: Random House.

Arnstein, S. (1969, July). A ladder of citizen participation. *Journal of American Institute Planners*, pp. 216–224.

Beauchamp, D. (1976). Public health as social justice. *Inquiry 12*, 2–14.

Becker, M. (1986). The tyranny of health promotion. *Public Health Review 14*, 15–23.

Bellah, R. N. (1991). *The good society*. New York: Knopf.

Berger, P. L., & Neuhaus, R. J. (1977). *To empower people: The role of mediating structures in public policy*. Washington, DC: American Enterprise Institute for Public Policy Research.

Binney, E. A., & Estes, C. L. (1988). The retreat of the state and its transfer of responsibility: The intergenerational war. *Journal of Health Services, 18*, 83–96.

Brown, E. R. (1983–1984). Roles for health educators in a time of health care cutbacks: Preventive and ameliorative approaches. *International Quarterly of Community Health Education, 4*, 298–302.

Brown, L. D. (1987). Small intervention for large problems: Reshaping urban leadership networks. *Journal of Applied Behavioral Science, 23*, 151–168.

Cottrell, L. S. (1983). The competent community. In R. Warren & L. Lyon (Eds.), *New perspectives on the American community*. Homewood, IL: Dorsey.

Driedger, F. D. (1989). *The last civil rights movement: Disabled peoples international*. New York: St. Martin's.

Duhl, L. (1986). The healthy city: Its function and its future. *Health Promotion 1*, 55–60.

Ehrenreich, B., & English, D. (1990) The sexual politics of sickness. In P. Conrad & R. Kern (Eds.), *The sociology of health and illness: Critical perspectives*. New York: St. Martin's.

Eng, E., Hatch, J., & Callan, A. (1985). Institutionalizing social support through the church and into the community. *Health Education Quarterly, 12*, 81–92.

Estes, C. L. (1984). Austerity and aging: 1980 and beyond. In M. Minkler & C. L. Estes (Eds.), *Readings in the political economy of aging*. Farmingdale, NY: Bay wood.

Farrant, W. L. (1991). Addressing the contradictions: Health promotion and community health action in the United Kingdom. *International Journal of Health Services, 21*, 423–439.

Foucault, M. (1977). *Knowledge/Power: Selected interviews and other writings*, 1972–1977. New York: Random House.

Freire, P. (1973). *Education for critical consciousness*. New York: Seabury Press.

Freire, P. (1988). *Pedagogy of the oppressed*. New York: Continuum.

French, M. (1986). *Beyond power: On women, men and morals*. London: Abacus.

Gallagher, D. A. (1989). Depression and other negative affects in family caregivers. In E. Light & B. D. Lebowitz (Eds.), *Alzheimer's disease treatment and family stress: Directions for research*. Rockville, MD: U.S. Department of Health and Human Services, Public Health Service.

Glendon, M. A. (1991). *Rights talk: The impoverishment of political discourse*. New York: Free Press.

Gruber, J., & Trickett, E. J. (1987). Can we empower others: The paradox of empowerment in the governing of an alternative public school. *American Journal of Community Psychology, 15*, 353–371.

Gutierrez, L. M. (1990). Working with women of color: An empowerment perspective. *Social Work, 35*, 149–153.

Haan, M., Kaplan, G. A., & Camacho, T. (1987). Poverty and health: Prospective evidence from the Alameda County study. *American Journal of Epidemiology, 125*, 989–998.

Hancock, T. (1986). Lalonde and beyond: Looking back at "a new perspective on the health of Canadians" *Health Promotion 1*, 93–100.

Health & Welfare Canada. (1986). *Achieving health for all: A framework for health promotion*. Ottawa: Government of Canada.

Hoffman, L. (1989). *The politics of knowledge in medicine and planning*. Albany, NY: State University of New York Press.

Jackson, T., Mitchell, S., & Wright, M. (1989). The community development continuum. *Community Health Studies, 13*, 66–73.

Kirp, D. (1989). *Learning by heart: AIDS and schoolchildren in America's communities*. New Brunswick, NJ: Rutgers University Press.

Labonte, R. (1986). Social inequality and healthy public policy. *Health Promotion 1*, 341–351.

Labonte, R. (1989). Community empowerment: Reflections on the Australian situation. *Community Health Studies, 13*, 347–349.

Labonte, R. (1990a). Community empowerment: The need for political analysis. *Canadian Journal of Public Health, 80*, 87–88.

Labonte, R. (1990b). Empowerment: Notes on professional and community dimensions. *Canadian Review of Social Policy, 26*, 1–12.

Labonte, R. (1992). *Empowerment*. Keynote address to American Public Health Association annual conference, October.

Leighton, D. C., & Stone, I. T. (1974). Community development as a therapeutic force: A case study with measurement. In P. M. Roman & H. M. Trice (Eds.), *Sociological perspectives on community mental health*. Philadelphia: Davis.

Marmot, M. G., Rose, G., Shipley, M., & Hamilton, P. J. S. (1978). Employment grade and coronary heart disease in British civil servants. *Journal of Epidemiology and Community Health, 3*, 244–249.

McKnight, J. (1987, Winter). Regenerating community. *Social Policy*, pp. 54–58.

McKnight, J. (1990). Politicizing health care. In P. Conrad & R. Kern (Eds.), *The sociology of health and illness: Critical perspectives*. New York: St. Martin's.

McKnight, J. (1992a). *Collaboration in the multicultural community: Turning adversity into empowerment*. Keynote presentation at the inaugural symposium for the Center for Community Health, Oakland, CA, October 2.

McKnight, J. L. (1992b). *Demedicalization and the possibilities of health*. Unpublished manuscript.

McLeroy, D., Steckler, A. B., Goodman, R. M., & Bordine, J. N. (1992). Health education research: Theory and practice, future directions. *Health Education Research, 7*, 1–8.

McMillan, D. W., & Chavis, D. M. (1986). Sense of community: A definition and theory. *Journal of Community Psychology, 14*, 6–23.

Milio, N. (1981). *Promoting health through public policy*. Philadelphia: F. A. Davis.

Miller, M. (1985). *Turning problems into actionable issues*. Unpublished report. Organize Training Center.

Miller, S. (1990). Race in America. In P. R. Lee & C. L. Estes (Eds.), *The nation's health*. Boston: Jones and Bartlett.

Mills, C. W. (1959). *The sociological imagination*. New York: Oxford University Press.

Minkler, M. (1990). *Public participation in health promotion*. Keynote address at the Summer Institute on Citizen Participation in Health Promotion, University of Manitoba, Winnipeg, Manitoba.

Moody, H. R. (1988). Abundance of life: Human development policies for an aging society. In A. Monk (Ed.), *Columbia studies of social gerontology and aging*. New York: Columbia University Press, 1988.

O'Neill, M. (1990). Community participation in Quebec's system: A strategy to curtail community empowerment? In *Proceedings of International Symposium on Community Participation and Empowerment Strategies in Health Promotion*. Bielefeld, Federal Republic of Germany, Center for Interdisciplinary Studies, University of Bielefeld, June 5–9.

Pilisuk, M., & Minkler, M. (1986). The social and economic constraints upon social support: Reexamining a panacea. *Health Education Quarterly, 12*, 93–106.

Pinderhughes, E. B. (1983, June). Empowerment for our clients and for ourselves. *Social Casework*, pp. 331–338.

Rappaport, J. (1985). The power of empowerment language. *Social Policy, 16*, 15–21.

Ratcliffe, J. (1978). Social justice and the demographic transition: Lessons from India's Kerala state. *International Journal of Health Services, 8*, 123–144.

Reynolds, C. H., & Norman, R. V. (eds.). (1988). *Community in America: The challenge of* Habits of the heart. Berkeley, CA: University of California Press.

Rifkin, S. B., Muller, F., & Bichmann, W. (1988). Primary health care: On measuring participation. *Social Science and Medicine, 29*, 931–940.

Schwartz, R. (1990). Commentary: Beware of the co-optation of self-help and empowerment. *SOPHE News Views, 17*, 3.

Shor, I., & Freire, P. (1987). *A pedagogy for liberation: Dialogues on transforming education.* South Hadley, MA: Begin & Garvey.

Siler-Wells, G. L. (1989). Challenge of the Gordian knot: Strengthening community health in Canada. In *Proceedings of International Symposium on Community Participation and Empowerment Strategies in Health Promotion.* Bielefeld, Federal Republic of Germany, Center for Interdisciplinary Studies, University of Bielefeld, June 5–9.

Simon, B. L. (1990). Rethinking empowerment. *Journal of Progressive Human Services, 1*, 27–39.

Syme, S. L. (1986). Social determinants of health and disease. In J. M. Last (Ed.), *Public health and preventive medicine.* Norwalk, CT: Appleton-Century-Crofts.

Syme, S. L., & Berkman, L. F. (1976). Social class, susceptibility and sickness. *American Journal of Epidemiology, 104*, 1–8.

Tesh, S. (1988). *Hidden arguments: Political ideology and disease prevention policy.* New Brunswick, NJ: Rutgers University Press.

Thomas, P. D. (1985). Effect of social support on stress-related changes in cholesterol level, uric acid level, and immune function in an elderly sample. *American Journal of Psychiatry, 142*, 735–737.

Wallerstein, N. (1992). Powerlessness, empowerment, and health: Implications for health promotion programs. *American Journal of Health Promotion, 6*, 197–205.

Wang, C. (1992). Culture, meaning and disability: Injury prevention campaigns and the production of stigma. *Social Science and Medicine, 35*, 1093–1102.

World Health Organization. (1984). *Report of the Working Group on the Concept and Principles of Health Promotion.* Copenhagen: WHO.

World Health Organization. (1986a). A discussion document on the concept and principles of health promotion. *Health Promotion, 1*, 73–78.

World Health Organization. (1986b). *Ottawa charter for health promotion.* Copenhagen: WHO.

Ann Robertson and Meredith Minkler, "New Health Promotion Movement: A Critical Examination," *Health Education & Behavior* (Volume 21, Issue 3), pp. 295–312, copyright © 1994 by SOPHE. Reprinted by Permission of SAGE Publications.

# CHAPTER

## 24

# POTENTIAL UNTAPPED: HEALTH EDUCATION AND HEALTH PROMOTION AS A MEANS TO PEACE

**DANIEL LEVITON**

Even before the terrorist attack by the al Qaeda on September 11th, the Four Horsemen of the Apocalypse (famine, pestilence, disease, and death) rode high in their saddle. Today, their threat to health is greater than ever before. The existence of and willingness to use weapons of mass destruction make it so. Today, the United States and its allies are in a conflict to bring to justice the murderers responsible for September 11th. Eventually, insuring the peace and the prevention of subsequent terrorist and similar killing events (peacekeeping) will take priority over peacemaking (that is, ending the conflict).

This article strongly suggests that health education and health promotion (HEHP) must contribute to peacekeeping and possibly peacemaking. With peace, health prevails. Terrorism, war, and other forms of people-caused, preventable deaths—what I call Horrendous Death (HD)—are antithetical to health and to peace. Peace is more than the absence of war. It is a way of living together in social harmony enhancing the health and well-being of the planet and its inhabitants. It is a natural and necessary undertaking for HEHP because "peace . . . simply and powerfully constitutes the only background under which human life can evolve and prosper" (Gonzalez-Vallejo & Sauveur, 1998, p. 17). It is in our best interest to do so if we wish our children and other loved ones to live both long and well.

The twentieth century has been characterized as the era of violence (Tuchman, 1981), and more recently by Kofi Annan, secretary-general of the United Nations, as a time of anxiety and insecurity (News Service, 2001). Anxiety implies a dread over what can be. It is future oriented. We think, "When will the other shoe drop?" People wonder if a subsequent terrorist attack will involve clean or dirty nuclear weapons, smallpox virus or worse. Will entire populations be annihilated? Will the future find us continually engaged in a "clash of civilizations" between modern, democratic, technology-oriented states, and states that are undeveloped and governed by extremist, fundamentalist, militant theocracies (Huntington, 1995) (1)? Will the twenty-first century be one of globalization in the very best sense of the word? That is, with a concern for establishing a peaceful environment and improving the quality of life for all? Or will the expansion of economic markets with their demand for increased productivity, and profits be the over riding goal? HEHP needs to be concerned with these questions.

My particular approach to peace is to prevent HD. I take the dogmatic position that anything that prevents premature mortality, morbidity, and suffering falls under the purview of HEHP, and is its responsibility (see Leviton, 1969a, 1969b, 1976a, 1976b, 1977). In May 1999 I placed the following on the HEDIR Internet discussion group:

> Let me offer an irreverent thought. Maybe if we health educators/health promoters took on the tough issues and problems plaguing our society, and the world in general, our image would be improved. For example, we say that we are concerned primarily with "prevention" of that which predicts ill health and premature mortality. Note that poverty, and the disparity between the economic haves and have nots predict a host of health problems ranging from [diseases such as tuberculosis, HIV/AIDS], premature mortality (say, homicide), morbidity, and suffering. They are "root causes." Yet it is rare to see our profession standing up and demanding that poverty and income inadequacy be eliminated. In fact, I haven't seen it raised as a national issue (and disgrace) since LBJ's War on Poverty .  . . . In my opinion, the public will better recognize and respect us [as a profession] when we make an impact on the tough but often controversial issues.

> Implicit in my remarks are the notions of "greatest health risk and/or threat," and "the greatest good for the greatest number." Anything that is a significant health risk/ threat should be cause enough for our involvement. One really doesn't need any specialized training to teach, research, and advocate in this area. In fact the methodology of health (that is, preventive intervention, epidemiology, etc.) provides a fine frame of reference. The people who have done the best writing, research, and/or been the most effective advocates on poverty, war, etc. do not have graduate degrees in these areas. For example, American Public Health Association leaders, Barry Levy and Victor

*Sidel, co-editors of War and Public Health (Levy & Sidel, 1997) are public health physicians. However, they are motivated, and knowledgeable in their area of interest. Believe me, if you wish to become knowledgeable the literature is out there.*

In this article I will discuss how awareness of HD (for example, death resulting from terrorism) might positively affect our view of health and our role as HEHP professionals. I will integrate themes of thanatology (2) (for example, denial of death, anticipatory grief, expectations of and for the future, and death as a motivator to action), public policy (for example, globalization, economics, and forms of governing), and public health, health education and health promotion (for example, epidemiology, education, prevention, and causation).

## WHAT IS HORRENDOUS DEATH (HD)?

Today [2002] we are threatened by terrorism. However, there are other threats to the quality of individual and global health, and peace. I group them under the heading Horrendous Death (HD) (Leviton, 2000b, 1991a, 1991b). HD is the umbrella term given to deaths caused by people. Hence, it is preventable. This is its crucial distinction compared to deaths caused by, say, Nature. There are two types: HD-1, where the motivation is to kill others, and HD-2, where the motivation to kill is absent. Examples of the first are deaths resulting from terrorism, war, intentional environmental assaults, intentional famine, intentional chronic hunger and poverty, and intentional racism (lynching) and murder of other minority groups. Examples of the second are deaths resulting from accidents, environmental degradation, unintentional famine, misuse of tobacco, alcohol, and other drugs, unintentional chronic hunger, and poverty, and indirectly as a result of racism, drug use, etc. The focus of this article is on the HD-1.

Two forms of HD-1 make their prevention a great, if not the greatest, challenge for all institutions designed to promote civil and civilized life including HEHP. They are (1) systematic thermonuclear or bio-chemical warfare or terrorist attack, and (2) environmental assault and/or the more insidious environmental degradation. Either could result in global devastation that would make all previous and ongoing epidemics including the bubonic plague of the fourteenth century, influenza in 1918–1919, HIV/AIDS, famines, and previous wars pale by comparison (Leviton, 2000b). HD is globalization ad absurdum, and must be prevented. A process for accomplishing this will be discussed later.

## LIFEGENIC FACTORS

With an understanding of HD and Lifegenic Factors, Quality of Global Health (QGH) will be defined. Lifegenic Factors (LF) increase the probability of living long and well. Examples are

1. Meaningful education
2. Meaningful employment

3. Meaningful love and friendship relationships

4. Financial security

5. Quality health care

6. Opportunity for self-actualization

7. Opportunity for enjoyable recreation and play

8. Purpose and meaning in life

9. Opportunity to achieve spirituality needs

10. Opportunity to maximize health

11. Opportunity for artistic and creative expression

Quality of Global Health (QGH) may be defined as an equation: $QGH = LFmax/HDmin\ or\ elim$ where high quality of global health and well-being is equated with a minimum or absence of HD, and a maximum of LF. One could arguably substitute *peace* for QGH.

## THE HD, GLOBAL HEALTH, AND WELL-BEING CONCEPT (HDC)

Conceptualizing HD as a preventable cause of mortality, morbidity and suffering led to the HDC. It was consonant with the World Health Organization's definition of health that was broadened beyond the "absence of disease to include the concept of well-being." To one degree or another the health professions and their professional organizations began to show interest in the *individual forms of HD* but not HD as an entirety, a gestalt. The approach of governments (certainly, the United States) in developing policies concerning terrorism, war, homicide, and environmental degradation tend to be fragmented, and characterized by crisis management rather than prevention. It became apparent that a systematic *process* was needed to expedite the selection, integration, implementation, testing, evaluation, and modification of such life enhancing policies.

The HDC is an example. It is a *unifying* process designed to expedite the implementation of policies that would prevent HD by dealing with underlying, root causes and outcomes. Solid, research-driven policies exist, but are gathering dust on the shelves of think tanks, the United Nations, academic centers, governmental agencies, and non-governmental organizations.

In what way is the HDC a unifying process? Since no one is immune from HD-1, working toward its prevention and elimination may be a way of uniting the country and perhaps the world in common purpose. We see this happening in the post September 11th era, for example, the coalition fighting the al Qaeda terrorists, high public approval rating for the President, and an increased trust in government and the military. The driving force? At least three motivations come to mind.

1.  To prevent acts of terrorism from reoccurring. The same phenomena occurred during World War II, generally regarded as a *just war*. The nation came together. Prior to that, from about 1936 to 1941, the U.S. was, essentially, isolationist in its foreign policy, trying hard to avoid involvement in the war against fascism.

2.  The desire for retribution.

3.  Fear of the dying and death of oneself and loved ones that is premature and torturous. Its reciprocal is the desire to live long and well.

## THE PROCESS

The first step in the process is to remove the denial of mortality and vulnerability concerning ourselves and our loved ones. As mentioned earlier, no one, I repeat, no one expects to die, or really "knows" that their loved ones can die in the next moment due to war, homicide, terrorist act, accident, or other forms of HD—until it happens. I hypothesize that once a person survives an HD, or is the survivor-victim of a loved one's HD, that person is more likely to act to prevent others (including oneself) from dying in similar fashion. HD has become real rather than an abstraction.

The HDC focuses on the beloved—usually the child or grandchild—due to the powerful, protective bond of love that exists between parent and child but it could be any beloved including oneself, mate, or companion animal. Secondly, the death of a child is untimely, unexpected, and otherwise inappropriate. I hypothesize that when denial of the possible HD of any loved one or oneself is high, action to prevent HD is low. It is this denial that oneself or loved ones, especially the beloved child, can die in such brutal ways, that reduces the probability of action to prevent HD. Most of us rationalize that if a child dies in war or is murdered it will be the amorphous other. It will not be, and cannot be his or hers.

Several years ago at a conference at King's College in London, Ontario, I asked the president of the organization Parents of Murdered Children whether, in her wildest imagination, she would have predicted the murder of her child. Her response was "Never!" After her child was murdered, she started the organization. Prevention of murder had become salient for her. The same holds true for the founder of Mothers Against Drunk Drivers, and survivors of those killed on September 11th.

A second hypothesis is that the more horrible the type or style of dying and/or death is perceived, the greater the fear; the greater the fear, the greater the denial; and, the greater the denial, the less chance of action to eliminate the very causes of such torturous deaths. Low and high fear of HD are associated with low probability of action. For example, I fear dying of cancer in old age. I deny any symptoms such as the mole on my face that has increased in diameter by six inches in two days (hyperbole—forgive me). I fail to go to my physician until my wife threatens me with divorce.

But there are more terrifying forms of death that may not even apply to me. I fear my wife and children dying in war or acts of terror by burning to death. Or death by means of rape-evisceration-murder. Here my fear is much greater. The denial is immense. It cannot happen to my beloved. I take no preventive action.

## THE POWER OF DENIAL OF VULNERABILITY AND MORTALITY

I see the removal of the denial of HD as prerequisite to individual and group action. It is obvious that this scenario hovers between reality and denial. This may be part of the explanation of the reaction of Americans and others to September 11th. Remove the denial, and the HD issue becomes salient. Salience follows when there is identification with the dead, the dead-who-might-have been, and/or the dead-who-will-be.

My surveys of over 300 students and others show that the removal of denial by means of discussion, videotapes and film and mental imagery of HD events, increases the probability of self-efficacy. Close to 90 percent of students and other participants agree to take action, such as signing a petition, sending a letter to a congressperson, and joining or donating money to relevant organizations.

Several writers have linked denial with aspects of HD, notably war. For example, World War I disillusioned Freud. He was horrified by the eradication of the rules of civilized moral and social conduct, and the brutality with which men could inflict death and suffering upon people whether soldiers or civilians (Freud, 1968). How could people be so barbaric? His answer was psychological denial of personal death. "Our own death is indeed unimaginable," he wrote. "[A]t bottom no one believes in his own death, or to put the same thing in another way, in the unconscious every one of us is convinced of his own immortality" (Rickman, 1968, p. 15).

But it was Herman Feifel, a psychologist and the father of the modern thanatological movement, who first helped me see the link between thanatology and HD (3). As Freud saw repressed sexuality as a powerful factor explaining human behavior, so Feifel saw our repressed meanings given death. Feifel felt that fear of death was a powerful factor contributing to our denial of reality. In 1959 he wrote, hopefully, "if we accept death as a necessity…. This might possibly mute some of the violence of our times, for energies now bound up in continuing attempts to shelve and repress the concept of death would be available to us for the more constructive aspects of living, perhaps even fortifying man's gift for creative splendor against his genius for destruction" (Feifel, 1959, p. 12). Ernest Becker (1973) agreed when he wrote, several years later, that "This narcissism is what keeps men marching into point-blank fire in wars: at heart one doesn't feel he will die, he only feels sorry for the man next to him" (p. 2).

Yet, Lifton (1979) is correct when he observes, "And our resistance to that knowledge, our denial of death, is indeed formidable…. But the denial can never be total; we are never fully ignorant of the fact that we die. Rather we go about life with a kind of 'middle knowledge' of death, a partial awareness of it side by side with expressions and actions that belie that awareness" (p. 17). Removal of denial of HD is central to motivating people to act to eliminate terrorism and other forms of preventable death.

## ANTICIPATORY GRIEVING THE HD OF THE FANTASIZED BELOVED CHILD OR BELOVED OTHER

Once denial of HD of the child (or other beloved including oneself) is removed, and the imagery of the torturous death confronted, intentional anticipatory grieving must follow to increase the odds of preventive action. I will focus on death resulting from terrorist attack.

Such a death is different from, say, death by means of childhood cancer. For our purposes, the difference between anticipatory grieving of the fantasized and actual terrorist-caused death of one's child lies in the modification and channeling of anger and vengeance. Anger is usually directed toward God or Medicine if one's child dies of cancer. If the child is literally killed by terrorism, vengeance would be directed toward the killer, Osama bin Laden, members of al Qaeda, or the Taliban in general. Some would be able to channel their need for retribution toward more civilized, less violent means such as forgiveness, working toward negotiation and reconciliation, and other peace making behavior. Most, however, have yet to achieve control over such primal drives.

On the other hand, *anticipatory* grieving over the *fantasized HD* of the beloved child elicits screams, fear and trembling of what might be. Themes of hatred and vengeance toward the fantasized killer become subordinate to the need to prevent such a death, and to subsequently survive well. Thus, in my conceptual framework the probability of personal action to eliminate HD is thought to increase if the actor experiences the anticipatory grieving resulting from the imagery of the beloved, dead child killed by terrorist act or other form of HD.

## REPRESENTATIVES OF DOMAINS OF INFLUENCE AND POWER

Who are the actors in this drama powerful enough to implement existing policies that would improve the prospects of peace and improve the quality of global health? They are the representatives of the domains of influence and power. The domains are government, politics and law; finance; commerce; labor; the military; medicine and public health; religion; the media; education; science; philanthropy; non-governmental organizations (NGOs); and, the community, that is, the grass roots representation. Some are as powerful as government-politics-law. For example, in the United States, it would be nice to have the support of President Bush, Tom Daschel, and Trent Lott. However, the project would have a greater chance of success if influential and powerful people were involved like Alan Greenspan (central banking and finance), Bill Gates (industry), George Soros (finance and philanthropy), the Pope, and Jesse Jackson and others from the community. Once motivated their task is to recommend to the leaders of nation-states preventive policies, and the means to test, evaluate, and modify them.

No one person has the answer on how to prevent terrorism or HD. Others do. The expertise is out there. It needs to be organized and focused on the task. Again, a reminder: HD or terrorism is *not* caused by God, naturally occurring bacteria or virus, or Nature. They are caused by people. Thus they are preventable.

## MOTIVATION OF THE ACTORS INVOLVED IN THE HDC

Any plan of action must consider motivation. Why should the representatives of the domains and others participate in the HDC? Their loved ones and themselves are as vulnerable to HD as anyone else. Presidents, popes, and CEOs of multinational corporations have been murdered, killed by terrorists, and are poisoned by contaminated drinking air and water. It is in the best interest of all people, institutions, and domains to have a healthy and peaceful physical, psychological and social environment free from the threat of terrorist or other HD attack. No one is immune or safe from HD.

One personality type or motivation that escapes the HDC is the death of war lover (Fromm, 1973). Another is the true believer or religious fanatic (Hoffer, 1966). It is difficult enough to deal with extremist religious groups like the Aum Shinrikyo in Japan who released Sarin gas in a downtown Tokyo subway. They believed that by destroying the world and its corruption they were making it a better place. This is the apocalyptic, Armageddon view of the world, a cornerstone of belief among extreme fundamentalists groups in any country, and of any religion. Combine religious fanaticism with hatred directed toward the non-believer and/or oppressor, and the problem is compounded. The members of al Qaeda, and most of the Taliban represent the latter.

On the other hand, the HDC should appeal to the motivation of nearly all others. For example, if one is motivated by altruism, that is, wishes to improve the world for future generations, the HDC should make sense. At the other extreme, the individual motivated by greed and the acquisition of possessions usually wishes to leave a legacy to his or her children and grandchildren. And if they are not alive? What, then, is the benefit of wealth and power? One has to be alive to use either. Similarly, if hedonism is the predominant drive, the individual must be alive and well to enjoy pleasure. Suppose one is motivated by fear of death or annihilation? Then removal of HD should offer some relief.

## UNDERLYING ROOT CAUSES

Policy and other action designed to prevent any form of HD-1 must recognize and address underlying root causes. Again, I focus on the al Qaeda. There is general agreement across the political spectrum that removing the underlying root causes are vital to preventing terrorism and other forms of HD-1 (Armstrong, 2002; Friedman, 2001; News Service, 2001; Rice, 2001; Useem, 2001; World Bank, 2001). They include poverty, hunger, illiteracy, and totalitarian and repressive regimes. Two related factors are a culture that sees modernity as anathema, and where the ruling class is a fanatical, fundamentalist theocracy.

Michael Renner (2000), writing about conflicts in general, also wrote of underlying causes.

> *The second challenge is to understand and address the underlying causes of today's conflicts. Those causes unquestionably included the continuing perpetuation of massive social and economic inequalities, ethnic tensions, population pressures, and environmental degradation. These phenomena appear to be accelerating in many societies, even as governance structures falter. Left unaddressed, it is likely that they will force heightened polarization and instability, which would trigger even more widespread violent conflict. (p. 39)*

Armstrong (2002) also emphasizes the need to address causes in the conflict against the al Qaeda.

> *Even as President Bush and our allies succeed in eliminating the threat posed by Osama bin Laden and his al Qaeda network, hundreds more terrorists will rise up to take their place unless we in the West address the* root cause *of this hatred [my emphasis]. This task must be an essential part of the war against terrorism. (pp. 45–46)*

I disagree. My view is that the hatred of al Qaeda and the Islamists toward the U.S. is so strong that the best policy is two pronged: Address historical grievances, but also speak softly and carry a big stick. I do not feel confident that redressing every perceived and real wrong would eliminate the enmity of the Islamists. On the other hand, if we are to develop permanent rapprochement and friendship with the larger Arab moderate majority, Armstrong's recommendations are a must.

In summary, the HDC is a unifying concept and process where the goal is improving the quality of global health by specifically preventing HD. The process involves removal of the denial of personal vulnerability and mortality, and anticipatory grieving of the beloved that lead to preventive actions. Actions that implement preventive policies sensitive to the underlying root causes of HD. Next to be considered are the barriers that inhibit the attainment of peace and the prevention of HD.

## BARRIERS TO PEACE AND THE PREVENTION OF HD

Barriers exist that reduce the probability of preventing HD. Before discussion a reminder that the world is made up of shades of gray. There is good, bad, and in between, and a waffling between the three. Some barriers are

1. Economic exploitation by the corporate domain at the expense of the health and well-being of people, and the ecosystem. Capitalism is responsible for improving

our standard of living, providing jobs, and earning income for corporation share-holders, in its charge to produce goods, services, and profit (4). I do not expect corporations to become humanitarian. Those that do are to be commended (for an example of one compassionate and caring company see McGrory, 2001). What can be done to control the exploitive, immoral and unethical aspects of the corpo-ration, and economic globalization? Enact preventive laws with teeth that would prevent malpractice at the national, international and global levels. An example? A global liveable wage.

Nationally, campaign financing and lobbying laws, and regulations reform should be welcomed. They would diminish the influence of the corporate world on lawmakers. At the international level, support for the United Nations to serve as an instrument of surveillance, and early warning, and conflict resolution would be beneficial. Globally? Provide teeth to the World Federalist slogan of "world peace through world law" by strengthening the World Court.

2.  If population growth, especially, in poor countries, is related to HD and dis-ease, then the Catholic Church needs to reformulate its dogma concerning birth control.

3.  If the media are increasingly owned and controlled by large corporations then news may become propaganda. The answer is to read and watch both main-stream and non-mainstream media. Read columnists who, themselves, are not celebrities and part of the establishment. For example, I find the commentary of Noam Chomsky, the MIT linguistics professor, to be brilliant. He publishes in Z *Magazine*.

4.  The herd effect, the failure to think independently, is another barrier to peace. Janis coined the expression *groupthink* (Janis, 1982a). His research showed how some advisors to the President Kennedy were afraid to counsel against the Bay of Pigs invasion even though they knew it would be disastrous. Another example: Once the war drums start beating the pressure to conform is tremendous. All German social classes participated in the conduct of the Holocaust with special reference to the "pillars of society": physicians, PhDs, lawyers, architects, and other professionals (Friedlander, 1995). Robert Lifton wrote of the psychological processes (such as psychic numbing, psychic splitting, conformity, and rational-ization) that allowed many Nazi physicians to participate in the torture and exe-cution of over six million people—to rationalize their Hippocratic Oath to save life and prevent suffering. Affectionate fathers and husbands, and accomplished in their professional field—on one hand, and on the other—mass killers (Lifton, 1986; Lifton & Markusen, 1990). They all conformed to Nazi ideology.

5.  The last barrier is faulty education. In my opinion the goals of education should be to learn a trade or profession; develop knowledge, insight, and wisdom; and encourage activism for the common good. Education benefits from a world rather

than a parochial view. Ignorance breeds ethnocentrism and jingoism, that, in turn are predictors of violence.

The present day movement toward service-learning is a step in the right direction. An example is The Adult Health & Development Program at the University of Maryland (AHDP), and its spread to fifteen other colleges and universities. They are intergenerational service-learning health promotion programs. One goal of the AHDP is to "contribute to peace, social harmony and well-being by bringing people together of diverse backgrounds, ethnic/racial roots, health and well-being and socio-economic status, to enjoy one another while reducing the probability of violence" (Leviton, 1998, 2000a; Leviton & Millar, 2002).

## PART OF THE PROCESS: UNDERSTANDING HISTORY AND CULTURE

If we would have a permanent peace the history and culture of other states must be understood. A crucial question is, Why are we hated? Karen Armstrong's suggestion is for people, Americans and others living in developed, modern states, to become more global in our view of the world and less isolationist. We need to understand the history of Islam, other states and their cultures (5). In my view that understanding comes about through knowledge, empathy, and results in ameliorative actions that insure peace.

In accepting the Nobel Peace Prize, Kofi Annan, the secretary-general of the United Nations, spoke of one world where each state's well-being is inextricably linked with others. He said:

> We have entered the third millennium through a gate of fire.... If today, after the horror of 11 September, we see better and we see further, we will realize that humanity is indivisible. New threats make no distinction between races, nations or regions. A new insecurity has entered every mind, regardless of wealth or status.... Today, no walls can separate humanitarian or human rights crises in one part of the world from national security crises in another...What begins with the failure to uphold the dignity of one life, all too often ends with a calamity for entire nations. (News Service, 2001)

## THE RISE AND HOPE OF GLOBALISM

Global trade policies and the search for markets, highly controversial as they are, killed isolationism. Early on President George W. Bush and his administration were perceived as advocating a unilateralist approach to international policy. It, too, became an anachronism as the need for international cooperation between states became urgent, that is, the Coalition. The formation of the Coalition exemplified an international response to a global problem. Globalism, in the best sense of the word, is similar to what Michael Hardt and Antonio Negri (2000) call "Empire":

> Our basic hypothesis is that sovereignty has taken a new form, comprised of a series of national and supranational organisms united under a single logic of rule. The new global form of sovereignty is what we call Empire . . . . The passage to Empire emerges from the twilight of modern sovereignty. In contrast to imperialism, Empire establishes no territorial center of power and does not rely on fixed boundaries or barriers. It is a decentered and deterritorializing apparatus of rule that progressively incorporates the entire global realm within its open expanding frontiers. Empire manages hybrid identities, flexible hierarchies, and plural exchanges through modulating networks of command. The distinct national colors of the imperialist map of the world have merged and blended in the imperial global rainbow. (pp. xiii–xiv)

Themes concerned with the development of global and international order and unity are not new. They can be traced back to the Peace of Westphalia and the Napoleonic Wars (Hardt & Negri, 2000). More contemporary examples are the short-lived League of Nations following World War I, the United Nations, the World Court, the World Federalist movement (still alive and espousing world peace through world law), and the Open Society founded by financier and philanthropist George Soros (1991, 2000) following World War II.

Eventually the present conflict will wind down. When it will end, who knows? The caveat—as long as Islamists feel that the United States and other secular states must be defeated regardless of its good intentions and reconciling, peaceful actions then the conflict will probably continue. Reconstruction, and a coming together of states, in peace, will likely occur as long as they see it as being in their best economic, health, religious, and well-being interests. To that end the wealthier, developed nations will have to cooperate to insure the well-being of underdeveloped and developing nations. Civilized states function best in a peaceful environment.

## UNDERSTANDING THE HISTORY OF ISLAM AND ISLAMISM

To wage peace insight and understanding of the "other's" history and culture are necessary for successful action. The history of Islam, itself, is one of constant wars, exploitation, and colonization. After the death of the Prophet Muhammad in 632, the Muslims ruled an empire that stretched from the Himalayas to the Pyrenees. By the fifteenth century, Islam was the greatest world power—similar to the United States (Armstrong, 2000).

Beginning in the twelfth century, the Christian nations of the West united to invade and ravage the Islamic states in one of the bloodiest eras known—the five holy wars known as the Crusades (Armstrong, 2000; Reston, 2001). They were initiated, in the name of Christianity, by Pope Urban II, in 1095 "as a measure to redirect the energies of warring European barons from their bloody, local disputes into a 'noble' quest to reclaim the Holy Land from the 'infidel'" (Reston, 2001, p. xiii).

Only the First Crusade managed to occupy Jerusalem—the rest were failures including the Third Crusade (1187–1192) that pitted Richard I of England (known as Lionheart) against Saladin, the sultan of Egypt, Syria, Arabia, and Mesopotamia (Reston, 2001). Saladin emerged a legend from that conflict. His heroic replacement is still awaited by Muslims to conquer the enemy. Every Muslim leader, including Gamal Abdel Nasser, Saddam Hussein, and Yasir Arafat, has evoked the image of Saladin in an effort to unite the Arab states in common purpose.

The Crusades, themselves, were a study of arrogance and religious fanaticism. James Reston Jr.'s description of the carnage sounds like the aftermath of Nazi Germany. He writes that "once unleashed, the passion could not be controlled. The violence began with the massacre of the Jews, proceeded to the wholesale slaughter of Muslims in their native land, sapped the wealth of Europe, and ended with the almost unimaginable death toll on all sides" (Reston, 2001, p. xiii). Centuries later, in 2000, Pope John Paul II issued a sweeping apology for all the sins committed by the Roman Church in the name of religion over the past 2000 years (Reston, 2001). For the Muslim population in the Middle East, the admission of horrible wrongdoing was cause for celebration because the Crusades had finally received equal billing with the Holocaust (Reston, 2001).

Reston explains that the Christian Holy War was evoked the Muslim response of *jihad*. It is, by definition, a defensive concept, provoked by an unbelieving aggressor. He notes with some irony that the word *jihad* strikes fear in the hearts of Westerners as it is associated with terrorism and Islamic fanaticism. "But," he writes, "there is nothing in Islamic history that rivals the terror of the Crusades or the Christian fanaticism of the twelfth century" (Reston, 2001, p. xix).

Another burr in the saddle of Muslims was the improvement in the quality of life of the West. Armstrong notes that the Islamic world could not keep up with the Great Western Transformation. The West had three hundred years to modernize; the Islamic world, fifty. Only Japan was able to modernize quickly but it had never been colonized. Most of the Islamic states remained agrarian, illiterate, and poor as the West embraced technology and development. Technology requires an educated population to man its machines, teach, and sell its products. An educated people demanded participatory democracy and democratic institutions.

With power, wealth, and modern armies, the West colonized the Arab states. In any master-subordinate relationship the self-concept of the latter is lessened, and characterized by smoldering hatred of the ruler (Armstrong, 2000).

The enmity toward secularism was exacerbated when, following World War II, the Allies agreed to the Zionist demand for a Jewish state, and partitioned Palestine as restitution for the horrible suffering of the Jews at the hands of the Axis powers (that is, the Holocaust). There was little concern that Palestine was the homeland of the Muslims living there, and their reverence for Jerusalem as a holy city. The price paid is that the United States, the chief sponsor of Israel, and the industrialized West in general, are seen as modern crusaders (6).

There are other wounds that promulgate hatred in the Islamic world such as the U.S.'s foreign policy, since the end of World War II. Our support of dictators and authoritarian, repressive regimes under two conditions come to mind. Our support was a given if access to oil was involved, and/or a policy of fervent anti-Communism was in place. Examples of our support of dictators include replacing the hated Shah Muhammad Reza Pahlavi on the throne after he had been deposed and forced to leave Iran in 1953. Saddam Hussein, who became the president of Iraq in 1979, was also a protégée of the United States, which literally allowed him to get away with the chemical attack against the Kurdish population (Armstrong, 2002).

Add to this our support of unpopular rulers, such as President Hosni Mubarak of Egypt, and the Saudi royal family. Indeed, Osama bin Laden was a protégée of the West, which was happy to support and fund his fighters in the struggle for Afghanistan against Soviet Russia. Too often the Western powers have taken a crudely short-term view without considering their long-term consequences. After the Soviets had pulled out of Afghanistan, for example, no help was forthcoming for the devastated country, whose ensuing chaos made it possible for the Taliban to come to power (Armstrong, 2002).

Our foreign policy comes back to haunt us. Armstrong (2002) writes

*When the U.S. supports autocratic rulers, its proud assertion of democratic values has at best a hollow right. What America seemed to saying to Muslims was "Yes, we have freedom and democracy, but you have to live under tyrannical governments." The creation of the state of Israel, the chief ally of the U.S. in the Middle East, has become a symbol of Muslim impotence before the Western powers, which seemed to feel no qualm about the hundreds of thousands of Palestinians who lost their homeland and either went into exile or live under Israeli occupation.*

*In their frustration many have turned to Islam. The secularist and nationalist ideologies, which many Muslims had imported from the West, seemed to have failed them, and by the late 1960s Muslims throughout the Islamic world had begun to develop what we call fundamentalist movements. (pp. 47–48)*

If you asked Armstrong her recommendations for peacemaking and prevention of subsequent acts of terrorism or other forms of HD-1, what would she say?

*What can be done to prevent a repetition of September 11th? We need to recognize and mitigate the plight of others…. [T]his tragedy can be turned to good, if we in the First World cultivate a new sympathy with other peoples who have suffered mass slaughter and experienced a similar helplessness: in Rwanda, in Lebanon, or in Srebrenica.*

*We cannot leave the fight against terrorism solely to our politicians or to our armies. In Europe and America, ordinary citizens must find out more about the rest of the world.*

*We must make ourselves understand, at a deep level, that it is not only Muslims who resent America and the West; that many people in non-Muslim countries, while not condoning those atrocities, may be dry-eyed about the collapse of those giant towers, which represented a power, wealth, and security to which they could never hope to aspire.*

*We must find out about foreign ideologies and other religions like Islam. And we must also acquire a full knowledge of our own governments' foreign policies, using our democratic rights to oppose them, should we deem this to be necessary. We have been warned that the war against terrorism may take years, and so will the development of this 'one world,' mentality, which could do as much, if not more, than our fighter planes to create a safer and more just world. (Armstrong, 2002, p. 71)*

The HDC assumes that drive to live is strong. However, as we have seen, the will to live can be subjugated to the will to die for a cause, hatred of the enemy, or combination of the two. If we would have peace we would be well served to understand the history, culture, and future expectations of the terrorist, warrior, or murderer. Karen Armstrong, the eminent scholar of world religions, makes the point well. I quote her for some length

*It is not only Islamic terrorists who feel this anger and resentment [toward the West], although they do so to an extreme degree. Throughout the entire Muslim world there is widespread bitterness against America, even among pragmatic and well-educated business men and professionals, who may sincerely deplore the recent atrocities, condemn them as evil, and feel sympathy with the victims, but who still resent the way the Western powers have behaved in their countries. Their atmosphere is highly conducive to extremism, especially now that potential terrorists have seen the catastrophe that is possible to inflict using only the simplest of weapons.*

Armstrong relates Osama bin Laden's hatred of the West, particularly the U.S. to the fundamentalist vision of the Egyptian ideologue Sayyid Qutb who was executed by President Nasser in 1966 (7). Armstrong (2002) shows that

*Qutb developed his militant ideology in the concentration camps in which he, and thousands of members of the Muslim Brotherhood were imprisoned. After 15 years of mental and physical torture in these ghastly prisons, Qutb and others became convinced that secularism was a great evil and that it was a Muslim's first duty to overthrow rulers such as Nasser, who paid only lip service to Islam. (p. 70)*

## IMPLICATIONS FOR HEHP AND SUGGESTED ACTION

Epictetus (AD 60–117) philosophized that for every evil there was a good, and for every good an evil. What could possibly be the *good* coming from September 11th?

The good is that we are more aware of our personal vulnerability and mortality than in the past. One result is that Americans and its allies have united against terrorism. The omniscient threat of HD can do that. Consider that for most of our history, wealth and station could postpone death. One could buy one's way out of a military draft, escape to less threatening environments, purchase armies and bodyguards. Today, no one is immune—rich man, poor man, beggar man, thief, politician, multinational corporation executive, child or adult, pope, or piker—all are at risk.

The "enemy" is at risk as well. While fear of death can be subjugated to dying for a cause or belief as has been shown life and living are always preferred. Does al Qaeda belie that proposition? Hard to tell. At bottom no parent wishes his or her child to die. The promise or martyrdom is that it works for the true believer. One has to reduce or remove the stimulus to die. On the other hand, moderate followers of Islam wish to live. Alexander the Great said that only a king can kill another king. Perhaps only moderate Islamic religious leaders can persuade the extremist mullahs, and subsequently the Mujahhedin, and others involved in jihad.

Another "good" is that HEHP now has an opportunity to become a global player in the quest for peace. Whether it will remains to be seen. HEHP has unusual assets. First, it is generally well-received. Its primary concern is the health and well-being of people and the ecosystem. Often their product is enlightening (in the case of health education), and fun (in the case of playful activities). Second HEHP is grounded in the scientific method as it considers cause and effect, and the process involving prevention (that is, epidemiology). Third, education is the primary venue for HEHP. By definition education is future oriented, that is, one learns today that which can be used tomorrow. Education is more, however, than book learning. Knowledge and insight must be applied to solving real world problems. Advocacy is one means. Service-learning and community outreach are others. HEHP professionals are usually nonthreatening, trustworthy, and function as reference persons (Janis, 1982b). No one is after the other's billfold or pocket book.

With such assets HEHP is well-suited to establish peace and the prevention of HD-1 as health issues, and part of the HEHP discipline. HEHP can be effective in two types of *prevention*:

- working to reduce the *underlying root causes* of terrorism and HD-1 nationally and globally. They include the elimination of poverty and inadequate income and illiteracy, while enhancing human rights, and the value of democratic processes, and should be included in curricula, research, and advocacy efforts. Implementation requires that the HEHP professional be knowledgeable in economics, politics, and foreign policy. This holds true especially in this age of globalization. Health is or will be affected by global treaties such as the General Agreement on Trade in Services, the Free Trade Area of the Americas, the General Agreement on Tariffs and Trade, and North American Free Trade Agreement. Organizations such as the World Trade Organization, International Monetary Fund, and World Bank provide useful information and initiate global policies affecting health. It is in the best interest of HEHP professionals to be informed. Again, to be effective our purview must be global, international, national, and local; catholic rather than provincial.

■   preventing the *acts* of terrorism, and HD-1 themselves, and mitigating their effects should they occur. Something as simple as educating about airline travel and airport safety comes to mind. Another example: As I write there is distrust and confusion in the U.S. about how to deal with the threat of anthrax. Are the vaccines effective? If so who will get them. What is the procedure and costs? HEHP professionals can serve as effective communicators of valid news. A third example concerns the apparent increase in manifestations of stress following September 11th. Post-traumatic stress reactions including depression, anxiety, grieving, and self-destructive behaviors are commonly reported. Serving as an effective on-site counselor or support person would be an appropriate role for HEHP professionals. Additional training should not be difficult to obtain.

What is the saying? Think globally, act locally? We can have it both ways. We can think and act globally and locally. How? A start is in modifying and adapting *The Guiding Principles for a Public Health Response to Terrorism* suggested by the American Public Health Association's Governing Council. A partial list follows. I comment, when necessary, on those that are particularly salient and efficacious for HEHP, and later give my own recommendations (Governing Council of the American Public Health Association, 2001). The principles are italicized:

In order to prevent future acts of terrorism and their adverse public health consequences, the public health community should support policies and programs that

1.  *Address poverty, social injustice and health disparities that may contribute to the development of terrorism.* These are root causes of most forms of HD-1, and should be included in HEHP curricula. Teach, research, and advocate the elimination of poverty in underdeveloped states by providing employment, government programs and subsidies when needed. In this way despair and hopelessness are minimized.

    Addressing these issues raises another concern certainly avoided by the media. What of the general welfare within the United States? Homeland Security should be concerned with increasing social cohesion, and domestic tranquility. How? A long conflict will increasingly drain money from health and other social programs. Those on the short end of the stick may join the domestic extremists who see the government as the enemy. Security implies future expectations. As unemployment and layoffs increase the prospects for the future become bleak. That is the stuff of social disintegration. HEHP should advocate and teach toward full employment at truly liveable wages.

2.  *Provide humanitarian assistance to, and protect the human rights of, the civilian populations that are directly or indirectly affected by terrorism.* I would especially include the rights of women, the elderly, and political dissidents. The topics are appropriate for HEHP.

3.  *Advocate the speedy end of the armed conflict in Afghanistan and promote nonvi-olent means of conflict resolution.* Other conflicts have to be prevented or ended. Already there is talk of spreading the conflict to Iraq, the Philippines, and other states allegedly harboring terrorists. The Arab-Israeli question must be resolved. If it were much of the overt and covert hostility, suspicions, and conflict between Arab and Western states would be reduced. Thankfully, as I write, there is some hope for resolution. Conflict resolution, like parent education, are topics not usu-ally associated with in HEHP but should be. Other means of resolving differences should be explored. One vexing problem is labeling. That is, what distinguishes a "terrorist" from a "freedom fighter" and vice versa?

4.  *Strengthen the public health infrastructure (which includes workforce, labora-tory and information systems) and other components of the public health system (including education, research, and the faith community) to increase the abil-ity to identify, respond to, and prevent problems of public health importance, including the health aspects of terrorist attacks.* There needs to be collaboration and coalition building *between health and other* organizations such as APHA, AAHE, ASHA, and others. Also *within* the same organizations. For example, on November 1, 2001, I sent the following email to several HEHP discussion groups on the web. The topic was the American Public Health Association's (APHA) top five public health priorities for the year 2002 with special reference to the listing of bio-terrorism but omission of other forms of HD:

    > Where is public health promotion/health education (PHPHE) in all of us— especially bio-terrorism, war and the other forms of HD? At the recent (2001) APHA conference the sessions having to do with bio-terrorism and war were mostly sponsored by the Peace Caucus. They were packed. I found nil spon-sored by PHPHE. I always thought that the purview of PHPHE was (or should be) preventing that which causes premature mortality, morbidity and suffering? . . . .

    > By the way, it does not take a genius to predict that another great problem looming on the horizon will be increasing, internal social fragmentation along class lines as the economy weakens and greater sums of money are spent on defense, corporate bailouts (that is corporate welfare), etc. As every-one knows the health and economic disparities were great before September 11th. Does anyone expect them to improve during the war and foreseeable future? And how will those on the short end of the stick respond? And where will HEHP be if this scenario happens?"

I tend to attend APHA conferences. As most readers know it is organized by sec-tions, caucuses, and interest groups. My experience has been that the Peace Caucus, International Health Section, and Socialist Caucus have consistently addressed the issues raised in this article. I suggest a continuous and systematic dialogue between those advo-cates, the Public Health Education and Health Promotion Section, and others.

Another organization that I respect is the *Association for Death Education & Counseling*. As explained in this article, thanatology and health are inextricably linked. Both organizations would benefit from collaboration. This concept of cross-fertilization, and working toward a common goal applies to other disciplines and advocacy groups. We need to become more catholic in our professional involvements. The pursuit of peace provides the nexus.

5. *Prevent hate crimes, ethnic, racial, and religious discrimination, including profiling; promote cultural competence, diversity training, and dialogue among peoples; and protect human rights and civil liberties.* One way is to integrate people from diverse backgrounds into programs and academic courses. Service-learning courses are well suited to this purpose. Our Adult Health and Development Program, mentioned earlier, does this as it matches students and older institutionalized and non-institutionalized adults to work on a one-to-one basis to improve health, well-being, and health knowledge status in a milieu of fun. Over 50 percent of the participants represent ethnic and racial "minority" groups.

6. *Advocate the immediate control and ultimate elimination of biologic, chemical, and nuclear weapons.* Another way of applying knowledge to resolve pressing social issues is through advocacy. In my opinion the academy could do more by organizing its intellectual and creative assets to address HD issues. A multidisciplinary team might take on a project like reducing homicide in a community. Such a team could involve disciplines such as education and health education, criminal justice, kinesiology, recreation, economics, psychology, sociology, cultural anthropology, philosophy, medicine, law, ecology, and the like. One gain for the university is that the project might unite the campus in common purpose.

That faculty, in general, might be challenged by such a project was suggested by a 1994 survey reported in the *Washington Post* (Jordan, 1994). It reported that the public's view toward higher education was low. Faculty, themselves, were discontented. Ernest L. Boyer, the late president of the Carnegie Foundation, said, "My interpretation is that there is a growing feeling that universities are not relevant to social issues and problems." Iris Molotsky, AAUP spokeswoman, said that faculty want to devote more time to service work but that the salary structure is skewed toward those who publish, not toward those who spend a lot of time with students or on community problems (Jordan, 1994). By integrating education, service, and research to improving the health and well-being of present and future generations, the function and utility of the academy might become meaningful in the eyes of the public.

HEHP professionals should serve as collaborator and consultants with other professions in the quest for peace. I was once asked to write a chapter integrating the HDC and diplomacy. The rationale was that most people, even one's enemy, share common death-related experiences, attitudes and beliefs. Could that shared experience help reduce hostilities and increase opportunity for negotiation? Suppose Israeli and

Palestinian parents came together to discuss their grief over the death of a child during war. Is it possible that the bond of mutual suffering could reduce hostility?

HEHP could be helpful to other professions and their endeavors. Politics is another example. Consider that health (as I define it) is highly valued by the public, and few politicians know anything about it. We should both collaborate with the political domain, and run for public office. Policies and laws are fashioned by politicians.

Lastly, I wish to legitimize *parent education* as an HEHP domain. Examination of the background of murderers and members of al Qaeda, for example, shows that most come from dysfunctional or nonexistent homes. Someone once said that any damn fool can occupy two of the most important professions known to mankind: Politics and parenthood. Neither *requires* a wit of training or education. For example, parents often beat their kids because that is how they were "disciplined." There are other ways to motivate children to behave in socially acceptable ways. The literature in child development is immense. Health and violence are strongly related to how we raise our children.

## CONCLUSION

My view is that all institutions, and professional endeavors, including that of HEHP, must proactively deal with the most profound health issue of our time: The attainment of peace, and the prevention of HD. However, the clock is ticking. The availability and willingness of people and their sponsors to use weapons of mass destruction make it so.

Facing the reality of the HD of self and loved ones is humbling and terrifying. It also reduces self-deception. For example, on the one hand I know that I have done some good works in my time. I also *know* my work has had no significant effect at all in preventing HD. The drama is almost Kafkaesque. How dumb can we mortals be? Policy makers, and others powerful enough to influence global monetary policies, wage wars, and make billion dollar deals do not see the urgency of preventing HD in general? They do not see "the clear and present danger" as someone once said? Absurd.

Professional, family, and other accomplishments are meaningless unless HD is eliminated. In this case, it is not enough how well one plays the game, but the outcome itself. One criterion of success is the ability to influence policy. But policy is only of value if it is implemented, and accomplishes its goals. Let me put it another way: Nuclear or bio-chemical-germ or environmental holocaust have the potential to destroy the planet. Such destruction will annihilate the past (that is, history and one's works), and the future (that is, expectations for oneself and loved ones). If this catastrophe were to come about, the legacy of Socrates, Beethoven, and Einstein would be dead.

However nihilism cannot and must not prevail. The great quest is to eliminate and prevent HD against the pressure of time and HD-related events. HEHP can do so much to increase the odds that present and future generations live long and well. Whether we take up the challenge remains to be seen.

## ENDNOTES

1. Thomas Friedman, the prize winning columnist for the *New York Times* distinguishes between Islamicists and Islam. The former distorts the religion of Islam for their own political purposes, and is characterized by militant, fanatical fundamentalism, authoritarianism, and repression of its own people and others.

2. I like Robert Kastenbaum's definition of thanatology as the study of life ending in death (2000).

3. I saw the linkage between the meaning given death and health-related behavior. If one really faced up to his own mortality as a result of smoking, for example, might it reduce the behavior—or contribute to it? Could the theories of health behavior change be improved by considering the meaning an individual or culture gives death? Certainly, it has affected my world view else I would not be pursuing the issue of HD since the late 1960s. Thanatology has prompted me to modify the WHO definition of health, i.e., *health is the process toward, and perception of acceptable physical, mental, and social well-being and not merely the absence of disease, Horrendous Death, and infirmity here and now, and as expected in the future*. Emphasis is on health as *a process* rather than a state. Also health is influenced by one's perception and meaning given the *future*. The person filled with "fear and trembling" and dread over what tomorrow might bring is not healthy according to this definition.

4. Recall the history of the tobacco industry, its duplicity before the Congress and public, and chronic lying regarding the deadly nature of its product (see Kessler, 2001). Also, the recent collapse of the giant corporation, Enron is another example of a total lack of morals or ethics. It declared bankruptcy in December 2001, and never forewarned its workers. Around 21,000 jobs were lost. Eleven thousand workers lost the large percentage of their retirement plans because they were forbidden to sell their stock in the company. Enron's CEO Kenneth Lay and his fellow executives were exempt from the lock down and sold, often at tremendous profits (McGrory, 2001). According to Mary McGrory (2001), the *Washington Post* columnist, "Enron lied about earnings, cooked its books and left its employees in the lurch, while its top brass made out like bandits.. On the other hand, Enron was one of those corporations that agreed that global climate change must be addressed (Pew Center on Global Climate Change, 1998).

5. Excellent references to better understand the historical, political, and religious basis of the present conflict are the works of Armstrong (1994, 2000), Bodansky (2001), and Friedman (1989).

6. President Bush was ill-advised to liken the military action following September 11th to a crusade. It is a buzz word among Arabs—as politically incorrect as they come. He has not used the term since the early days of the conflict.

7. Yossef Bodansky (2001), author of the definitive work on Osama bin Laden, describes him "as a man not to be ignored, for he is at the core of Islamist international terrorism…. Bin Laden has always been—and still is—part of a bigger system, a team player and a loyal comrade in arms. The terrorist operations in several parts of the world now attributed to bin Laden were actually state-sponsored operations perpetrated by dedicated groups of Islamists" (p. x).

## REFERENCES

Armstrong, K. (1994). *A History of God*. New York: Alfred A. Knopf.

Armstrong K. (2000). *Islam: A Short History*. New York: Modern Library.

Armstrong, K. (2002, January/February). Ghosts of our past. *Modern Maturity, 45*, 44+.

Becker, E. (1973). *The Denial of Death*. New York: Free Press.

Bodansky, Y. (2001). *Bin Laden: The Man Who Declared War on America*. Roseville, CA: Prima Publishing.

Feifel, H. (1959). *The Meaning of Death*. New York: McGraw-Hill.

Freud, S. (1968). Thoughts for the times on war and death. In J. Rickman (Ed.), *Civilisation, war and death: Sigmund Freud* (p. 125). London: Hogarth Press.

Friedlander, H. (1995). *The origins of Nazi genocide*. Chapel Hill: University of North Carolina Press.

Friedman, T. L. (1989). *From Beirut to Jerusalem*. New York: Anchor Books.

Friedman, T. L. (2001, December 9). Ask not what. *New York Times*.

Fromm, E. (1973). *The anatomy of human destructiveness*. New York: Holt, Rinehart and Winston.

Gonzalez-Vallejo, C., & Sauveur, G. B. (1998). Peace through economic and social development. In H. J. Langholtz (Ed.), *The psychology of peacekeeping* (pp. 18–30). Westport, CT: Praeger.

Governing Council of the American Public Health Association. (2001). *Governing Council Directives to the Executive Board on Public Health and Terrorism*, [web page]. American Public Health Association. Retrieved from http://www.apha.org/legislative/policy/policysearchndex.cfm?fuseaction=view&id=266

Hardt, M., & Negri, A. (2000). *Empire*. Cambridge, MA: Harvard University Press.

Hoffer, E. (1966). *The true believer*. New York: Harper and Row.

Huntington, S. P. (1995). *The clash of civilizations and the remaking of world order*. New York: Simon & Schuster.

Janis, I. (1982a). *Groupthink: Psychological studies of policy decisions and fiascoes* (2nd ed.). Boston: Houghton Mifflin.

Janis, I. (1982b). Psychological effects of warnings. In C. D. Spielberger (Ed.), *Stress, attitudes, and decisions* (pp. 57–91). New York: Praeger.

Jordan, M. (1994, June 20). Respect is dwindling in the hallowed halls. *Washington Post*, p. A3.

Kastenbaum, R. J. (2000). *Death, society, and human experience* (7th ed.). Boston: Allyn and Bacon.

Kessler, D. (2001). *A question of intent*. New York: Public Affairs.

Leviton, D. (1969a). Critical issues in health education. *School Health Review* (November), 2–4.

Leviton, D. (1969b). Speaking out. *Journal of Health, Physical Education, and Recreation* (September), 41–42.

Leviton, D. (1976a). Education toward love and peace behaviors. *Journal of Clinical Child Psychology, 2*, 14–17.

Leviton, D. (1976b). The stimulus of death. *Health Education, 7*(2), 17–20.

Leviton, D. (1977). The scope of death education. *Death Education, 1*(1), 41–56.

Leviton, D. (Ed.). (1991a). *Horrendous death and health: Toward action*. New York: Hemisphere Publishing.

Leviton, D. (Ed.). (1991b). *Horrendous death, health, and well-being*. New York: Hemisphere Publishing.

Leviton, D. (1998). What university students learn in an intergenerational, holistic, service-learning health promotion program. *International Electronic Journal of Health Education, 1*(3), 157–162. Retrieved from http://www.iejhe.org

Leviton, D. (2000a). Linking aging, death, global health and university based community service-learning. *Journal of Public Service and Outreach, 4*(2), 19–26.

Leviton, D. (2000b). The need and challenge to address the greatest threat to health and well-being in our time. *Health Education Monographs, 18*(2), 27–32.

Leviton, D., & Millar, M. (2002). *AHDP manual for staffers* (4th ed.). College Park, MD: University of Maryland.

Levy, B. S., & Sidel, V. W. (Eds.). (1997). *War and public health.* New York City: Oxford University Press in cooperation with the American Public Health Association.

Lifton, R. J. (1979). *The broken connection.* New York: Simon & Schuster.

Lifton, R. J. (1986). *The Nazi doctors: Medical killing and the psychology of genocide.* New York: Basic Books.

Lifton, R. J., & Markusen, E. (1990). *The genocidal mentality: Nazi Holocaust and nuclear threat.* New York: Basic Books.

McGrory, M. (2001, December 20). A CEO who lives by what's right. *Washington Post,* p. A3.

News Service. (2001, December 11). Accepting Peace Prize, Annan speaks of "new insecurity." *Washington Post,* pp. A27.

Pew Center on Global Climate Change. (1998). *Pew Center on Global Climate Change* [www]. Retrieved from http://www.pewclimate.org

Renner, M. (2000). How the prospects for world peace have grown brighter. *WorldWatch, 13*(1), 37–39.

Reston, J., Jr. (2001). *Warriors of God.* New York: Doubleday.

Rice, S. E. (2001, December 11). The Africa battle. *Washington Post,* p. A33.

Rickman, J. (Ed.). (1968). *Civilisation, war and death: Sigmund Freud.* London: Hogarth Press.

Soros, G. (1991). *Underwriting democracy.* New York: Free Press.

Soros, G. (2000). *Open society: Reforming global capitalism.* New York: Public Affairs.

Tuchman, B. (1981). *Practicing history.* New York: Ballantine Books.

Useem, J. (2001, October 15). Is it a small world after all? *Fortune, 144,* 38–40.

World Bank. (2001, October 1). Poverty to rise in wake of terrorist attacks in U.S. [Web site]. *Development News—The World Bank's daily webzine.*

# 25

# PUTTING POLITICS BACK IN PUBLIC HEALTH EDUCATION

MARTHA L. COULTER

TERRANCE ALLBRECHT

ELIZABETH GULITZ

MARY FIGG

CHARLES MAHAN

Preparation of leaders in the field of public health is one of the many responsibilities of graduate education in the field. There is renewed interest in public health education in the use of a practice internship as a routine part of masters education and closer attention to this internship by the Council on Education in Public Health, the accrediting body for public health programs. There has been a call for the inclusion of practice components that are integral parts of the entire curriculum and that are not limited to either the practice internship or to masters students (Legnini, 1994). Traditionally, doctoral student preparation has been viewed as a research-based curriculum, with limited attention to practice components. However, doctorally prepared students are also expected to provide leadership in the field in a variety of settings.

Public health leadership entails an understanding of the political nature of the field. Since the field is focused on the health of the population, the translation of new research findings into public policy must often take place through the political process. Leaders in the field have an obligation to be advocates and to lead in efforts to assure that the health of the public is protected and improved. Although doctoral students are well prepared in their scientific roles to conduct sound research and contribute to the development of new knowledge, they are often less well prepared to assume advocacy roles in translating this knowledge into practice. This article contends that not only is professional preparation for advocacy a necessity, but also that it requires the participation of the students, the faculty, and of the politicians themselves.

The following article describes a program designed to provide exposure to, and practice in, the presentation of a scientific position in a political arena. The forum used was that of a mock legislative committee hearing. This hearing was conducted as part of a course that is required for all doctoral students. A model was developed that would ensure that the students had sound academic and practical preparation for legislative advocacy. The model included four components: (1) issues preparation, (2) communication skills, (3) political environment exposure, and (4) application (the mock hearing).

This article will describe the conceptual and skill-based issues included in each part of the model. It is intended to provide guidance to those public health educators or educators in other applied fields who wish to enhance the leadership skills of their students.

## ISSUE PREPARATION

The selection of issues and topics to be argued before the mock legislative hearing was based on a series of learning objectives that were perceived to be critical to the political process. Students worked collaboratively, in groups of three to four students, on a presentation that could be of two types: (1) an argument for or against legislation currently being considered by the state legislature or (2) initiation of new legislation to be presented to the legislative committee.

The learning objectives that were part of issue selection were to be able to select issues that have a public health population impact, defend policy and practice recommendations using actual data, articulate the values underlying political positions, and identify and work with constituency groups.

### Public Health Impact

In their initial selection of topics, the student groups were encouraged to identify topics in which they had an interest and were also of significant public health concern. They were encouraged to select issues from a population-based perspective. That is, what would the effect of this legislation be on the broad population? Within these parameters, they were free to select policy or practice areas of concern, such as mental health legislation, health insurance policy, and maternal and child health policy.

## Use of Data

After selecting their topic, students began an analysis of available data regarding their legislative issue. The group reviewed and critiqued the literature and developed its final position based on these data. Students were encouraged to think through the process of interpreting data for its relevance to practice, such as whether statistical significance is equal to clinical (or practical) significance. They were also helped to understand that political decisions are made based on both scientific and value bases and that an in-depth presentation of data is not always possible.

## Values

Students were asked to use a value-based policy analysis approach to consider what values underlie decision-making processes in the area of their selected topic. They discussed and considered the possible value orientations of those who were in policy-making positions and their own value positions in regard to their topic.

### Constituent Groups

Each working group identified the relevant constituent groups in the community who might have an interest in their position statement. In some cases students identified themselves as members of a constituent group, such as professional or community groups.

## COMMUNICATION

### Development and Practice of Communication Skills

Public health students increasingly want and need communication training across the curriculum to support their advocacy and education roles. The students in this program receive didactic and interactive instruction in presentation and argumentation principles prior to the mock legislative hearing. The objectives of such training are to assist students in (1) recognizing and developing propositions, (2) identifying the elements of the Toulmin model and being able to adapt it as a guide for structuring arguments, and (3) being able to apply tests for sources of evidence.

The following is a brief overview of each content area.

### Proposition Framing

Students were guided to clarify their purposes for speaking, generally to specify the types of claims they were advancing based on their issues. They focused on either propositions of fact or designative claims that posed and answered the question "was it, is it, will it be true?" or propositions of values, or evaluative claims related to the question "of what worth is it?"

## Toulmin Argumentation Model

Stephen Toulmin's classic model has been widely used to plan and structure the elements of a logical, though parsimonious and compelling argument. The students reviewed the model and adapted portions of it to plan their own persuasive strategies. The elements were helpful for assisting students with specifying the claims they were making, the data they were providing, the warrant (the justification for why the data support the claim), and the possible rebuttals to the claim, which, if the issue is controversial, inoculate the audience by anticipating possible objections and offering persuasive and disarming counterarguments.

## Test for Sources of Evidence

Students used multiple sources to support their claims that would best appeal to the legislators. Suggested tests for determining the quality and quantity of evidence included the reliability test (Is the source objective and competent?), the recency test (Is the information current?), the completeness test (Are as many sources as possible used?), and the accuracy test (Is the information redundant and verifiable?).

# POLITICAL ENVIRONMENT

## Legislative Observation

Some students were able to participate in the trip to the state capital. This experience provides insight into legislative activities by giving students opportunities to interact with local and state politicians, participate in select political activities, actively support a political agenda/bill, and demonstrate good communication skills suitable in a political environment. The following components are integral to this experience: (1) discussion about practical aspects of the political process, such as presentation of information to politicians, key sources, tracking proposed bills, and advocacy; (2) selection and support of a public health issue that may be affected by proposed legislation; (3) discussions with local and state political leaders about the politicians' experiences, how to effectively present the issue to a legislator, and their view of the critical issues facing politicians; (4) participation in select local-level political and legislative activities, such as the "Governor's Conference on Children"; and (5) participation in select state-level political and legislative activities, including a trip to the state capitol with a faculty member and former state representative that involves participation in a statewide "Healthy Baby Day" and enables students to attend committee meetings, observe the House or Senate, and speak with individual legislators and/or their aides about a public health issue.

## APPLICATION

### Rationale and Objectives

Testifying before a congressional or state legislative committee can be an intimidating experience. Public health professionals who present a factual and compelling case have high credibility with legislators and government staff members. There are, however, communication and procedural land mines awaiting inexperienced public health spokespersons. Objectives of this part of the program include (1) teaching the students communication in context; the mode, tone and rhetorical style of speaking must fit the genre of the audience; and (2) allowing panelists to illustrate the types of arguments, questions, and biases exhibited by legislators and to demonstrate the reasons behind the legislative perspective.

### Legislative versus Public Health Professional Perspectives

Professionals from an academic or medical background tend to expect professionals in other areas to respond to the types of reasoned arguments and factual appeals that elicit a positive response from their colleagues. While the legislative process may appear to deal in reason and facts, actually legislators may pay more attention to parochial interests than carefully constructed logic. Communication, then, must be at the level of those "back home" regional interests. Additionally, legislators must deal with hundreds of different areas of legislation and have neither the time nor tolerance to become familiar with all of the issues. Therefore, the information being presented to legislators should be technical enough to explain the issue, but not so detailed that the audience loses interest.

### Process and Outcomes

The students' training in the political nature of public health culminated in their presentations to a mock legislative panel. The panel was made up of former legislators and individuals who had prior experience in giving legislative testimony. Although the students had been advised on the content of their presentations and coached in their stylistic approach, the actual presentations to the panel were their own. It was evident that they had invested considerable time and effort in the content and delivery of their presentations. However, they did not make a sufficient audience adjustment from giving a paper in a graduate class to addressing a legislative panel.

The students were repeatedly interrupted by the panelists' seemingly irrelevant questions and rude remarks, such as, "This sounds like another liberal give-away program to me." The students were unprepared for the panelists' seemingly unprofessional and inconsiderate behavior.

The students did have a chance to express their concerns and vent their feelings at an extensive debriefing session following the hearing. Public health faculty members were present to reassure the students but also to underscore the realistic nature of the process that they had just experienced.

## Closure

After the students had time to reflect on the panelists' responses to their presentations, they appreciated the aims of those panelists. The shock value stemming from the "outrageous" behavior of the panelists effectively underscored the importance of using communication techniques that are appropriate for a particular audience, in a way that a typical lecture could not.

## CONCLUSIONS

This article has described a program that assures practice in presenting public health information in a political environment. This program enables students to experience the political nature of public health and the various aspects of the political process. It is based on the premise that although a sound research and knowledge base are necessary for public health practitioners, they are not sufficient for developing leadership skills applicable to public health.

Through description of the model that provides the structure for the program, this article has highlighted the process of preparing students to assume public health leadership positions. The importance of issues preparation, communication, exposure to the political environment, and the application of these skills in a political context has been illustrated.

Opportunities to interact with local and state politicians, participate in political activities, and to support a political agenda provide students with essential political experience. This interaction also enables local and state political leaders to share first-hand knowledge and experience with the students, and demonstrates the reality of the political process. It demonstrates to students the importance of political survival and the inability of legislators to focus on all of the important public health issues.

## REFERENCE

Legnini, M. W. (1994). Developing leaders vs. training administrators in the health services. *American Journal of Public Health, 84*, 1569–1573.

# 26

# HEALTH CARE REFORM: INSIGHTS FOR HEALTH EDUCATORS

**THOMAS O'ROURKE**

Health care reform continues to be a topic on the public agenda. Nothing new there. It probably always will be, regardless of whatever reforms are initiated. Health educators are affected by the debate in their roles as health professionals, citizens, taxpayers, and consumers of service. The problem is that the current paradigm guiding health care reform is flawed. It eliminates the possibility of improving health, while consuming huge resources in the process. This article challenges some current paradigms and suggests another for consideration.

A decade ago, soaring health care costs and increasing numbers of uninsured pushed health care reform onto center stage. The collapse of the Clinton health reform effort in 1994, a strong economy, and a lower rate of health care inflation moved health care from the spotlight but kept it warm on the back burner. The recent economic downturn and an accelerated rate of health care cost increases are sure to bring the issue to the front burner. For example, the health insurance program for federal government employees and retirees (the largest purchaser of private insurance) recently disclosed a 13.3 percent premium increase, the largest increase since the 1980s. Some outcomes are obvious. Many employers (especially in a labor market favorable to employers) have already or are likely to respond by either reducing benefits or shifting more premiums or health care costs to employees. In the process, the underlying limitations of how health care is viewed narrows our perspective of the nature of the problem and what reform options to consider, debate, and implement.

## MEDICAL CARE DOES NOT EQUAL HEALTH

In any policy debate (or put another way, a war of economics, politics, and ideology), how an issue is framed is all-important. Success in framing the issues determines the focus of the debate, the possible options, and the eventual outcome. Health care is no exception. The current paradigm guiding much of health care reform is straightforward. It is based on the premise that expenditure of resources results in health care services that lead to improved health as measured by crude indicators such as infant mortality and longevity. Within the framework, health care reform is debated primarily within the context of costs and access, and to a lesser extent on quality. Certainly, these issues are related. Many legislators; business; industry, and labor leaders; health care providers; and policy wonks have bought into the equation that medical care equals health care equals health.

Once this simple paradigm is accepted, it follows that if one wants to improve health, one needs to address the cost, accessibility, and quality of medical care services. In turn, the popular gestalt is that this is achieved by increasing medical care expenditures. These increased resources may be in the form of increases in the infrastructure (buildings, equipment, and so on), size, or quality of the workforce, or simply paying more for services. Even when concerns about costs are expressed, they are usually within the context of this paradigm. Efforts to address the concern may take many forms such as controlling the costs, reducing administrative waste, utilization review, and so forth. The important point is that the debate, options, and initiatives are all done within the existing paradigm where medical care is equated with health care and health care is equated with health.

But here's the rub and why a new paradigm is needed. The previous paradigm isn't true (Lamarche, 1995). Never was, most likely never will be. We have come to substitute the words *health care* for *medical care* as if they were synonymous. As Turnock notes, the word *health* is an adjective and not a noun. He asks, Shouldn't the focus be on healthy people and not medical care? That is simply not the case now. Fully 99 percent of the current annual "health care" expenditure is focused on medical care. According to the 1979 *Surgeon General's Report on Health Promotion and Disease Prevention* (Department of Health, Education, and Welfare, 1979), "Medical care begins with the sick and seeks to keep them alive, make them well, or minimize their disability" (p. 119). The focus of medicine and where the "health care" resources are spent, is the diagnosis and attempted treatment of illness, disease, and disability. The classic 1979 *Surgeon General's Report* "suggests that perhaps as much as half of U.S. mortality was due to unhealthy behavior; 20 percent to environmental factors; 20 percent to human biological factors; and only 10 percent to inadequacies in health care" (p. 9).

## MEDICAL EXPENDITURES AND HEALTH STATUS

It would be one thing if it could be shown that increased medical care expenditures resulted in improved health status as measured by crude indicators such as infant mortality and longevity. Such is not the case. Research fails to show any clear relationship between the resources countries spend on medical care and the health of their populations. For this article a correlation was run on medical care expenditures and health status indicators for twenty-nine Organization for Economic Cooperation and Development (OECD) countries (Anderson & Poullier, 1999). Results indicated an insignificant negative correlation of –.32 between expenditures and infant mortality, suggesting not only wasn't there a positive relationship, but also that if anything, it showed that higher spending was inversely and insignificantly related. For longevity, the relationship was an insignificant .24 for men and an insignificant .33 for women.

The United States is an excellent case study for the lack of any relationship. In 1998 the United States spent far more (13.6 percent of the gross domestic product [GDP]) than most other OECD industrialized countries, where spending is about 8 percent of GDP. U.S. per capita health care expenditures in 1998 were $4,178 or 134 percent higher than the OECD median of $1,783. Per capita U.S. expenditures were 50 percent higher than the next highest country, Switzerland, where per capita cost was $2,794 (Anderson & Hussey, 2001). Meanwhile U.S. health status indicators historically have been and continue to be poorer (Anderson, Hurst, Hussey, & Jee-Hughes, 2000). In the midst of an increased rate of medical care spending compared with other OECD countries, the relative position of the United States continues to decline. If there were a relationship between medical care spending and health status indicators, one might expect that the United States would have the best health status in the world by far, for we not only spend the highest GNP but also have the largest economy from where that percentage is derived. Again, such is not the case.

Another way of noting the absence of a positive relationship between medical care and health is the relative ranking expressed as the percentile rank of the United States compared with other OECD countries; Anderson and Hussy (2001) report interesting findings over a nearly forty-year period in Table 26.1. In reviewing these data, a percentile rank of 100 is given to the country with the highest value for each indicator, except for infant mortality, potential years of life lost, and alcohol consumption, where a percentile rank of 100 is given to the country with the lowest value.

Results of Table 26.1 evidence that for no indicator did the relative performance of the United States improve from 1960 to 1998. Although the relative ranking of health status indices worsened, health spending per capita and as a percentage of GDP remained consistently highest. During that period medical expenditures as a percentage of GDP nearly tripled from 5.2 to 13.6 percent.

One might argue that U.S. spending of considerably more on medical care than any other country—more than double the amount spent by the median OECD country in 1998—is explained by the average wealth of the country as measured by GDP per capita.

**TABLE 26.1**  **Relative Ranking of the United States on Selected Indicators, 1960, 1980, and 1998**

| Indicator | 1960 | 1980 | 1998 |
|---|---|---|---|
| Life expectancy at birth, females | 54 | 58 | 35 |
| Life expectancy at birth, males | 38 | 44 | 39 |
| Life expectancy at age 60, females | 85 | 85 | 45 |
| Life expectancy at age 60, males | 46 | 73 | 55 |
| Infant mortality | 61 | 39 | 19[A] |
| Potential years of life lost | 42 | 19 | 31 |
| Average annual alcohol intake per capita | 56 | 64 | 63[A] |
| Practicing physicians per 1,000 population | 88 | 52 | 53 |
| Acute hospital beds per 1,000 population | 50 | 29 | 29[A] |
| Hospital acute care days per capita | NA | 11 | 16[A] |
| Average length of acute inpatient stay | NA | 10 | 32[A] |
| Health spending per capita | 100 | 100 | 100 |
| Health spending, percentage of gross domestic product | 94 | 92 | 100 |

*Source:* OECD, 2000. Reprinted with permission from Anderson & Hussey, 2001, p. 229.

Note: NA = not available.
[A]1997

Not so. It is known that countries with higher average wealth spend proportionally more on medical care. However, Anderson and Hussey (2001) report that, taking the average wealth of U.S. citizens into account, the expected level of U.S. health spending is $2,868 per capita. This is still $1,301 less than the actual spent per person in the United States, or $370 billion when multiplied by the approximately 281 million Americans (Anderson & Hussey, 2001).

## HEALTH MORE THAN MEDICAL CARE

In 1945 the renowned medical historian Henry E. Sigerist commented, "Health is promoted by providing a decent standard of living, good labor conditions, education, physical culture, and means of rest and relaxation" (1946, p. 127). Building on this idea, Milton Terris (1986) noted:

> Many areas of health promotion, such as nutrition, physical exercise, housing, employment, income, and education, have major impacts also on disease prevention. The logic of our discipline makes it necessary to support a healthful standard of living through full employment and adequate family income; improved working conditions; decent housing, including the elimination of urban and rural slums and the grim spectacle of thousands of homeless Americans; effective protection from environmental discomforts such as excessive heat and cold, smog, noise and noxious odors; good nutrition that will foster optimal physical and mental development; increased financial support to public education and elimination of financial barriers to higher education; improved opportunities for rest, recreation, and cultural development; greater participation in community activities and decision-making; an end to discrimination against minority groups based on race, gender, age, social class, religious belief, national background or sexual preference; and freedom from the pervasive fear of violence, war, and nuclear annihilation. A healthful standard of living is one of the three basic components of a national health program, along with greatly expanded preventive services and a comprehensive medical care system. Failure to understand this will narrow our horizons, limit our success in improving the health status of the population, and impede our ability to forge meaningful alliances with the citizen groups whose understanding and support are essential to our efforts. (pp. 150–151)

## HEALTH AND MEDICAL CARE—A NEW PARADIGM

At present medical care predominates the "health care" budget to such an extent that "health care" has become a surrogate for medical care. Medical care is dominated by powerful economic interests such as insurers, provider groups, the pharmaceutical industry, and the medical supply/equipment industry. They are more than content to capture the term *health care* for what is really medical care. As Terris (1986) mentions, medical care is a component of, but not synonymous with either health or health care. A new paradigm would include a distinction between health and medical care both organizationally and functionally.

A rational paradigm could include a Department of Health with a focus as broadly outlined in earlier paragraphs and a Department of Medical Services that would include programs consistent with what it is—keeping sick people alive, making them well, or minimizing their disability. Both would be funded by private (business, industry, consumers, and patients) and public sources. Certainly there is some relationship between health and medical care, just as there is between health and programs by the Department of Agriculture (nutrition, food safety, and so on) and the Department of Labor (occupational health and safety) and many other agencies. Very importantly, both departments would have separate budgets. In this way legislators, policy makers and, importantly, the citizenry would (1) get a clearer picture of the functions of each department, (2) be far less likely to confuse the terms or consider medical care synonymous with health, and (3) be able to see the amount of resources devoted and the impact of each. However, as long as health care continues to be subsumed under medical care, efforts at improving health will not be optimized. Once the organizational and functional separation is made, society will be in a much better position to enhance health. It also is quite likely that once the two areas are differentiated, consistent with patterns in other countries resources will be reallocated more rationally from medical care to health. Health educators and public health professionals would benefit from this paradigm change. For it is health educators who would be focusing on health and doing the things necessary to make positive and cost-effective improvements in the health status of the population. Support for this approach can be found in the recent excellent publication *Health & Health Care 2010—The Forecast, the Challenge* (Institute for the Future, 2000), which mentions that the first shift should be from rigid adherence to the biological model to an expanded, multifactorial view of health that expands and goes beyond the biological model and includes social, mental, and spiritual as well as physical health. Review of this publication not only highlights the limitations of our current paradigm but also suggests new and exciting directions Such a change, including the necessary organizational and functional changes suggested here, would go a long way toward a true health care system.

## REFERENCES

Anderson, G., & Hussey, P. S. (2001). Comparing health system performance in OECD countries. *Health Affairs, 20*, 219–232.

Anderson, G., & Poullier, J. (1999). Health spending, access, and outcomes: Trends in industrialized countries. *Health Affairs, 18*, 178–192.

Anderson, G., Hurst, J., Hussey, P. S., & Jee-Hughes, M. (2000). Health spending and outcomes: Trends in OECD countries, 1960–1998. *Health Affairs, 19*, 150–157.

Department of Health, Education, and Welfare. (1979). *Healthy People, the Surgeon General's Report on Health Promotion and Disease Prevention*. Washington, DC: U.S. Government Printing Office.

Institute for the Future. (2000). *Health & health care 2010: The forecast, the challenge*. San Francisco: Jossey-Bass.

Lamarche, P. (1995). Our health paradigm in peril. *Public Health Report, 110*, 556–560.

Organization for Economic Cooperation and Development (OECD). (2000). *OECD Health Data 2000*. Paris: OECD.

Sigerist, H. E. (1946). *The university at the crossroads: Address & essays*. New York: Henry Schuman.

Terris, M. (1986). What is health promotion? *Journal of Public Health Policy, 7*, 147–151.

# 27

# THE ROLE OF HEALTH EDUCATION ASSOCIATIONS IN ADVOCACY

**M. ELAINE AULD**
**ELEANOR DIXON-TERRY**

Professional societies and associations provide an important function by advancing the knowledge of and providing support for a particular occupation or field of study. Traditionally, many health professional organizations were organized to provide a nexus around scientific research and practice issues of their particular disciplines. In the latter part of this century, however, health professional societies have become more visible and vocal public policy advocates. Unlike the labor movement, which recognized the political advantage of "power in numbers" in the early 1800s, most professional societies were not organized solely to influence legislation. The purpose of this article is to review issues affecting an association's type and scope of advocacy efforts, describe the recent [1999] movement of the health education profession toward policy advocacy, provide examples of recent health education advocacy efforts, and suggest future advocacy challenges for the health education profession.

## ORGANIZATIONAL CONSIDERATIONS IN ADVOCACY

An organization's tax-exempt status from the Internal Revenue Service (IRS) significantly affects the types and level of its political activities. While there are a variety of IRS categories, most health or trade groups have either a 501(c)(3) or 501(c)(6) tax status (Henson, 1996). IRS defines a 501(c)(3) organization as one that is organized and operated exclusively for charitable, religious, education, or safety purposes, or for fostering national or international amateur sports competition, prevention of cruelty to children and animals, or a private foundation (Henson, 1996). The main benefits of 501(c)(3) tax status are that such groups are eligible to receive grants from public and private sources, donations from its contributors are tax-deductible, and the association can apply to receive an exemption from paying state sales tax. Organizations designated as 501(c)(4) are designed for the promotion of social welfare, with their net earnings devoted exclusively to charitable, educational, or recreational purposes. Although contributions to a 501(c)(6) organization is one in which persons or entities have some common business interest, the purpose of which is to promote such common interest and not to engage in a for-profit business. While 501(c)(3) organizations cannot participate directly or indirectly in a campaign for public office, 501(c)(6) groups are not limited in their endorsement of political candidates (Ernstthal & Jones, 1996). Furthermore, a 501(c)(3) organization's political activities must comprise an "unsubstantial" portion of its overall program, which by various inurement tests is considered roughly 20 percent of its total operating budget (Henson, 1996). In contrast, the IRS does not restrict the amount of lobbying by 50l(c)(6) organizations, except that its members cannot consider the portion of member dues attributable to lobbying a tax-deductible contribution.

Both 501(c)(3) and 501(c)(6) tax-exempt designations are common among health groups. Many groups that apply for 501(c)(6) status to provide flexibility in their political pursuits also have companion 501(c)(3) foundations to be eligible for the attractive tax-exempt benefits, for example, the American Dietetic Association and the American Dietetic Association Foundation. Many health-related organizations such as the American Medical Association (AMA) have formed political action committees (PACs) to enhance their political effectiveness. AMA's political action committee, AMPAC, was formed in 1961 "to advance the goals of medicine at the federal level by supporting candidates who share basic philosophies and similar views on health care issues" (AMAPAC, n.d.). AMPAC is solely supported by voluntary, non-dues contributions by members from the state level up.

In addition to forming PACs, many of the larger, better-established health groups operate government relations departments that include registered lobbyists. According to the Lobbying Disclosure Act of 1995, a lobbyist is a person paid by another, whether a client or employer, to make lobbying contacts, unless that person spends less than 20 percent of his or her time on lobbying activities for the employer or a particular clients during a six-month period (Ballantine & Ross, 1996). A lobbying contact is an oral or written communication with members of Congress, congressional staff, political appointees, or other senior executive-branch officials regarding federal legislation, federal rules or regulations, the administration of a federal program or policy, or the nomination or confirmation of a person subject confirmation by the Senate. Lobbying activities are broadly defined to include any lobbying contacts with persons covered under the Lobbying Disclosure Act of 1995, as well as any preparation, planning or research, and background work originally intended for use in contacting there persons. If lobbyists make lobbying contacts, they must register under the Act and report information about the contacts to the Internal Revenue Service and information about any lobbying activities. If a person engages in lobbying without contacts, however, no registration or reporting is required (Ballantine & Ross, 1996).

In addition to the legal issues governing the amount of political activity an organization may undertake, many other considerations will affect a group's policy advocacy involvement, such as

- *Budget*—Amount of funds committed to advocacy versus other organizational priorities;

- *Office location*—Accessibility to policymakers, which may require having a satellite office if the organization is not headquartered in Washington, DC or state/local seat of government;

- *Staffing*—Employing lobbyists or trained government relations staff to maintain ongoing contacts with policymakers and their staffs, monitor legislation and policies, draft positions on proposed legislation based on organizational policy, plan and implement strategies to influence policy, form coalitions, and the like;

- *Organizational structure for policy development*—Clarifying the role of advocacy within the organization's mission and strategic plan and establishing internal structures/committees for developing resolutions or other papers to guide organizational policy;

- *Communication support*—Developing a communications plan with members, Congress, the media, and general public to support the advocacy goals; and

- *Advocacy priorities*—Identifying what issues are important to the organization's leaders and members and making strategic decisions about which issues to pursue (Golden, 1996).

One of the most difficult but important tasks for any association is establishing priorities among the myriad of important issues related to its mission. To help set priorities, it is vital to conduct an environmental scan on each potential issue that includes information on the (1) importance of the issue to the organization and its membership; (2) economic, social, environmental, health, or other impact of the proposed issue; (3) existing science-base supporting the proposed policy or issue; (4) current organizational resolutions or policy statements on the issue; (5) likelihood of being successful at this time on the issue given the current political climate; (6) nature of the opposition to the organization's stance; (7) availability of resources needed for success; and (8) organizational allies on the issue or groups which might be contacted to form coalitions. Although the authority or process for selecting advocacy priorities may vary by association, each group's final list of priorities should be congruent with its mission and strategic plan (Golden, 1996).

## THE EVOLVING ROLE OF ADVOCACY IN HEALTH EDUCATION

Prior to the social movements affecting the latter part of [the twentieth] century, health professional organizations in general often assumed an indirect role in policy advocacy, such as serving as an information resource for legislators or providing expert testimony. One of the most notable examples was in 1976, when the Society for Public Health Education's (SOPHE) president, Dr. William Griffiths, presented testimony to the President's Committee on Health Education, the Task Force on Health Education, and the Policy Committee of the National Center for Health Education Project (Bloom, 1999). Direct lobbying for political candidates or legislation generally was viewed as a more appropriate role for trade associations, rather than scientific professional groups.

Social movements in the 1960s and 1970s eventually led to enactment of legislation calling for increased direct citizen participation in the decision-making process (Schwartz, Goodman, & Steckler, 1995). By the late 1970s, articles in SOPHE's journal *Health Education Quarterly* and other professional publications began to recognize policy advocacy as a form of health promotion and called for increased participation of health educators in the political process. Over the next decade, research in the application of ecological approaches to health education as well as the role of health educators in community coalitions led to further recognition of health educators' roles as policy advocates. Writing about emerging roles for health education in policy advocacy in 1987, Steckler, Dawson, Goodman, and Epstein concluded, "As members of a profession, health educators must actively endeavor to influence those policies that not only determine the kind and amount of resources allocated for health education programs, but also consider the large policy framework under which health education is subsumed" (Steckler & Dawson, 1982). In 1995, a theme issue of *Health Education Quarterly* on "policy advocacy interventions for health promotion and education" highlighted examples of successful environmental and policy interventions in cardiovascular disease, tobacco control, physical activity, and other program areas (Schwartz, Goodman, & Steckler, 1995).

The essential role of policy interventions in health education programs eventually paved the way for changes in health education professional curriculum and the competencies expected of new health education graduates. *Standards for the Preparation of Graduate-Level Health Educators* enumerated numerous advocacy-related competencies (American Association for Health Education, National Commission for Health Education Credentialing, & Society for Public Health Education, 1999). A report commissioned by the Health Resources and Services Administration, *Health Education in the 21st Century*, identified advocacy as one of four critical areas for improving graduate education in the next millennium (Merrill, Chen, Gielen, McDonald, Auld, & Mulrooney, 1998). Policy advocacy is also cited as one of the critical areas for future education and training of the public health education workforce (Allegrante, Moon, Auld, & Gebbie, 1999).

## CURRENT ADVOCACY ROLES OF HEALTH EDUCATION ASSOCIATIONS

With the increased recognition of advocacy in the profession and practice of health education, today [1999] most health education groups include a specific reference to policy involvement in their mission statements or organizational goals. Many groups have offices in or near the nation's capital to facilitate their involvement: American Association for Health Education, Association Public Health Association (APHA, which includes the Public Health Education & Health Promotion Section and the School Health Education and Services Section), Association of State and Territorial Directors of Health Promotion and Public Health Education, SOPHE, and the Society of State Directors of Health, Physical Education, and Recreation. Although SOPHE was headquartered for more than forty-five years in New York and California, the Society relocated to Washington, DC, in 1995 explicitly for the purposes of increasing its policy advocacy efforts (Bloom, 1999). The American School Health Association, based in Kent, Ohio, retains a part-time registered lobbyist to represent its views in Washington, DC.

In addition to organizing individual advocacy efforts, health education organizations have been working collectively since 1972 as part of the Coalition of National Health Education Organizations (CNHEO) to "facilitate national level coordination, collaboration, and communication among member organizations; provide a forum to identify and discuss health education issues, formulate and take action on issues affecting the members' interest; serve as a resource for external agencies; and serve as a focus for the collaborative exploration and resolution of issues pertinent to professional health educators" (Coalition of National Health Education Organizations, n.d.). Recent examples of political issues that the CNHEO has addressed on behalf of the health education profession include tobacco legislation, Healthy People 2010, and proposed regulations for identifying health educators as part of the Standard Occupational Classification (SOC) used by the Departments of Labor and Commerce.

All CNHEO members have advocacy committees or mechanisms in place for issuing action alerts to their leadership and members as well as resolution processes to form the basis for their political positions. The availability of electronic communications, including Web sites and listservs, has greatly enhanced the timeliness of groups' political responsiveness and helped ease financial barriers of advocacy-focused communications programs. Advocacy priorities span the broad range of issues from funding of research in the behavioral and social sciences, to education/training of future health educators, to appropriations of major health programs (such as Centers for Disease Control and Prevention, Health Resources and Services Administration, National Institutes of Health).

In 1995, the CNHEO and the National Commission for Health Education Credentialing sponsored an invitational meeting in Atlanta, titled "The Health Education Profession in the Twenty-first Century: Setting the Stage," to address the future of the health education profession (National Commission for Health Education Credentialing & Coalition of National Health Education Organizations, 1995). Advocacy emerged as one of six priority areas, with participants identifying fifteen actions needed with the profession and fourteen actions needed external to the profession to move it into a significant role within the United States. Many of these advocacy goals are being addressed, in part, through sponsorship of an annual Health Education Advocacy Summit.

The First and Second Annual Health Education Advocacy Summits were conducted during the spring of 1998 and 1999. The Summits provided health education organizations the opportunity to come together for the first time to develop a common advocacy agenda and to collectively advocate for these issues on Capitol Hill. They also provided the catalyst for participating groups to subsequently provide training, materials, and other resources to their leaderships, members, and chapters on key health education issues. This has been accomplished through special sessions of the groups' annual meetings, newsletter articles, Web pages, and targeted mailings. Particularly exciting is the role of students and new professionals from Eta Sigma Gamma in the Summit and in encouraging grassroots follow-up through its chapters. The Summit provides the students an opportunity to "practice what is preached" in the classroom.

Support for the Summit grew from 1998 to 1999, both financially and in terms of the number of participating organizations, and appears to be gaining momentum for future years as an ongoing mechanism for the profession's advocacy goals. The Summits also have helped forge new partnerships and coalitions with organizations such as the National Education Association, Effective National Action for Control of Tobacco, the Campaign for Tobacco-Free Kids, and the Centers for Disease Control and Prevention Coalition. Planning is now [1999] underway for the third Health Education Advocacy Summit in March 2000.

Health education organizations have also made significant progress in recent years in terms of developing external systems to influence public policy and affecting policy changes in support of health education. Almost all groups have had input into broad policy-related documents such as the proposed Healthy People 2010 Objectives, which, in part, provide the basis for policy and resource allocation at the state and local levels. In 1997–98, SOPHE spearheaded an effort involving the CNHEO to obtain recognition by the Departments of Labor and Commerce for the distinct occupational classification of "health educator," which was a major victory (Auld, 1997). For the first time, the federal government and states will begin gathering data about the geographic distribution, salaries, and other essential data for the profession. In addition, the Association of State and Territorial Directors of Health Promotion and Public Health Education (ASTDHPPHE), SOPHE, and the Society of State Directors of Health, Physical Education, and Recreation (SSDHPER) are collaborating on a Public Health Education Leadership Institute, a year-long program to develop leadership skills of their members (Capwell, 1998).

## FUTURE CHALLENGES

Although health education organizations have made significant advocacy strides in recent years, many challenges are ahead for the twenty-first century. First, health education groups must have a sustained presence on Capitol Hill, not just a barrage of visits once per year. Relationships built during the Summits with Congressional representatives and their staffs must be sustained for long-term political impact.

Second, the groups need to narrow and better focus their annual political objectives. Although there are many worthwhile public health issues, taking on too many complex and difficult issues only decreases the likelihood of political victory on any one of them.

Third, health education associations need to expand ways of effectively mobilizing their memberships "outside the Beltway" (including chapters, regional groups, and districts) and continue developing their advocacy skills. Likewise, such groups must encourage members to run for leadership positions or political offices at the local, state, or national levels. Currently [1999], a formally trained health educator, Robert Patton, is serving his second term in the Tennessee legislature.

Fourth, health education groups must continue advocating for funds to expand the research base of the health education discipline. A richer science-base on the effectiveness of health education interventions will, in turn, strengthen our arguments for health education programs in Congress.

Finally, because the occupation of health educator and the issues important to the profession are still relatively obscure to policymakers, health education organizations must make a long-term commitment to advocacy. They must budget the financial and human capital to maximize the effectiveness of their advocacy efforts, while still acting within IRS restrictions of their tax-exempt status.

## REFERENCES

Allegrante, J. P., Moon, R., Auld, M. E., & Gebbie, K. (1999). Future training needs of the public health education workforce. Submitted for publication to *Health Promotion Practice*.

American Association for Health Education, National Commission for Health Education Credentialing, & Society for Public Health Education. (1999). *A competency-based framework for graduate-level health educators.*

American Medical Association Political Action Committee (AMPAC). (n.d.). AMPAC [Web site]. Retrieved from http://www.ampaconline.org

Auld, E: (1997). SOC approves new occupational category for "Health Educator." *CHES Bulletin, 8*, 61–62.

Ballantine, R., & Ross, J. L. (1996, February). *Government relations newsletter*. American Society of Association Executives.

Bloom, F. K. (1999). *The Society for Public Health Education: Its development and contributions, 1976–1996*. Doctoral dissertation. UMI Dissertation Services, 88–379.

Capwell, E. (1998). Public Health Education Leadership Institute. *News & Views, 25*(2), 5.

Coalition of National Health Education Organizations. (n.d.). About us. [Web site]. Retrieved from http://www.cnheo.org/.

Ernstthal, H. L., & Jones, B. (1996). *Principles of association management* (3rd ed.). Washington, DC: American Society of Association Executives.

Golden, M. (1996). *Government relations in the association environment*. Presented at the American Society of Association Executives School of Association Management: Government Relations, June 4–5, Washington, DC.

Henson, J. A. (1996). *The ABCs of non-profit status*. Society for Public Health Education annual meeting, November 15–17, New York, NY.

Merrill, R., Chen, D. W., Gielen, A., McDonald, E., Auld, M. E., Mulrooney, S. J., et al. (1998). The future health education workforce. *Journal of Health Education 29*(5), S59–S64.

National Commission for Health Education Credentialing and Coalition of National Health Education Organizations. (1996). The health education profession in the twenty-first century: Setting the stage. *Journal of Health Education 27*(6), 357–364.

Schwartz, R., Goodman, R., & Steckler, A. (1995). Policy advocacy interventions for health promotion and education: Advancing the state of practice. *Health Education Quarterly, 22*(4), 421–527.

Steckler, A., & Dawson, L., (1982). The role of health education in public policy development. *Health Education Quarterly, 9*(4), 275–292.

Vernick, J. S. (1999). Lobbying and advocacy for the public's health: What are the limits for nonprofit organizations? *American Journal of Public Health 59*(89), 1425–1429.

28

# THE ROLE OF HEALTH EDUCATION ADVOCACY IN REMOVING DISPARITIES IN HEALTH CARE

**JOHN P. ALLEGRANTE**

**DONALD E. MORISKY**

**BEHJAT A. SHARIF**

Since the founding of the Centers for Disease Control and Prevention over fifty years ago, people in the United States have experienced unprecedented improvements in health status. There are now almost one million fewer cases of measles compared to 1941, and two hundred thousand fewer cases of diphtheria. Average blood-lead levels in children are now less than one-third of what they were in 1976. More than two million Americans are alive today who otherwise would have died from tobacco-attributable heart disease and stroke because of the landmark announcement by the Surgeon General in 1964 regarding the threat posed by tobacco. Moreover, efforts to protect the blood supply have now prevented more than two million Hepatitis B and C infections and more than fifty thousand HIV infections, resulting in savings of more than $3.5 billion in medical costs associated with these three diseases (Turnock, 1997).

Despite these notable achievements in disease control and prevention, there is mounting evidence that disparities in health care have grown unacceptably wide in American society. The disparities between minorities and the white population have increased in the last decade [1989–1999] on virtually every measure of health status (U.S. Department of Health and Human Services, 1998a). Consequently, the *Healthy People 2010 Objectives* (U.S. Department of Health and Human Services, 1998b) calls for the elimination of health disparities in six major areas—infant mortality, cardiovascular disease, diabetes, and HIV/AIDS, as well as cancer screening and management and childhood and adult immunizations. Health education advocacy can play an important role in eliminating such health disparities (Montes & Johnson, 1998). Advocacy constitutes the development of coalitions and partnerships, as well as working with the media, to influence political, regulatory, and environmental policies that can improve community health. There are numerous examples of health promotion policy initiatives that have relied on advocacy efforts to influence the tobacco, alcohol, and environmental issues (Green & Kreuter, 1999). Although there is not extensive literature on the use of advocacy to reduce health disparities among disadvantaged populations, Braithwaite and Lythcott (1989) and Thomas (1990) have argued that community empowerment strategies are critical to health promotion for African Americans and other minorities.

This paper will first summarize the mounting evidence of disparities in health status and access to health services across disadvantaged American populations. Next, we review some of the major contributing factors to these health disparities. We then highlight selected examples of advocacy approaches that have been conceptualized and implemented in health education efforts. Finally, we conclude by discussing the role of advocacy aimed at eliminating the health disparities that persist among the disadvantaged.

## DISPARITIES IN HEALTH STATUS AND ACCESS TO HEALTH SERVICES

Despite notable progress in achieving many of the national goals and objectives for the improvement of overall health status, there are persistent disparities in the burden of illness and death experienced by African Americans, Hispanics and Latinos, American Indians and Alaskan Natives, and Pacific Islanders. According to the U.S. Department of Health and Human Services (1998c), these disparities are even greater when comparisons are made between each racial and ethnic group and the U.S. population as a whole.

- Infant mortality rates are two and a half times higher for African Americans and one and a half times higher for Native Americans than for Caucasian Americans.

- African American men under 65 years of age suffer from prostate cancer at nearly twice the rate of Caucasians.

- Heart disease, the leading cause of death and a common cause of morbidity in the U.S., occurs at nearly twice the rate in African American men compared to Caucasian men. The age-adjusted death rate for coronary heart disease for the total population declined by 20 percent from 1987 to 1995, but for blacks, the overall decrease was only 13 percent. Compared with rates for whites, coronary heart disease mortality was 40 percent lower for Asian Americans but 40 percent higher for blacks in 1995.

- Native Americans suffer from diabetes at nearly three times the average rate, while African Americans suffer 70 percent higher rates than Caucasians; the prevalence of diabetes in Hispanics is nearly double that of Caucasians.

- Racial and ethnic minorities constitute approximately 25 percent of the total population, yet they account for nearly 54 percent of all AIDS cases.

Such disparities in health status, however, are not constrained to racial and ethnic minority groups. The disparities have become increasingly evident for women, people with low incomes, people with disabilities, and specific age groups, including children, adolescents, and the elderly, as well as by geographic location.

## MAJOR CONTRIBUTING FACTORS TO HEALTH DISPARITIES

The causes of health disparities have long been of interest to epidemiologists, sociologists, and public health professionals. Among the major contributing factors to these disparities are race and ethnicity, socioeconomic status, gender, age, geographic location, insurance coverage, and political will.

### Race and Ethnicity

Health disparities by race and ethnicity are especially pronounced among Americans (Council on Ethical and Judicial Affairs, 1990). For example, studies have found that African American men living in Harlem have a life expectancy that is less than that of men living in Bangladesh (McCord & Freeman, 1990); that there are dramatic racial differences in preventable deaths in the Medicare population (Woolander et al., 1985); that race can influence the stage at diagnosis for endometrial cancer (Barrett et al., 1995), as well as colon cancer survival (Mayberry et al., 1995); and that the prevalence of arthritis and other potentially disabling musculoskeletal conditions is higher in African Americans than other groups (Charlson, Allegrante, & Robbins, 1993).

In addition, numerous studies have documented disparities in access to health services. Studies of access by African Americans to emergency room services (Perkoff & Anderson, 1970), health and hospital services (Gornick et al., 1996; Yergan, Flood, LoGerfo, & Diehr, 1987), organ transplantation (Kasiske et al., 1991), total joint replacement (Katz, Freund, Heck, & Dittus, 1996), and treatment for chest pain and recommendations for cardiac catheterization (Schulman et al., 1999) have all suggested that race independently influences access to health services that can reduce morbidity and mortality and prevent disability.

Disparities also exist in the prevalence of risk factors. For example, racial and ethnic minorities have higher rates of hypertension, tend to develop hypertension at an earlier age, and are less likely to undergo treatment to control their high blood pressure. From 1988 to 1994, 35 percent of black males ages 20 to 74 had hypertension compared with 25 percent of all men. When age differences are taken into account, Mexican American men and women also have elevated blood pressure rates. However, the results of recent studies (Morisky & Ward, 1999; Ward, Morisky, Lees, & Fong in press) have demonstrated that both African American and Hispanic populations can benefit dramatically from community-based educational programs that utilize targeted and tailored approaches to blood pressure control.

Similarly, although significant effort has been made to reduce the overall U.S. infant mortality rate, a significant indicator of a nation's overall health status, marked disparities between minority groups and Caucasians persist. Puerto Rican, Hawaiian, American Indian, and African American infants suffer higher mortality rates, 26%, 33%, 55%, and 112% respectively, compared to Caucasian infants.

While the mechanism by which race and ethnicity influence health status may not be clear, it is entirely possible that perceived systematic discrimination may play an important causative role in diseases such as hypertension. Ren, Amick, and Williams (1999) have noted that the experiences of discrimination tend to have a strong negative association with health and that much more work needs to be done to specify the social distribution of discrimination and assess its consequences for health status in people of color.

## Socioeconomic Status

The contribution of socioeconomic status to health disparities has been well documented (Adler, Boyce, Chesney, Folkman, & Syme, 1993; Pappas, Queen, Hadden, & Fisher, 1993). Socioeconomic factors, including education, income, and occupation, are strongly associated with health and trends in health status in both individuals and populations (Kaplan, 1998). For example, maternal education and family income both inversely affect infant mortality (Singh & Yu, 1995). In addition, income inequality is not only a major determinant of infant mortality, but also life expectancy at birth (Smith, 1996).

Navarro (1997) states that differences in morbidity and mortality rates are related to social class and, in fact, these differentials are much larger by class than by race. For example, blue-collar workers' mortality rate for heart disease has been found to be 2.3 times higher than that of Caucasian-collar professionals. However, mortality rates for heart disease in African American males and females were respectively 1.2 and 1.5 times higher than their Caucasian counterparts. Those making $10,000 or less per year encountered 4.6 times more morbidity than those making over $35,000, while African Americans' morbidity rate was 1.9 times higher than that of Caucasians (Navarro, 1997).

Generally, minorities, who are among the lowest-paid, poorly educated working class, continue to have morbidity and mortality rates higher than those who are well-educated and well-paid. In addition, the low-paid population's standard of living has been deteriorating due to the growing inequity in income and wealth between the upper and lower classes. Navarro (1997) reports that the lower class of the population (40 percent) received 15.7 percent of the total income while the wealthiest of the population (20 percent) received 42.9 percent of total income. Thus, the growing gap in the nation's health clearly cannot be understood and remedied by examining individual differences by race and ethnicity alone.

The relationship of poverty to poor health is well established (Kawachi, Kennedy, Lochner, & Prothrow-Smith, 1997; Wilkinson, 1997). Being impoverished, however, not only results in destruction of individual health, but also in the social, physical and mental decay of generations. High mortality rates for both children and adults are directly related to poverty as well as income inequality. For example, the population death rate in North America attributable to poverty increased between the early 1970s and early 1990s. Moreover, the surge in the local incidence of some diseases, such as tuberculosis in New York City, during the last decade has been linked to poverty (Hamburg, 1993). Hence, it is not surprising to find observers such as Poland, Coburn, Robertson, & Eakin, (1997) and Tesh (1988) arguing that the political economy is a major determinant of health and illness.

Choice of occupation may also influence health (Karasek & Theorell, 1990; Tesh, 1988). For example, occupations that are characterized as high demand and low control have been correlated with coronary heart disease. In addition, low-paying jobs often involve exposure to harmful substances, require potentially repetitive motion or entail exposure to potentially dangerous equipment and machinery, or other unhealthy situations. Thus, improvements in occupational health should not only focus on redesigning jobs but examine why many current work designs generally result in such an excessive demand and insufficient level of job control.

Unfortunately, the scientific, multi-causal approach to analyzing the etiology of diseases often does not specify the contribution of fundamental factors, such as social condition, in the causal nexus of poor health (Tesh, 1988). Historical records support the notion that the origins of diseases have been largely social in nature. In the case of epidemics, what data are available suggest a clear linkage between disease and the conditions under which people live. For example, Lantz, House, Lepkowski, Williams, Mero, & Chen (1990) indicate that socioeconomic differences in mortality are due to social-structural factors and that high mortality could persist despite improved health behaviors among the poor. Similarly, Minkler (1999) has argued that while we need not abandon concepts of personal responsibility for health, focusing on the broader social responsibility for health is necessary if we are to improve health.

The foregoing suggests that effective disease prevention not only seeks to identify the specific agent, web of causation, or personal actions, but also the more fundamental political and economic causes of disease and those factors that may result in an unequal distribution of power and resources. Those with secure employment, a good education, adequate medical care, and regular leisure activities do not develop diseases that plague the impoverished. Consequently, satisfying jobs, decent housing, and good schools serve as strong factors in disease prevention and should be targets of intervention if we are to reduce disparities in health.

## Gender

Women are more likely than men to bear a significantly greater proportion of the burden of disease and illness in American society. Since the 1970s there has been considerable interest in the relative health of women and men and the extent to which gender differences play a role in determining the health status of Americans and Western Europeans (Hunt & Annandale, 1999). While there is consensus that gender disparities in health continue to be mediated to some degree by women's unequal status in society (Cook, 1994; Doyal, 1995; Fee & Krieger, 1994), in addition to the inherent physiological differences that influence their proclivity to greater disability and morbidity than males (Arber & Cooper, 1999; Belgrave, 1993; Graham, 1998), a noteworthy recent finding by Kawachi, Kennedy, Gupta, and Prothrow-Smith (1999) is that indices of American women's health status strongly predict both American male and female mortality rates. Severe marital violence is also highest in those states where gender inequality is the highest.

Another important observation documented by Bayne-Smith and McBarnette (1996) is that among women in the United States, the particular disparities that have limited the intellectual growth of minority women, arguably account, in part, for their inferior health status, both physical and mental, when compared to their more well-endowed Caucasian counterparts and males who live in poverty. Indeed, Roberts (1999) found African American female adolescents who were poor and living in inner cities to bear a disproportionate burden of poor health outcomes compared to white women. As such, interdisciplinary collaborations examining the structural inequities and combined consequences of sexism, racism, and inner-city poverty for young women of color are necessary to inform public health interventions designed to improve the health of African American female adolescents.

In addition to societal-wide inequities in health status generated by gender discrimination, gender inequities in access, particularly to quality prenatal care, have a strong bearing on the health status of infants. There is a two-fold risk of sudden infant death in American minority populations (Hill, 1999). Moreover, gender may also influence access and exposure to material and other resources differentially and inequitably (Stacey & Olesen, 1993).

## Age

An excess of morbidity with more severe domains of poor health is likely to be found among elderly people. Work by Fitzpatrick and Van Tran (1997), who have studied the effects of age, gender, and health among African Americans, found both the objective and subjective dimensions of health to vary according to age, but that the effects of age on health status were not the same for men and women at any age. Older women are, however, substantially more likely to experience functional impairment in mobility and self-care than men of the same age (Arber & Cooper, 1999; Belgrave, 1993).

Inner-city older blacks also have higher levels of functional disability than whites of a comparable age and black adults in other regions, regardless of gender, as well as increased body fat, and lower levels of dental care, along with high levels of visual and hearing impairments (Miller et al., 1996). However, age disparities in medical treatment are more likely to affect females because they are less likely than males to receive available treatments for cardiac, renal, and other conditions (Belgrave, 1993).

In addition, economic inequities are extremely detrimental to older females. This is supported by Smith and Kington (1997), whose research demonstrated health outcomes at old age with respect to race and ethnicity are influenced by economic differences. Similarly, there are striking inequalities in susceptibility of minority children to infectious diseases whose consequences may stretch into adulthood (Reading, 1997). This finding supports the view that environmental and material factors have a strong influence on health. Consequently, Reading favors an emphasis on structural and community-wide policy interventions that remove disparities, rather than intervention directed solely at changing individual behavior.

## Geographic Location

Geographic location may also play a role in contributing to health disparities. For example, there is growing evidence that urban populations bear a significantly greater proportion of disease burden due to problems such as asthma (Crain et al., 1994), HIV infection (Holmberg, 1996), and lead poisoning (Sargent et al.,1995), than do those living in suburban or rural areas. In addition, studies of the delivery of health services, including the treatment of acute myocardial infarction (O'Connor et al., 1999), total hip replacement (Peterson et al., 1992), and other common surgical procedures (Birkmeyer, Sharp, Finlayson, Fisher, & Wennberg, 1998) have shown dramatic variations in access to preventive services, medical treatment, and surgical procedures by geographic location.

## Insurance Coverage

According to Blendon, Donelan, Hill, Carter, Beatrice, and Altaian (1994), research has documented that decreased access to health care services, increased burden of economic hardship, poor health, and excess mortality are experienced by the uninsured and underinsured. Moreover, wide gaps in insurance coverage between racial and ethnic groups in America exacerbate the experience for minorities. For example, in a recent study conducted in California, rates of uninsured residents in 1997 amounted to 15 percent for Caucasians, 19 percent for African Americans, 24 percent for Asian Americans, and 38 percent for Latinos. Just 41 percent of Latinos in California were found to have job-level coverage, compared to 69 percent of Caucasians. The major reason for the high uninsured rates by ethnicity is affordability. The response most often given by the majority of Caucasians and Latinos when asked why they are not insured is that it was too expensive (Brown, 1996). In addition, despite the role that Medicaid has played in improving access to care, minority children still have a poorer quality of life than whites (Hall, 1998). Thus, improving access to health services will require eliminating the gaps in insurance coverage that still persist for the one out of four Americans who is either uninsured or underinsured.

## Political Will

Unfortunately, the basic questions that characterized the debate on health-care reform of the early 1990s have remained unanswered. Unlike the historical lack of understanding about public health, Americans have recently raised questions about effectiveness, efficiency, and cost of the health-care system. However, policy makers appear to take their cues from other sources and may not have the political will to do what is necessary to eliminate the disparities in health. Lee and Estes (1997) have argued that the most powerful constituencies in health care continue to be physicians, hospitals, insurance companies, and pharmaceutical industries. Although these groups appear to be concerned about the quality of care, they are generally more interested in surviving in the increasingly market-driven health care system than changing the system to make it more responsive to the health needs of an increasingly diverse America

To make matters worse, although there is a consensus about the nature of the problems in the health-care system, there is little agreement on what should be done to correct them (Lee & Estes, 1997). At the federal and state level, prevention has emerged as an important goal of health policy, yet prevention is still competing for a more equitable share of national resources (Allegrante, 1999). Whether policy makers will have the political will to shift resources from the investments that have historically been made in medical care to creating the community capacity and other resources necessary to eliminate the disparities in health status between poor and those who have considerably greater economic means remains to be seen.

## SOME EXAMPLES OF HEALTH EDUCATION ADVOCACY

Health educators have pioneered the use of advocacy to improve health and social conditions. The role of political advocacy in shaping public policies that can influence health can be found in the seminal writings of Freudenberg (1978), McKinlay (1993), Minkler and Cox (1980), Steckler and Dawson (1982), Steckler, Dawson, Goodman, and Epstein, (1987), and Wallerstein and Bernstein (1988). In addition, media advocacy, which is designed to alter the way in which the media frames its coverage of health issues and to provide a means by which a social or public policy initiative can be advanced, has been conceptualized by Jernigan and Wright (1996) and Wallack (1997; Wallack & Dortman, 1996). Below we review some examples of advocacy from the health education literature.

## Environment

A number of efforts have been made by health educators and others to use advocacy to bring about community-based political change and support for environmental policies. These have included health education advocacy and community coalitions to reduce lead poisoning in New York City (Freudenberg & Golub, 1987), improve the housing conditions in an urban, low-income neighborhood through community development (El-Askari et al., 1998), and prevent urban arson at Halloween (Maciak, Moore, Leviton, & Guinan, 1998).

## Tobacco Control

Recent tobacco control initiatives in several states, including California, Minnesota, Texas, and Florida, have been the result of intense advocacy by public health groups. These initiatives have stimulated activities at the local, county, and state levels through community coalitions and partnerships, which have resulted in legislative initiatives supporting the regulation and control of tobacco products. Such advocacy efforts have led to public information, building community awareness of the tobacco problem, and policy and ordinance development within establishments (Blaine et al., 1997), as well as media advocacy related to cardiovascular disease risk reduction (Schooler, Sundar, & Flora, 1996).

## Alcohol

Advocacy has been especially effective in a number of health education efforts to promote responsible use of alcohol and to prevent alcohol-related motor vehicle deaths (DeJong, 1996) and alcohol-related violence against women (Woodruff, 1996). This work has demonstrated that media advocacy can be an effective means by which to increase public awareness of alcohol-related issues and to advance the cause of alcohol-related prevention efforts in the community (Holder & Treno, 1997).

## Elderly

One of the first advocacy efforts in health education was Minkler's work to reduce the poor health conditions, social isolation, and powerlessness of low-income elderly residents living in single-room occupancy hotels in the Tenderloin section of San Francisco (Minkler, 1985, 1992; Minkler, Franz, & Wechsler, 1982). The Tenderloin Senior Outreach Project utilized individual and community empowerment strategies to build self-reliance and community cohesion among inner-city disadvantaged elderly. Subsequent work by Roe and Minkler and their colleagues has extended the use of concepts of community organizing and advocacy that proved so successful with grandparents in this project (Minkler, Driver, Roe, & Bedeian, 1993; Roe, Minkler, & Saunders, 1995).

## HIV/AIDS

Advocacy efforts have been utilized for more than two decades to inform the public about the risk of HIV/AIDS and to foster public support for prevention programs in schools (Krieger & Lashof, 1988) and the general community (Rundall & Phillips, 1990). More recent advocacy approaches have focused on developing consortium approaches to the delivery of HIV services (McKinney, 1993), and have been used to develop community-based HIV prevention programs for Americans of Asian and Pacific Islander backgrounds (Wong, Chng, & Lo, 1998). Targeted educational interventions, which have included organizational change policy, directed at female bar workers and the managers of the establishments in which they are employed have demonstrated significant reductions in STD and prevention of HIV infection (Morisky et al., 1998).

### Racial and Ethnic Minorities

Advocacy approaches have been used in numerous efforts by health educators and other professionals to reduce health disparities for racial and ethnic minorities. These include reducing teenage pregnancy (Liburd & Bowie, 1989), improving access to health services for the Latino population in St. Louis (Baker et al., 1997), mobilizing minority communities in Indiana to facilitate enactment of legislation for a minority health initiative to reduce preventable disease (Russell, 1997), and developing improved community-wide asthma care for low-income minority populations (Wilson et al., 1998).

### Youth Violence

Advocacy has been used as a public health strategy in the prevention of youth violence (Cohen & Swift, 1993). These efforts have resulted in laws being passed at the local and state levels that make it more difficult for young people to purchase handguns and other firearms. A model program that relies heavily on advocacy, and that has been effective in bringing about changes in media coverage of the issues, as well as community and policy change, is the California Violence Prevention Initiative (California Wellness Foundation, 1994). This multiple-component advocacy effort was designed to reduce violence among youth and young adults. The initiative included policy development, community action programs, leadership development, public education, and research. Through such advocacy, communities throughout California have been able to promote and enact gun-control legislation at both the state and local levels (RAND and Stanford Center for Research in Disease Prevention, 1997).

## CONCLUSION

Despite the overall decline in mortality rates in recent decades, there is persuasive evidence (only a small portion of which could be reviewed here) that disparities in health are increasing along the lines of race and ethnicity. This is especially troubling given that America's population is projected by demographers to grow even more racially and ethnically diverse in the next century. Advocacy will become increasingly necessary if we are to stimulate the community political action and economic and environmental changes that promise to address the health needs of such a diverse population, in order to eliminate the disparities in health status and access to health services that now exist, however, new knowledge concerning the influence of socioeconomic factors in the causation of disease and the effectiveness of policy-related interventions to alter such factors is required In the meantime, if we are to have any hope of eliminating disparities in health we need to address the broad socioeconomic determinants of disease that we already know influence health, and we must seek to eliminate those inequities in power and wealth that all available evidence suggests is still at the root of the problem. Health educators can be at the vanguard of this effort by expanding their work to influence community-level and national policy development through advocacy.

## REFERENCES

Adler, N., Boyce, T, Chesney, M., Folkman, S., & Syme, L. (1993). Socioeconomic inequalities in health. *Journal of the American Medical Association, 269*, 3140–3145.

Allegrante, J. P. (1999). 1998 SOPHE Presidential Address: SOPHE—At the intersection of education, policy, and science and technology. *Health Education & Behavior, 26*, 457–464.

Arber, S., & Cooper, H. (1999). Gender differences in health in later life: The new paradox? *Social Science and Medicine, 48*, 61–76.

Baker, E. A., Bouldin, N., Durham, M., Lowell, M. E., Gonzalez, M., Jodaitis, N., et al. (1997). The Latino health advocacy program: A collaborative lay health advisor approach. *Health Education & Behavior, 24*, 495–509.

Barrett, R. J., Harlan, L. C, Wesley, M. N., Hill, H. A., Chen, V. W., Clayton, L. A., et al. (1995). Endometrial cancer: Stage at diagnosis and associated factors in black and white patients. *American Journal of Obstetrics and Gynecology, 173*, 414–422.

Bayne-Smith, M., & McBarnette, L. S. (1996). Redefining health in the 21st century. In M. Bayne-Smith (Ed.), *Race, gender and health*. Thousand Oaks, CA: Sage.

Belgrave, L. L. (1993). Discrimination against older women in health care. *Journal of Women and Aging, 5*, 181–199.

Birkmeyer, J. D., Sharp, S. M., Finlayson, S. R., Fisher, E. S., & Wennberg, J. E. (1998). Variation profiles of common surgical procedures. *Surgery, 124*, 917–923.

Blaine, T. M., Forster, J. L., Hennrikus, D., O'Neil, S., Wolfson, M., & Pham, H. (1997). Creating tobacco control policy at the local level: Implementation of a direct action organizing approach *Health Education & Behavior, 24*, 640–651.

Blendon, R. J., Donelan, K., Hill, C. A., Carter, W., Beatrice, D., & Altaian, D. (1994). Paying medical bills in the United States: Why health insurance isn't enough. *Journal of the American Medical Association, 271*, 949–951.

Braithwaite, R. L., & Lythcott, N. (1989). Community empowerment as a strategy for health promotion for black and other minorities. *Journal of the American Medical Association, 261*, 282–283.

Brown, E. R. (1996). Trends in health insurance coverage in California, 1989–1993. *Health Affairs, 15*, 118–130.

California Wellness Foundation. (1994). *The California Wellness Foundation violence prevention initiative: A new direction for improving health and well-being in California*. Woodland Hill, CA: Author.

Charlson, M. E., Allegrante, J. P., & Robbins L. (1993). Socioeconomic differentials in arthritis and its treatment. In D. E. Rogers, & E. Ginzburg (Eds.), *Medical care and the health of the poor* (pp. 77–89). Boulder, CO: Westview Press.

Cohen, L., & Swift, S. (1993). A public health approach to the violence epidemic in the United States. *Environment and Urbanization, 5*, 50–66.

Cook, R. J. (1994). *Women's health and human rights*. Geneva, Switzerland: World Health Organization.

Council on Ethical and Judicial Affairs. (1990). Black-white disparities in health care. *Journal of the American Medical Association, 263*, 2344–2346.

Crain, E. E. Weiss, K. B., Bijur, P. E., Hersh, M., Westbrook, L., & Stein, R.E.K. (1994). An estimate of the prevalence of asthma and wheezing among inner-city children. *Pediatrics, 94*, 356–362.

DeJong, W. (1996). MADD Massachusetts versus Senator Burke: A media advocacy case study. *Health Education Quarterly, 23*, 318–329.

Doyal, L. (1995). *What makes women sicker: Gender and the political economy of health*. New Brunswick, NJ: Rutgers University Press.

El-Askari, G., Freestone, J., Irizarry, C., Kraut, K. L., Mashiyana, S. T., Morgan, M. A., et al. (1998). The healthy neighborhood project: A local health department's role in catalyzing community development. *Health Education & Behavior, 25*, 146–159.

Fee, E., & Krieger, N. (1994). *Women's health, politics, and power*. New York: Baywood Publishing.

Fitzpatrick, T. R., & Van Tran, T. (1997). Age, gender and health among African-Americans. *Social Work in Health Care, 26*, 69–85.

Freudenberg, N. (1978). Shaping the future of health education: From behavior change to social change. *Health Education Monographs, 6*, 372–377.

Freudenberg, N., & Golub, M. (1987). Health education, public policy and disease prevention: A case history of the New York City coalition to end lead poisoning. *Health Education Quarterly, 14*, 387–401.

Gornick, M. E., Eggers, P. W., Reilly, T. W., Mentaeck, R. M., Fitterman, L. K., Kucken, L. E., et al. (1996). Effects of race and income on mortality and use of services among Medicare beneficiaries. *New England Journal of Medicine, 335*, 791–799.

Graham, R. J. (1998). The relationship between sex, gender, and disability: Do women really tend to be more disabled than men? Paper presented at the meeting of the American Sociological Association.

Green, L. W., & Kreuter, M. W. (1999) *Health promotion planning: An educational and ecological approach* (3rd ed.). Mountain View, CA: Mayfield.

Hall, A. G. (1998). Medicaid's impact on access to and utilization of health care services among racial and ethnic minority children. *Journal of Urban Health, 75*, 677–692.

Hamburg, M. A. (1993). Poverty, public health, and tuberculosis control in New York City: Lessons from the past. In D. E. Rogers & E. Ginzburg (Eds.), *Medical care and the health of the poor* (pp. 33–41). Boulder, CO: Westview Press.

Hill, W. C. (1999). Jumping the broom toward eliminating health disparities: Presidential address. *American Journal of Obstetrics and Gynecology, 180*, 1315–1321.

Holder, H. D., & Treno, A. J. (1997). Media advocacy in community prevention: News as a means to advance policy change. *Addiction, 2*, S189–S199.

Holmberg, S. D. (1996). The estimated prevalence and incidence of HIV in 96 large U.S. metropolitan areas. *American Journal of Public Health, 86*, 642–654.

Hunt, K., & Annandale, E. (1999). Relocating gender and morbidity: Examining men's and women's health in contemporary Western societies. Introduction to special issue on gender and health. *Social Science and Medicine, 48*, 1–5.

Jernigan, D. H., & Wright, P. A. (1996). Media advocacy: Lessons from community experiences. *Journal of Public Health Policy, 17*, 306–330.

Kaplan, G. A. (1998). Socioeconomic considerations in the health of urban areas. *Journal of Urban Health, 75*, 228–235.

Karasek, R., & Theorell, T. (1990). *Healthy work: Stress, productivity and the reconstruction of working life*. New York: Basic Books.

Kasiske, B., Neylan, J., Riggio, R., Danovitch, G., Kahana, L., Alexander, S., et al. (1991). The effect of race on access and outcome in transplantation. *New England Journal of Medicine, 324*, 302–307.

Katz, B. P., Freund, D. A., Heck, D. A., & Dittus, R. S. (1996). Demographic variation in the rate of knee replacement: A multi-year analysis. *Health Services Research, 31*, 124–140.

Kawachi, I., Kennedy, B. P., Gupta, V., & Prothrow-Stith, D. (1999). Women's status and the health of women and men: A view from the states. *Social Science and Medicine, 48*, 21–32.

Kawachi, I., Kennedy, B., Lochner, K., & Prothrow-Smith, D. (1997). Social capital, income inequity, and mortality. *American Journal of Public Health, 87*, 1491–1497.

Krieger, N., & Lashof, J. C. (1988). AIDS, policy analysis, and the electorate: The role of schools of public health. *American Journal of Public Health, 78*, 411–415.

Lantz, P., House, J., Lepkowski, J., Williams, D., Mero, R., & Chen, J. (1990). Socioeconomic factors, health behaviors, and mortality: Results from a nationally representative prospective study of U.S. adults. *Journal of the American Medical Association, 279*, 1703–1708.

Lee, P. R., & Estes, C. L. (Eds.). (1997). *The nation's health*. Sudbury, MA: Jones and Bartlett.

Liburd, L. C., & Bowie, J. V. (1989). Intentional teenage pregnancy: A community diagnosis and action plan. *Health Education, 205*, 33–38.

Maciak, B. J., Moore, M. T., Leviton, L. C., & Guinan, M. E. (1998). Preventing Halloween arson in an urban setting: A model for multisectoral planning and community participation. *Health Education & Behavior, 25*, 194–211.

Mayberry, R. M., Coates, R. J., Hill, H. A., Click, L. A., Chen, V. W., Austin, D. F., et al. (1995). Determinants of black/white differences in colon cancer survival. *Journal of the National Cancer Institute, 87*, 1686–1693.

McCord, C., & Freeman, H. (1990). Excess mortality in Harlem. *New England Journal of Medicine, 322*, 173–177.

McKinlay, J. B. (1993). The promotion of health through planned sociopolitical change: Challenges for research and policy. *Social Science and Medicine, 36*, 109–117.

McKinney, M. M. (1993). Consortium approaches to the delivery of HIV services under the Ryan White Care Act. *AIDS and Public Policy Journal, 8*, 115–125.

Miller, D. K., Carter, M. E., Philip, M. J., Fornoff, J. E., Bentley, J. A., Boyd, S., et al. (1996). Inner-city older blacks have high levels of functional disability. *Journal of the American Geriatric Society, 44*, 1166–1173.

Minkler, M. (1985). Building supportive ties and sense of community among the inner-city elderly: The Tenderloin Senior Outreach Project. *Health Education & Behavior, 12*, 303–314.

Minkler, M. (1992). Community organizing among the elderly poor in the United States: A case study. *International Journal of Health Services, 22*, 303–316.

Minkler, M. (1999). Personal responsibility for health? A review of the arguments and the evidence at century's end. *Health Education & Behavior, 26*, 121–140.

Minkler, M., & Cox, C. (1980). Creating critical consciousness in health: Applications of Freire's philosophy and methods to the health care setting. *International Journal of Health Services, 20*, 311–322.

Minkler, M., Driver, D., Roe, K. M., & Bedeian, K. (1993). Community intervention to support grandparent caregivers. *Gerontologist, 33*, 807–811.

Minkler, M., Franz, S., & Wechsler, R. (1982). Social support and social action organizing in a "grey ghetto": The Tenderloin experience. *International Quarterly of Community Health Education, 3*, 3–15.

Montes, J. H., & Johnson, L. L. (1998). Eliminating health disparities for vulnerable populations through health education intervention within health services programs. *Journal of Health Education, 29*, 6–9.

Morisky, D. E., Tiglao, T. V., Sneed, C. D., Tempongko, S. B., Baltazar, J. C., Detels, R., et al. (1998). The effects of establishment practices, knowledge and attitudes on condom use among Filipina sex workers. *AIDS Care, 70*, 213–220.

Morisky, D. E., & Ward, H. J. (1999). Contrasting approaches and experiences for improving hypertension control among inner city minorities: The Los Angeles program. Paper presented at the meeting of the American Society of Hypertension, New York, NY.

Navarro, V. (1997). Race or class versus race and class: Mortality differentials in the United States. In P. R. Lee, & C. L. Estes (Eds.), *The nation's health* (pp. 32–36). Sudbury, MA: Jones and Bartlett.

O'Connor, G. T., Quinton, H. B., Traven, N. D., Ramunno, L. D., Dodds, T. A., Marciniak, T. A., et al. (1999). Geographic variation in the treatment of acute myocardial infarction: The cooperative cardiovascular project. *Journal of the American Medical Association, 281,* 627–633.

Pappas, G., Queen, S., Hadden, W., & Fisher, G. (1993). The increasing disparity between socioeconomic groups in the United States, 1960–1986. *New England Journal of Medicine, 329,* 103–109.

Perkoff, G., & Anderson, M. (1970). Relationship between demographic characteristics, patient's chief complaint and medical care destination in an emergency room. *Medical Care, 8,* 309–323.

Peterson, M.G.E., Hollenberg, J. P., Szatrowski, T. P., Johanson, N. A., Mancuso, C. A., & Charlson, M. E. (1992). Geographic variations in the rates of elective total hip and knee arthroplasties among Medicare beneficiaries in the United Suites. *Journal of Bone and Joint Surgery, 74,* 1530–1539.

Poland, B., Coburn, D., Robertson, A., & Eakin, J. (1997). Wealth, equity and health care: A critique of a "population health" perspective on the determinants of health. *Social Science and Medicine, 46,* 785–796.

RAND and Stanford Center for Research in Disease Prevention. (1997). *The California Wellness Foundation violence prevention initiative mid-initiative assessment,* vol. I. Santa Monica, CA: RAND Corporation.

Reading, R. (1997). Social disadvantage and infection in childhood. *Sociology of Health and Illness, 19,* 395–414.

Ren, X. S., Amick, B. C., & Williams, D. R. (1999). Racial/ethnic disparities in health: The interplay between discrimination and socioeconomic status. *Ethnic Diseases, 9,* 151–165.

Roberts, L. (1999). Creating a new framework for promoting the health of African-American female adolescents: Beyond risk taking. *Journal of the American Medical Women's Association, 54,* 126–128.

Roe, K. M., Minkler, M., & Saunders, F. F. (1995). Combining research, advocacy, and education: The methods of the grandparent caregiver study. *Health Education Quarterly, 22,* 458–475.

Rundall, T. G., & Phillips, K. A. (1990). Informing and educating the electorate about AIDS. *Medical Care Review, 47,* 3–13.

Russell, K. M. (1997). Public policy analysis of Indiana's minority health initiatives. *Ethnicity and Health, 2,* 105–116.

Sargent, J. D., Brown, M. J., Freeman, J. L., Bailey, A., Goodman, D., & Freeman, D. H., Jr. (1995). Childhood lead poisoning in Massachusetts communities: Its association with sociodemographic and housing characteristics. *American Journal of Public Health, 85,* 528–534.

Schooler, C., Sundar, S. S., & Flora, J. (1996). Effects of the Stanford five-city project media advocacy program. *Health Education Quarterly 23,* 346–364.

Schulman, K. A., Berlin, J. A., Harless, W., Kerner, J. F., Sistrank, S., Gersh, B. J., et al. (1999). The effect of race and sex on physicians' recommendations for cardiac catheterization. *New England Journal of Medicine, 340,* 618–626.

Singh, G. K., & Yu, S. M. (1995). Infant mortality in the United States: Trends, differentials, and projections, 1950 through 2010. *American Journal of Public Health, 85,* 957–964.

Smith, G. D. (1996). Income inequality and mortality: Why are they related? *British Medical Journal, 312,* 987–989.

Smith, J. P., & Kington, R. (1997). Demographic and economic correlates of health in old age. *Demography, 34,* 159–170.

Stacey, M., & Olesen, V. (1993). Introduction. *Social Science and Medicine, 36,* ii-4.

Steckler, A., & Dawson, L. (1982). The role of health education in public policy development. *Health Education Quarterly, 9,* 275–292.

Steckler, A., Dawson, L., Goodman, R. M., & Epstein, N. (1987). Policy advocacy: Three emerging roles for health education. In W. B. Ward, & S. K. Simonds (Eds.), *Advances in health education and promotion*, vol. 2 (pp. 5–28). Greenwich, CT: JAI Press.

Tesh, S. N. (1988). *Hidden arguments: Political ideology and disease prevention policy*. New Brunswick, NJ: Rutgers University Press.

Thomas, S. B. (1990). Community health advocacy for racial and ethnic minorities in the United States: Issues and challenges for health education. *Health Education Quarterly, 17*, 13–19.

Turnock, B. T. (1997). *Public health: What it is and how it works*. Rockville, MD: Aspen Publishers.

U.S. Department of Health and Human Services. (1998a). *Closing the gap, healthy people 2010 and beyond*. Washington, DC: U.S. Government Printing Office.

U.S. Department of Health and Human Services. (1998b). *Healthy people 2010 objectives: Draft for public comment*. Washington, DC: U.S. Government Printing Office.

U.S. Department of Health and Human Services. (1998c). DHHS aims to eliminate racial disparities in health status. *Health Care Financing Review, 20*, 136.

Wallack, L. (1997). Media advocacy: A strategy for empowering people and communities. In M. Minkler (Ed.), *Community organizing & community building for health* (pp. 339–352). New Brunswick, NJ: Rutgers University Press.

Wallack, L., & Dorfman, L. (1996). Media advocacy: A strategy for advancing policy and promoting public health. *Health Education Quarterly, 23*, 293–317.

Wallerstein, N., & Bernstein, E. (1988). Empowerment education: Freire's ideas adapted to health education. *Health Education Quarterly, 15*, 379–394.

Ward, H. I., Morisky, D., Lees, N. B., & Fong, R. (2000). A community based approach to hypertension control for an underserved minority population: Design and methods. *American Journal of Hypertension, 13*, 177–183.

Wilkinson, R. G. (1997). Comment: Income, inequality, and social cohesion. *American Journal of Public Health, 87*, 1504–1506.

Wilson, S. R., Scamagas, P., Grado, J., Norgaard, L., Starr, N. I., Eaton, S., et al. (1998). The Fresno asthma project: A model intervention to control asthma in multiethnic, low-income inner-city communities. *Health Education & Behavior, 25*, 79–98.

Wong, F. Y., Chng, C. L., & Lo, W. (1998). A profile of six community-based HIV prevention programs targeting Asian and Pacific Islander Americans. *AIDS Education and Prevention, 10*, 61–76.

Woodruff, K. (1996). Alcohol advertising and violence against women: A media advocacy case study. *Health Education Quarterly, 23*, 330–345.

Woolander, S., Himmelstein, D., Silber, R., Bader, M., Harnely, M., & Jones, A. (1985). Medicare and mortality: Racial differences in preventable deaths. *International Journal of Health Services, 15*, 1–15.

Yergan, J., Flood, A. B., LoGerfo, J., & Diehr, P. (1987). Relationship between patient race and the intensity of hospital services. *Medical Care, 25*, 592–603.

# CHAPTER

# LESSONS FROM DEVELOPING COUNTRIES: HEALTH EDUCATION IN THE GLOBAL VILLAGE

**HELDA PINZON-PEREZ**

The need for cross-cultural interaction and the acknowledgment of the potential for learning from each other have never been so clear as they are today, thanks to the Internet and other electronic means, which have practically erased the communication limits imposed by borders between countries. Immigration issues have become a major concern for health care systems in industrialized nations. In the United States, the number of foreign-born residents has reached the highest level in U.S. history. Immigrants account for 11 percent of the U.S. population, which translates into 28 million residents of foreign origin (U.S. Census Bureau, 2000).

Gambescia (2002) indicated that health care systems around the world are undoubtedly affected by each other. In the words of this author, health educators and health promotion specialists "must move beyond simply learning about and being responsive to local culture and ideas and learn how a seemingly distant parochial problem, from pestilence to war, becomes everyone's global health problem" (p. 443). In this context, global and multicultural health issues have become priorities for health educators in the United States. Some of you may be thinking, "Oh, no! the 'm' word again!" Given the recent events in our nation, we talk over and over about "multiculturalism" but perhaps what we need is less "talk" and more "listening." Maybe we now need to open our ears and our hearts to various experiences and lessons from international settings. There is so much that those of us who live in industrialized nations can learn from those living in developing countries. The purpose of this article is to share with you some of the lessons I have learned from my work in international settings.

The first lesson I have learned is that developing healthy lifestyles is a universal priority; however, the pursuit of a healthy lifestyle often comes into direct conflict with daily struggles lived by many populations around the world, for whom "survival" is the main priority. Day-to-day issues such as dealing with safety and food supply make the development of healthy lifestyles a luxury that not even those who are economically privileged can afford. On this matter, it may be pertinent to recall Maslow's hierarchy of human needs. According to the pyramid proposed by Maslow, the physiological needs (food, oxygen, water, sleep) are the very core of survival These needs are followed by safety (security, stability, freedom from threat or danger), belongingness and love (acceptance, affiliation, relations, identification), esteem (recognition, status), and self-actualization (ideal development, self-fulfillment, full power of self) (Seaward, 2002). Many populations around the world are still struggling with satisfying their physiological and security needs and may, therefore, see exercising three to five times a week or engaging in relaxation techniques as superfluous goals.

What September 11, 2001, brought to many U.S. residents was the need to revisit and reflect on their security needs. To live in the United States gave many people a sense of relative security and a feeling of being protected. I say "relative" because I know this feeling may not be applicable to many groups in the United States, especially those economically disadvantaged who have to struggle with the reality of unsafe neighborhoods.

Many people around the world emigrate to the United States to satisfy their security needs. They have migrated to escape a reality of fear, threat, and risk of being kidnapped in their native lands. Since September 11th, that reality has become part of many lives again. Often migrants are the ones who call their family members in other countries to check on their security and to ensure they are doing fine. Since September 11th many find their family members calling them in the United States, worried about their safety.

This situation has major implications for health educators. One question to address is whether health education has something to offer to people who are still struggling with the basic physiological and security needs. The answer is definitely yes; otherwise many of us would not be in this field. A better question would be "How can health education contribute to the populations who struggle with survival issues?"

Annan (2001) stated that "today's real borders are not between nations, but between powerful and powerless, free and fettered, privileged and humiliated." The paradigm of healthy lifestyles, which involves physical fitness, occupational health, stress management, nutrition education, and environmental protection seems to practitioners and academicians in the United States intrinsically related to the satisfaction of physiological and security needs; yet this relationship is not obvious for economically underprivileged individuals. Health educators working with these populations in the United States and abroad are called to advocate for employment opportunities, to emphasize the importance of generating grass-roots programs, and to train community members to become self-sufficient and active role-players. Green and Jones (2002), commenting on Kofi Annan's statement, indicated that a major role of health educators is to participate in the process of "conscience raising" by motivating people to reflect on these conditions and to take an active stand against disparities in health care.

A different view of our health paradigm may be achieved by being directly exposed to some of the realities of developing countries. Health educators in the United States need to interact with foreign-born populations and should take advantage of opportunities for a foreign work experience. One way to accomplish this is by participating in international exchange programs, traveling during sabbaticals, promoting scholarly activities under programs such as the Fulbright Academic Exchange Initiative and the Peace Corps, among others, and establishing partnerships with international organizations (Pinzon-Perez & Perez, 2002).

A second lesson I have learned is that poverty is definitely not foreign to industrialized nations. In the United States poverty is a major concern, especially for immigrants. Immigrants constitute 22 percent (9.2 million) of the 42 million uninsured people in the United States (Hoffman & Pohl, 2000). Based on my own research in the area of multicultural health, I can theorize that most people who migrate to the United States, in search of better economic opportunities, tend to experience a sense of "improvement" in their living conditions once they arrive in the United States.

This is true in the economic sense because generally at the beginning, immigrants observe better housing conditions, better sanitation, and better opportunities for employment. This "sense of improvement," however, may be short-lived. Generally, after two years people abandon their parameter of reference they had for comparison (how they lived in their countries of origin) and adopt a new standard: a comparison with the lifestyle lived by most in their new host country.

Following this short-lived period of "sense of improvement," immigrants may encounter "relative poverty." They may start seeing that many others around them have greater material items such as three or four television sets in their homes, large swimming pools, and two or three cars per household, whereas they are still struggling to ensure money for food, housing, and education. Fertman (2002) proposed that health education interventions ought to promote individual, family, and community involvement in the planning, implementation, and evaluation of health education programs. This premise is of special relevance when dealing with economically disadvantaged groups. Health educators are challenged to promote an equitable distribution of the resources and emphasize the value of education as an essential tool for economic prosperity.

A third lesson I have learned is that environmental health is a core issue for health education, not only in the United States but also around the world. Environmental pollution, industrial contamination, lack of drinkable water, and adequate sewage disposal are daily occurrences in many developing countries (Baffigo et al., 2001; Makutsa et al., 2001). In developing countries health educators play an essential role in providing guidance about environmental protection measures. As a matter of fact, due to economic limitations, in many countries health educators may be the only healthcare personnel with the responsibility to educate about environmental health issues. More training for health educators is needed in the area of environmental health.

The United States needs to become an active partner in ensuring an adequate utilization of resources and the rational use of worldwide environmental sources. At the United Nation's World Summit on Sustainable Development, held in South Africa from August 26 to September 4, 2002, world leaders made an agreement to collaborate in the provision of clean water for all the nations around the world, invest in renewable energy sources, and reduce the production of harmful chemicals (United Nations, 2002). In this effort the United States is expected to have a major commitment. Making environmental health a priority for foreign policy in the United States is based not only on altruistic principles, but also on a sense of self-preservation. Fox and Kassalow (2001) described three major principles that support the need for U.S. involvement in worldwide health issues. The first principle is that people in the United States face growing danger from emerging diseases around the world; the second principle is that health risks around the world affect economic and security interests in the United States, and the third principle is that the United States has an important opportunity and moral responsibility to participate in the creation of incentives for constructing a healthier world population.

In my opinion, many of us living in the United States waste too much. Our houses are beautifully decorated for the holiday season even while we use an incredible amount of electricity; our yards are perfect, at the cost of possibly using water in an irrational way; and we tend to waste food in the "all you can eat buffets." Please don't get me wrong. It is good to have luxuries; we work hard for them, but we also need to think about the long-term implications of our actions, which are related to how we are affecting the rest of the world. For health educators this represents a challenge. We need to lead the way in becoming more rational users of resources and incorporating this teaching into the academic programs for our students. Our lifestyles should be congruent with our thoughts. In other words, health educators need to model a rational utilization of environmental resources.

A fourth lesson I have learned is the relevance and real-life value of concepts related to cultural competence in health education. Cross, Bazron, Dennis, and Isaacs

(1989) listed six major steps professionals should take toward achieving cultural proficiency. These steps have been depicted in a graphical representation in the form of a ladder. In the first step, called "cultural destructiveness," one cultural group is seen as superior to others. Professionals in this step adopt attitudes and practices that dehumanize those who are seen as inferior. The second step is called "cultural incapacity." In this step, practitioners promote racist policies and perpetuate the maintenance of stereotypes about particular groups. The third phase is called "cultural blindness," and it is characterized by an oversimplified attitude of treating everybody in the same way without acknowledging historical and cultural specificities. The fourth step is "cultural precompetence." In this phase, practitioners become aware that they have gaps and weaknesses in regard to providing services to culturally and ethnically diverse groups. The following step is "cultural competence" in which health care personnel actively engage in learning processes and adopt practices that denote respect for others who are "different" from them. The last step, called "advanced cultural competence" previously known as "cultural proficiency," is characterized by an attitude that values difference and by an action-oriented lifestyle in which respect and high esteem are provided to ethnically and culturally diverse populations (Cross et al., 1989).

I have found this ladder very useful in understanding the complexity of multicultural issues involved in health education. Practitioners in health education have the responsibility to move up this ladder and to achieve a state of advanced cultural competence. In this context it is also very important that those of us who have been seen as "minorities" actively strive to become culturally competent, too. We need to learn how to respect and appreciate the value of those called "majority." Many times I have seen how someone of my own ethnicity treats a White person in a disrespectful way just because that person is White. I have seen many White people who are very culturally competent and who are trying very hard to acquire a proper level of cultural proficiency in their personal and professional lives. Culturally diverse populations need to give credit to them. We cannot continue to cover ourselves with the "shield" of the past. We cannot continue to generalize about how we have been mistreated. It is important to recognize the historical events that document the mistreatment of certain ethnic and cultural groups and may serve as the basis for distrust, but we need to move beyond. We need, however, to realize that cultural competency is a two-way street. We ought to become examples of cultural acceptance and respect for others who are different from us. Health educators need to fight discrimination, but we need to fight it in our own homes, through educating our children, through promoting cultural competence, and through advocating for social justice here in the United States and around the world. Our behavior can teach more than our words.

I am very glad to have been given the opportunity to share my personal perspective on these issues. This represents an attempt to provide a small contribution to the development of our profession. Opening this dialogue is, in my view, a healthy way to ensure prosperity in our profession.

# REFERENCES

Annan, K. (2001). Nobel Lecture: *We can love what we are, without hating what—and who—we are not*. Retrieved from www.un.org/News/Press/docs/2001/sgsm807Ldoc.htm

Baffigo, V., Albinagorta, J., Nauca, L., Rojas, P., Alegre, R., Hubbard, B., et al. (2001). Community environmental health assessment in Peru's desert hills and rainforest. *American Journal of Public Health, 91*, 1580–1582.

Cross, T. L., Bazron, B. J., Dennis, K. W., & Isaacs, M. R. (1989). *The cultural competence continuum. Toward a culturally competent system of care: A monograph on effective services for minority children who are severely emotionally disturbed*. Washington, DC: Child and Adolescent Service System Program (CASSP), Georgetown University.

Fertman, C. (2002). Behavioral health and health education: An emerging opportunity. *American Journal of Health Education, 33*, 115–117.

Fox, D., & Kassalow, J. (2001). Making health a priority of U.S. foreign policy. *American Journal of Public Health, 91*, 1554–1555.

Gambescia, S. (2002). Message from the editor. *Health Promotion Practice, 3*, 443–446.

Green, J., & Jones, K. (2002). Health promotion, equity and access to information. *IUHPE-Promotion and Education, IX*(2), 42–43.

Hoffman, C., & Pohl, M. (2000). *Health insurance coverage in America: 1999 data update*. Washington, DC: Kaiser Commission on Medicaid and the Uninsured.

Makutsa, P., Nzaku, K., Ogutu, P., Barasa, P., Ombeki, P., Mwaki, A., et al. (2001). Challenges in implementing a point-of-use water quality intervention in rural Kenya. *American Journal of Public Health, 91*, 1571–1573.

Pinzon-Perez, H. L., & Perez, M. A. (2002). *International academic exchange programs: The globalization of health*. Paper presented at the AAHPERD National Convention, San Diego, CA.

Seaward, B. (2002). Toward a psychology of stress. In *Managing stress. Principles and strategies for health and well-being* (pp. 71–93). Boston: Jones and Bartlett.

United Nations. (2002). World summit on sustainable development. Retrieved from htt://un.org/events/wssd/summaries/envdevj31.htm

U.S. Census Bureau. (2000). *United States Census 2000*. Retrieved from http://www.census.gov/main/www/cen2000.html

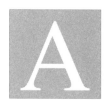

# PHILOSOPHY OF HEALTH EDUCATION GRID

| Philosophy | Purpose of Health Education | Role of Learner | Role of Teacher | Educational Method | Content |
|---|---|---|---|---|---|
| **Cognitive-based** | Facts are necessary, no matter what; appeals to the intellect; factual info as base; deepen content understanding; produce quickest results; present basic information | Individual need to know facts; maturity level a concern; content appropriate to age level; people need guidelines | To educate; dispense facts; stay current with content; educator can teach to teacher's beliefs | Written literature; group discussions; structured programs | Meets the needs of employer; justify approach by citing research |
| **Decision-making** | Critical thinking & decision-making skills more effective; overall ability to make healthy decisions, teaching skills to utilize info; learned skills stay w/student longer; giving usable skills | Learner consciously decides on own; critical thinking impacts the clients' understanding of why they do what they do; client takes control of situation; practice skills | Facilitator; observer; to give feedback | Practice skills; practice in roles | Process evaluation; AIDS—an area where bad decisions can kill |
| **Behavior Change** | Goal setting; changes needed; seek to make tangible changes; present lifestyle changes; reinforce positive behaviors; knowing alternatives | Actively initiate change; set goals; incorporate behavior changes into personal lifestyle; students may become hopeless or blame self for failure | Positive role models; motivator, encourager | Goal setting; reward system; contract; "sandwich" approach—positive reinforcement, change, positive reinforcement | Specific health content area (depends on the targeted behavior) |

| | | | | | |
|---|---|---|---|---|---|
| **Freeing/ Functioning** | Highly personalized; not content oriented; self-directed learning; empowering; incorporate knowledge into present lifestyle; tailor to individual; individual differences must be respected | Individual choices; not everyone learns the same way; patient variation requires flexibility; ownership; values assessment | Help students develop their own goals; support students in decisions | Workshops; self-directed support groups; alternative teaching formats; experience the "how to" of an activity | Offer program as a service; holistic and humanistic |
| **Social Change** | Individual choices affect society; legislative process to reduce risks; link person to bigger picture; work at root of underlying causes to health problems | Passage of laws to protect individuals who cannot protect themselves | Agitator, instigator, organizer | Class discussion, sales package; use success stories; advocacy, political change | Health policy, laws, ethics |

*Source:* H. M. Welle. (1995). *An exploration of philosophical trends and preferences in health education.* Unpublished doctoral dissertation, Southern Illinois University at Carbondale, Carbondale, IL.

# APPENDIX

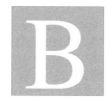

# PHILOSOPHY OF HEALTH EDUCATION: A POSITION STATEMENT OF THE AMERICAN ASSOCIATION OF HEALTH EDUCATION (AAHE)

**ADOPTED 1991**
**REVISED 2005**

Health education is a unique and separate academic discipline. It influences individual, family and societal development, knowledge, attitudes and behavior. It seeks the improvement of individual, family and community health. Because the emphasis is upon health, both the process and the program may be said to originate in an understanding of the nature of health as it relates to humans as individuals or in groups.

The contemporary concept of health embraces the entire being. The individual is not a composite of separate entities, such as body, mind and spirit, arranged in presumed ascending order of importance. The individual is a multi-dimensional entity, with each component—chemical, physical, spiritual, intellectual or emotional—existing as an element within a complex of interrelationships. The individual is not a passive participant in the wellness process. Good health requires positive efforts directed toward total well-being. These efforts have larger potential for success when operating in a socio-political system that values individual, family and societal well-being. Individual attempts to enhance one's own well-being should be joined by a commitment to enhance societal well-being. Conversely, society as well bears a responsibility to promote the well-being of all individuals.

Education in health helps individuals seek that which moves them toward optimal stages of wellness. It means also to aid individuals and families in overcoming the debilitating effects of economic deprivation, the lack of balance, disease and accidents of life.

The ultimate goal of health education is to enable individuals to use knowledge in ways that transform unhealthy habits into healthy habits. It is difficult to expect that individuals can accomplish this end in a societal framework that provides confusing and mixed messages. It thus is an objective for health education to provide learners with the skills to judge messages received in terms of their potential benefit to self and society. It is also an objective to provide criticism of such mixed messages in public forums.

Paradoxically, educators in general or health educators in particular must teach individuals to look beyond health as an end or goal and to utilize health enhancing skills as a means for achieving life's goals. Though health itself may be quantitatively evaluated bio-chemically, health status can only be used as a qualitative measure of functional ability. Wellness is, in this functional sense, a means, not an end. Thus, the end should involve greater societal well being.

Health is a personal and societal matter. Health education, therefore, must become a part of the experience of each learner and extend itself into the surrounding society. For health education to occur health must eventually become a directing factor in one's ever-present lifestyle. The subject matter and health-enhancing skills of health education must be established and taught within the context of individuals' lives, not treated as something to be transmitted simply because it is available.

This makes health education a hazardous undertaking in some respects but no more so than any other form of formal education. There are risks involved in having learners treat subject matter as personal and relevant to current situations. They may focus to a greater than appropriate extent on themselves and their ills. They may become critical of their elders, of government policy, of business practices. If, as noted, the subject matter of health education is established and taught in the context of the lives the learners live and the society within which they live, the educational process will contribute to the development of social values which should maximize the development of individuality and independent thinking. The risk seems worth taking. The principal purpose and direction of health education should be to equip students to cope with the elements of change and cultivate the ability to resolve the problems produced by change, through knowledge and skills-based learning.

Knowledge should be taught in a manner that facilitates an understanding of current realities and fosters a willingness among students to accept today's information as usable, but anticipate that later discoveries, perceptions or political realities may significantly change the usefulness of that knowledge. Learners will gain their security, finally, not in given and fixed bodies of knowledge, but in the skill of knowledge acquisition and the ability to analyze and apply it. Individuals must be given an opportunity to choose which information to believe, and which behaviors to perform. If not given such opportunities they may revolt, become apathetic, or deliberately live in opposition to what is known and what is taught. They need to be informed, not threatened. Learners need to be aided in the solution of their problems, not forced to accept an imposed solution. Of equal importance is that they be equipped to do problem solving for themselves and society as new situations confront them. Thus, health educators must help learners use knowledge in making their choices, which in turn will encourage them to engage in experimentation and evaluation throughout their life span.

The ultimate value of health education cannot be measured by ordinary standards or in ordinary periods of time. One bit of health information properly applied may save a life in the present or forty years later. That single life may be so valuable to society that this health education learning may be of greater value than any other learning that an individual may have experienced.

American Association of Health Education. (2005). *Philosophy of Health Education: A Position Statement of the American Association of Health Education (AAHE)*. Retrieved from http://www.aahperd.org/aahe/pdf_files/pos_pap/Philosophy.pdf.

# APPENDIX

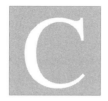

# HEALTH LITERACY: A POSITION STATEMENT OF THE AMERICAN ASSOCIATION OF HEALTH EDUCATION (AAHE)

**ADOPTED 2008**

Health literacy is the degree to which individuals have the capacity to obtain, process, and understand basic health information and services needed to make appropriate health decisions.[1] An estimated excess cost for the US healthcare system of 50 billion to 73 billion dollars per year is attributable to low literacy.[2] In addition, low levels of health literacy have been directly linked to increased hospitalization rates.[3,4]

An estimated 90 million adults in the United States are unable to adequately comprehend health information.[5] *The Health Literacy of America's Adults* is the first release of the results of a national assessment of adult health literacy. Health literacy was reported using four performance levels: Below Basic, Basic, Intermediate, and Proficient. The majority of adults (53 percent) had Intermediate health literacy; 22 percent of adults had Basic and 14 percent had Below Basic health literacy.[4]

Health literacy includes quantitative abilities, e.g. determining correct doses of medication and comprehending nutrition labels.[7] People with low health literacy often misunderstand information about the human body and how diseases develop.[7]

Facts about health change constantly, and health-related information people have learned is often out of date, forgotten or obsolete. In addition, health information given in stressful or unfamiliar circumstances may not be remembered.[7] *Health literacy skill development is an essential component of health education instruction. The National Health Education Standards, a framework for health education curriculum development, instruction and assessment of student performance, benchmark health literacy skill development for students enrolled in pre-K – secondary education. The overall goal of these standards is improved educational achievement for students and improved health in the United States.*[8]

Therefore, the American Association for Health Education actively supports the development, implementation, and evaluation of health education and promotion programs wherein health literacy concepts are incorporated and, thereby, enhance decision making for health-related choices.

## REFERENCES

1.  Selden, C. R., Zorn, M., Ratzan, S., et al., eds. (February 2000). *Health Literacy, January 1990 through 1999*. NLM Pub. No. CBM 2000-1. Bethesda, MD: National Library of Medicine, p. vi.

2.  Friedland, R. B. (1998). *Understanding Health Literacy: New Estimates of the Cost of Inadequate Health Literacy.* Washington, DC: National Academy on an Aging Society.

3.  Baker, D. W., Parker, R. M., Williams, M. V., Clark, W. S. (1998). Health literacy and the risk of hospital admission. *Journal of General Internal Medicine 13*, 791–798.

4.  Baker, D. W., Gazmararian, J. A., Williams, M.V., Scott, T., Parker, R. M., Green, D., et al. (2002). Functional health literacy and the risk of hospital admission among Medicare managed care enrollees. *American Journal of Public Health 92*, 1278–1283.

5.  Kindig, D., Affonso, D., Chudler, E., Gaston, M., Meade, C., Parker, R., et al. (April 2004.) *Report brief. Health literacy: A prescription to end confusion.* Retrieved from http://www.iom.edu/Object.File/Master/19/726/health%20literacy%20final.pdf. Accessed June 27, 2008.

6.  National Center for Education Statistics, Institute of Education Science, U.S. Department of Education. (September 2006). *The Health Literacy of America's Adults: Results from the 2003 National Assessment of Adult Literacy.* Retrieved from http://nces.ed.gov/pubsearch/pubsinfo.asp?pubid=2006483

7.  U.S. Department of Health and Human Services. (n.d.). *Health Literacy Basics: Fact Sheet.* Retrieved from http://www.health.gov/communication/literacy/quickguide/factsbasic.htm

8.  National Health Education Standards. (n.d.). *An Introduction to Student Standards.* Retrieved from http://www.aahperd.org/aahe/template.cfm?template=natl_health_education_standards.html

9.  Johnston-Lloyd, L., & Yun, S. (March 2007). *Health Literacy Outreach Paper.* Rockville, MD: U.S. Department of Health and Human Services, Health Resources and Services Administration.

American Association of Health Education. (2008). *Health Literacy: A Position Statement of the American Association of Health Education (AAHE).* Retrieved from http://www.aahperd.org/aahe/pdf_files/pos_pap/HealthLiteracy.pdf.

# APPENDIX

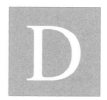

# CODE OF ETHICS FOR THE HEALTH EDUCATION PROFESSION

## PREAMBLE

The Health Education profession is dedicated to excellence in the practice of promoting individual, family, organizational, and community health. Guided by common ideals, Health Educators are responsible for upholding the integrity and ethics of the profession as they face the daily challenges of making decisions. By acknowledging the value of diversity in society and embracing a cross-cultural approach, Health Educators support the worth, dignity, potential, and uniqueness of all people.

The Code of Ethics provides a framework of shared values within which Health Education is practiced. The Code of Ethics is grounded in fundamental ethical principles that underlie all health care services: respect for autonomy, promotion of social justice, active promotion of good, and avoidance of harm. The responsibility of each health educator is to aspire to the highest possible standards of conduct and to encourage the ethical behavior of all those with whom they work.

Regardless of job title, professional affiliation, work setting, or population served, Health Educators abide by these guidelines when making professional decisions.

## ARTICLE I: RESPONSIBILITY TO THE PUBLIC

A Health Educator's ultimate responsibility is to educate people for the purpose of promoting, maintaining, and improving individual, family, and community health. When a conflict of issues arises among individuals, groups, organizations, agencies, or institutions, health educators must consider all issues and give priority to those that promote wellness and quality of living through principles of self-determination and freedom of choice for the individual.

**Section 1**: Health Educators support the right of individuals to make informed decisions regarding health, as long as such decisions pose no threat to the health of others.

**Section 2**: Health Educators encourage actions and social policies that support and facilitate the best balance of benefits over harm for all affected parties.

**Section 3**: Health Educators accurately communicate the potential benefits and consequences of the services and programs with which they are associated.

**Section 4**: Health Educators accept the responsibility to act on issues that can adversely affect the health of individuals, families, and communities.

**Section 5**: Health Educators are truthful about their qualifications and the limitations of their expertise and provide services consistent with their competencies.

**Section 6**: Health Educators protect the privacy and dignity of individuals.

**Section 7**: Health Educators actively involve individuals, groups, and communities in the entire educational process so that all aspects of the process are clearly understood by those who may be affected.

**Section 8**: Health Educators respect and acknowledge the rights of others to hold diverse values, attitudes, and opinions.

**Section 9**: Health Educators provide services equitably to all people.

## ARTICLE II: RESPONSIBILITY TO THE PROFESSION

Health Educators are responsible for their professional behavior, for the reputation of their profession, and for promoting ethical conduct among their colleagues.

**Section 1**: Health Educators maintain, improve, and expand their professional competence through continued study and education; membership, participation, and leadership in professional organizations; and involvement in issues related to the health of the public.

**Section 2**: Health Educators model and encourage nondiscriminatory standards of behavior in their interactions with others.

**Section 3**: Health Educators encourage and accept responsible critical discourse to protect and enhance the profession.

**Section 4**: Health Educators contribute to the development of the profession by sharing the processes and outcomes of their work.

**Section 5**: Health Educators are aware of possible professional conflicts of interest, exercise integrity in conflict situations, and do not manipulate or violate the rights of others.

**Section 6**: Health Educators give appropriate recognition to others for their professional contributions and achievements

## ARTICLE III: RESPONSIBILITY TO EMPLOYERS

Health Educators recognize the boundaries of their professional competence and are accountable for their professional activities and actions.

**Section 1**: Health Educators accurately represent their qualifications and the qualifications of others whom they recommend.

**Section 2**: Health Educators use appropriate standards, theories, and guidelines as criteria when carrying out their professional responsibilities.

**Section 3**: Health Educators accurately represent potential service and program outcomes to employers.

**Section 4**: Health Educators anticipate and disclose competing commitments, conflicts of interest, and endorsement of products.

**Section 5**: Health Educators openly communicate to employers, expectations of job-related assignments that conflict with their professional ethics.

**Section 6**: Health Educators maintain competence in their areas of professional practice.

## ARTICLE IV: RESPONSIBILITY IN THE DELIVERY OF HEALTH EDUCATION

Health Educators promote integrity in the delivery of health education. They respect the rights, dignity, confidentiality, and worth of all people by adapting strategies and methods to the needs of diverse populations and communities.

**Section 1**: Health Educators are sensitive to social and cultural diversity and are in accord with the law, when planning and implementing programs.

**Section 2**: Health Educators are informed of the latest advances in theory, research, and practice, and use strategies and methods that are grounded in and contribute to development of professional standards, theories, guidelines, statistics, and experience.

**Section 3**: Health Educators are committed to rigorous evaluation of both program effectiveness and the methods used to achieve results.

**Section 4**: Health Educators empower individuals to adopt healthy lifestyles through informed choice rather than by coercion or intimidation.

**Section 5**: Health Educators communicate the potential outcomes of proposed services, strategies, and pending decisions to all individuals who will be affected.

## ARTICLE V: RESPONSIBILITY IN RESEARCH AND EVALUATION

Health Educators contribute to the health of the population and to the profession through research and evaluation activities. When planning and conducting research or evaluation, health educators do so in accordance with federal and state laws and regulations, organizational and institutional policies, and professional standards.

**Section 1**: Health Educators support principles and practices of research and evaluation that do no harm to individuals, groups, society, or the environment.

**Section 2**: Health Educators ensure that participation in research is voluntary and is based upon the informed consent of the participants.

**Section 3**: Health Educators respect the privacy, rights, and dignity of research participants, and honor commitments made to those participants.

**Section 4**: Health Educators treat all information obtained from participants as confidential unless otherwise required by law.

**Section 5**: Health Educators take credit, including authorship, only for work they have actually performed and give credit to the contributions of others.

**Section 6**: Health Educators who serve as research or evaluation consultants discuss their results only with those to whom they are providing service, unless maintaining such confidentiality would jeopardize the health or safety of others.

**Section 7**: Health Educators report the results of their research and evaluation objectively, accurately, and in a timely fashion.

## ARTICLE VI: RESPONSIBILITY IN PROFESSIONAL PREPARATION

Those involved in the preparation and training of Health Educators have an obligation to accord learners the same respect and treatment given other groups by providing quality education that benefits the profession and the public.

**Section 1**: Health Educators select students for professional preparation programs based upon equal opportunity for all, and the individual's academic performance, abilities, and potential contribution to the profession and the public's health.

**Section 2**: Health Educators strive to make the educational environment and culture conducive to the health of all involved, and free from sexual harassment and all forms of discrimination.

**Section 3**: Health Educators involved in professional preparation and professional development engage in careful preparation; present material that is accurate, up-to-date, and timely; provide reasonable and timely feedback; state clear and reasonable expectations; and conduct fair assessments and evaluations of learners.

**Section 4**: Health Educators provide objective and accurate counseling to learners about career opportunities, development, and advancement, and assist learners secure professional employment.

**Section 5**: Health Educators provide adequate supervision and meaningful opportunities for the professional development of learners.

 *Approved:* Coalition of National Health Education Organizations, November 8, 1999, Chicago, IL

Coalition of National Health Education Organizations (1999). *Code of Ethics for the Health Education Profession.* Retrieved from http://www.cnheo.org/code2.pdf.

# APPENDIX

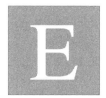

# CHES QUESTIONS

The American Association for Health Education (AAHE) is pleased to provide professional development/continuing education units (CEUs) through the chapters in this text. Twenty-five of the twenty-nine chapters have been prepared for CEUs with questions in this appendix. These include Chapter 4 and Chapter 6 through Chapter 29. It is anticipated that readers will be able to:

- Identify various philosophical approaches to health education and promotion

- Compare and contrast philosophical approaches

- Determine the relationship between philosophical approaches and behavioral outcomes.

This appendix contains ten questions for each of the twenty-five CEU articles. The downloadable response form for the CEU questions can be purchased online at http://www.aahperd.org/bookstore/. Search under "Philosophical Foundations of Health Education CEU Response Form."

Twenty-five Category I credit hours for Certified Health Education Specialists (CHES) are available. However, participants who may wish to complete the hours for non-CHES professional development credit will also receive a certificate of completion for submission to other settings or with other allied health professions.

The cost for up to twenty-five CEU credits is $35.00 for AAHE/AAHPERD members and $55 for non-AAHE/AAHPERD members. Certificates of completion will be emailed back from AAHE to each participate upon receipt of the completed response form. Participants may complete and submit question responses for as many as twenty-five chapters or as few as they like. The cost remains the same as noted above. For additional questions please contact AAHE at mailto:aahe@aahperd.org.

## CHAPTER 4: HEALTH EDUCATION AS A BASIC (WILLGOOSE)

1. This article states that there is general agreement on the basic need to educate people of all ages about healthful living and that the focus should be on:

   a. improved medical and surgical techniques

   b. well-being

   c. urban dehumanization

   d. prevention

   e. biomedical advances

2. Which one of the following is NOT identified as a public health concern by this article:

   a. rising health care costs

   b. environmental health concerns

   c. gullibility of health consumers

   d. leading causes of death

   e. changing patterns of illness

3. According to a study conducted by the Center for Health Promotion and Education, health professionals were interested in which of the following topics:

   a. risk reduction

   b. stress management

   c. nutrition

   d. exercise

   e. all of the above

4. Which one of the following was NOT identified as a shortcoming in educational practices and curricula in the nation's schools:

   a. graduates who cannot read properly

   b. graduates who cannot write a check

   c. students who do not graduate

   d. graduates who cannot construct an appropriate sentence.

   e. none of the above

5. This article asks the question "Is not health education a basic need?" Who supports this position?

   a. Horace Mann

   b. Aldous Huxley

   c. Rene Dubos

   d. Joseph Krutch

   e. none of the above

6. According to this article, Comprehensive School Health Education includes the following components:

   a. consumer health

   b. personal health

   c. growth and development

   d. family health

   e. all of the above

7. According to this article, Comprehensive School Health Education does NOT include the following components:

   a. school health services

   b. healthful school environment

   c. physical education

   d. stress management

   e. none of the above

8. This article states that the long-range goal of health education is to:

   a. have the vitality to meet life's challenges

   b. prepare persons with the wherewithal to work toward their life objectives

   c. narrow the gap between what is known and what not known

   d. change attitudes and values in a positive manner

   e. make better health decisions

9. This article calls for the health dimension in a school curriculum to be divided up among science, physical education, and social studies.

   a. true

   b. false

10. According to this article, the topic of health and wellness are:

    a. subtle and dramatic

    b. obvious and hidden

    c. mean different things to different people

    d. requires in-depth treatment

    e. all of the above

# CHAPTER 6: THE HOLISTIC PHILOSOPHY AND PERSPECTIVE OF SELECTED HEALTH EDUCATORS (THOMAS)

1. The primary focus of this article is the:

    a. emergence of the holistic health movement

    b. ideological struggle between philosophical viewpoints

    c. concept of health and primary prevention

    d. problem-oriented health care

    e. all of the above

2. Who was responsible for the formulation of the philosophy of holism?

    a. Stephen B. Thomas

    b. Jan C. Smuts

    c. Charles Darwin

    d. Jesse F. Williams

    e. Howard Hoyman

3. Which of the Health Educators' published work was examined and discussed in this article:

    a. Jesse F. Williams

    b. Delbert Oberteuffer

    c. Howard Hoyman

    d. all of the above

    e. none of the above

4. Which one of the following categories was NOT used in the comparative analysis in this article?

    a. nature of the universe

    b. evolution of man

    c. nature of man

    d. relationship of mind to body

    e. human personality

5. According to Smuts, creative evolution provides the best explanation of the whole-making tendency in the universe.

    a. true

    b. false

6. Smuts and Hoyman share the view of the universe as:

    a. dynamic

    b. static

    c. mechanical

    d. organic

    e. fundamental

7. Hoyman emphasizes the relationship between human beings, other life forms and the environment.

    a. true

    b. false

8. According to Oberteuffer, man is essentially a unified integrated whole organism, not just the sum of his parts.

    a. true

    b. false

9. Who supported the idea that personality is the evolutionary outgrowth of the integrated mind and body of the individual?

    a. Aldous Huxley

    b. Socrates

    c. Jan C. Smuts

    d. John Dewey

    e. Abraham Maslow

10. According to this article, the holistic perspective can be synthesized into a philosophical framework for health education that is not counter to the concept and science of evolution.

    a. true

    b. false

# CHAPTER 7: CONNECTING A PERSONAL PHILOSOPHY OF HEALTH TO THE PRACTICE OF HEALTH EDUCATION (SMITH)

1. "A state of complete physical, mental, and social well-being and not merely the absence of disease or infirmity" as a definition of health is attributed to:

   a. National Institutes of Health

   b. Centers For Disease Control and Prevention

   c. World Health Organization

   d. Pan American Health Organization

   e. American Heart Association

2. One of the first renowned scientists to acknowledge the need for studying the human organism in relation to its environment was:

   a. Edward Jenner

   b. Charles Darwin

   c. Joseph Lister

   d. Alexander Fleming

   e. Jonas Salk

3. One of the challenges inherent to implementation of a holistic approach to health and health education is:

   a. language

   b. lack of research

   c. credentialing

   d. needs assessment

   e. body of knowledge

4. Who stated in 1960 that, "Above all, health is not and cannot be static or compartmentalized":

    a. Delbert Oberteuffer

    b. Howard Hoyman

    c. Ann Nolte

    d. Mabel Rugen

    e. J. Keogh Rash

5. Reward and punishment and aversion therapy are examples of:

    a. relaxation techniques

    b. operant conditioning

    c. behavior modification

    d. affective training

    e. psychomotor learning

6. The individual best described as a professor of anatomy and physical anthropology, educator, and author would be:

    a. Abraham Maslow

    b. Ashley Montagu

    c. Paul Tillich

    d. Becky Smith

    e. Erich Fromm

7. The various definitions of health described in this article all support the concept that health is an expression of quality of life:

    a. true

    b. false

8. Which early leader in the field of health and physical education developed a perspective of health as "the quality of life that renders the individual fit to live most and serve best":

    a. Mabel Rugen

    b. David K. Brace

    c. Delbert Oberteuffer

    d. Jesse F. Williams

    e. none of the above

9. Who develops measures for the physical dimensions of health:
   a. psychologists
   b. neurologists
   c. psychiatrists
   d. kinesiologists
   e. none of the above

10. The individual best described as a microbiologist, environmentalist, educator and author would be:
    a. Rene Dubos
    b. Erich Fromm
    c. Paul Tournier
    d. Ashley Montagu
    e. Howard Hoyman

# CHAPTER 8: HEALTH EDUCATORS AND THE FUTURE: LEAD, FOLLOW OR GET OUT OF THE WAY (CLARK)

1. Clark states that the fastest growing minority groups in the country are:
   a. African Americans and Asian Americans
   b. White non-Latinos and African Americans
   c. Latinos and Asian Americans
   d. African Americans and Latinos
   e. none of the above

2. Two examples of successful multi-faceted health education programs that were mentioned in the article include:
   a. diabetes prevention and smoking cessation
   b. AIDS education and teenage pregnancy prevention
   c. asthma education and STI prevention
   d. weight loss programs and diabetes programs
   e. smoking cessation and asthma education

3.  Estimates show that by the year 2025 over 40 percent of New York City residents will be African American:

    a.  true

    b.  false

4.  The article states that the American Association of Retired Persons (AARP) has a current membership in excess of _____ million members:

    a.  30

    b.  40

    c.  50

    d.  60

    e.  70

5.  Which of the following issues does this article NOT address:

    a.  ethnic minorities

    b.  aging

    c.  nature of American families

    d.  the environment

    e.  all of the issues above are addressed

6.  The core of health education practice in the future will be:

    a.  helping people locate information

    b.  helping people establish positive health habits

    c.  helping people avoid addictive behaviors

    d.  helping people learn how to learn

    e.  helping people relate to others

7.  The article states that the measure of successful health education in the future will be whether or not people judge the quality of their lives to be better because of it:

    a.  true

    b.  false

8.  By the year 2030 estimates predict that one in every _____ people will be 65 years of age or older:

    a.  two

    b.  three

    c.  four

    d.  five

    e.  six

9. Clark indicates that our country is not effective in running television ads about:

   a. deodorant

   b. feminine protection

   c. AIDS

   d. hemorrhoids

   e. all of the above

10. Examples of new channels for getting health education into action include all of the following EXCEPT:

    a. activism

    b. the workplace

    c. health care organizations

    d. peer education

    e. secondary school health education programs

## CHAPTER 9: HEALTH EDUCATION AND HEALTH PROMOTION: A LOOK AT THE JUNGLE OF SUPPORTIVE FIELDS, PHILOSOPHIES, AND THEORETICAL FOUNDATIONS (TIMMRECK, COLE, JAMES, & BUTTERWORTH)

1. This article makes the claim that health education and promotion have become more associated with:

   a. medical science

   b. behavioral science

   c. fitness

   d. physical education

   e. nutrition science

2. Holism, lifestyle, and wellness are being embraced by many segments of the helping professions, medicine and business:

   a. true

   b. false

3. Changing a person's behavior after a crisis occurs (such as when a heart attack victim stops smoking) is considered:

   a. primary prevention

   b. secondary prevention

   c. tertiary prevention

   d. none of the above

   e. all of the above

4. Which of following is NOT a licensed clinical field:

   a. social workers

   b. psychiatrists

   c. marriage counselors

   d. health educators

   e. all of the above are licensed clinical fields

5. One of the first areas where preventive medicine and health education have been moderately well received is in the area of:

   a. communicable disease prevention

   b. nutrition education

   c. first aid

   d. community health analysis

   e. substance abuse

6. Timmreck, Cole, James, and Butterworth claim that graduating health educators face the real world and the job market lacking in what area:

   a. needs assessment skills

   b. infectious disease knowledge

   c. administrative skills

   d. chronic disease knowledge

   e. community health knowledge

7. Behavioral science is a broad field encompassing all of the following EXCEPT:

   a. psychology

   b. anthropology

   c. sociology

   d. education

   e. all of the above are included in behavioral science

8. An analysis of publication activity showed that the category with the LEAST number of published articles was:

   a. content

   b. process

   c. research

   d. history

   e. theory

9. Which major area of focus is given the most attention in health education:

   a. theory

   b. process

   c. teaching

   d. research

   e. content

10. Health education has had only limited success in the field of patient education:

   a. true

   b. false

## CHAPTER 10: PHILOSOPHICAL TRENDS IN HEALTH EDUCATION: IMPLICATIONS FOR THE 21ST CENTURY (WELLE, RUSSELL, AND KITTLESON)

1. Historically the most well-rooted philosophy would be:

   a. decision making

   b. social change

   c. cognitive based

   d. behavior change

   e. freeing/functioning

2. The instrument used to collect data in this study was:

   a. Multiple Philosophy Scale (MPS)

   b. Health Education Philosophy Inventory (HEPI)

   c. Newberry Philosophy Rating Scale (NPRS)

   d. Philosophy Inquiry Inventory (PII)

   e. Adult Education Philosophy Inventory (AEPI)

3. Content analysis determined the philosophical preference in educational settings was:

   a.  decision making

   b.  social change

   c.  cognitive based

   d.  behavior change

   e.  freeing/functioning

4. Which adult education philosophy matches up to the cognitive-based health education philosophy:

   a.  liberal

   b.  behaviorist

   c.  progressive

   d.  humanistic

   e.  radical

5. The highest ranked health education philosophy in this study was:

   a.  social change

   b.  decision making

   c.  behavior change

   d.  freeing/functioning

   e.  cognitive-based

6. Which adult education philosophy matches up to the decision-making health education philosophy:

   a.  liberal

   b.  behaviorist

   c.  progressive

   d.  humanistic

   e.  radical

7. In this study practitioners preferred social change, while academicians demonstrated stronger agreement with behavior change:

   a.  true

   b.  false

8. Which adult education philosophy matches up to the social change health education philosophy:

   a. liberal

   b. behaviorist

   c. progressive

   d. humanistic

   e. radical

9. Decision-making philosophy encompasses all of the following EXCEPT:

   a. problem solving

   b. lifelong learning

   c. pragmatic knowledge

   d. inductive methodologies

   e. all of the above are included in decision-making philosophy

10. Health educators, regardless of stated philosophical beliefs, often change philosophy according to health education setting:

    a. true

    b. false

## CHAPTER 11: TEACHING FOR UNDERSTANDING IN HEALTH EDUCATION: THE ROLE OF CRITICAL AND CREATIVE THINKING SKILLS WITHIN CONSTRUCTIVISM THEORY (UBBES, BLACK, & AUSHERMAN)

1. The main purpose of this article was to:

   a. explore how critical and creative thinking can extend our understanding of health content

   b. explore how people learn

   c. explore the role of health education

   d. explore educational theory

   e. explore teaching strategies

2. Ubbes, Black, and Ausherman suggest that the following is a needed component of health pedagogy:

   a. being a subject expert

   b. knowledge acquisition

   c. frequent testing of subject material

   d. understanding theory

   e. decision-making

3. Providing health information does not often enlighten learners unless equal time is spent:

   a. using pictures/illustrations of issues

   b. testing learner on knowledge

   c. teaching learner how to use Internet

   d. reducing misinformation and misconceptions

   e. organizing and categorizing information

4. Ubbes, Black, and Ausherman suggest ways to teach for understanding in health education, these include all of the following EXCEPT:

   a. the need for systems thinking in addition to linear thinking to develop multiple perspectives

   b. use of collaborative learning

   c. use of charts and diagrams

   d. focus on the developmental needs and interests of the learners

   e. none of the above

5. Learners in health education classes should be encouraged to use the following:

   a. logical, critical thinking

   b. use of the Internet

   c. frequent testing

   d. memorization of factual information

   e. practice of skills

6. A method used to teach for understanding in health education is to:

   a. assist the learner to recognize the limitations in their thinking

   b. use illustrations to make point

   c. incorporate multiple choice tests

   d. emphasize cultural diversity of learners

   e. build the self-esteem of the learner

7. According to the National Health Standards, a health-literate person is:

    a. a critical thinker

    b. a responsible citizen

    c. an effective communicator

    d. a self-directed learner

    e. all of the above

8. Constructivist theory implies that health educators would do the following:

    a. keep knowledge to themselves

    b. teach only content

    c. teach only process

    d. educators will do more than teach content

    e. none of the above

9. Which of the following is suggested as a helpful technique for probing what learners know and understand about health-related topics, issues, and problems?

    a. use of Internet

    b. pop quizzes

    c. use of questioning techniques and writing narratives

    d. asking learner to write down what he or she knows

    e. none of the above

10. A suggestion for teaching for understanding included all of the following EXCEPT:

    a. focus on the developmental needs of learner

    b. focus on background of learner

    c. focus on learners interests

    d. focus on learner outcomes

    e. focus on how a learner feels

# CHAPTER 12: THE PARADIGM SHIFT TOWARD TEACHING FOR THINKING: PERSPECTIVES, BARRIERS, SOLUTIONS, AND ACCOUNTABILITY (KEYSER & BROADBEAR)

1. The primary focus of this article is to:

   a. serve as the definitive resource for literature irrelevant to critical thinking

   b. serve as a resource of all known literature on critical thinking

   c. highlight all educational literature relevant to critical thinking

   d. highlight past and recent educational literature most relevant to critical thinking

   e. none of the above

2. The historical roots of critical thinking is thought to originate in ancient Greece with the teachings of the following:

   a. Socrates, Plato, and Aristotle

   b. Socrates, Aristotle, and Titus

   c. Socrates, Plato, and Archimedes

   d. Socrates, Plato, and Caesar

   e. Socrates, Caligula, and Zeus

3. The term "critical thinking" emphasized the skills of

   a. analysis, argument, and psychology

   b. analysis, judgment, and argument

   c. analysis, argument, and thinking

   d. analysis, psychology, and judgment

   e. none of the above

4. Barriers often cited for impeding teachers being able to shift toward teaching for thinking include all but the following:

   a. large class sizes

   b. faculty reward systems

   c. time and effort required

   d. small class sizes

   e. teaching to the test

5. One of the solutions to overcoming barriers to include more critical thinking in classroom lessons include:

    a. provide training to teachers

    b. forget about critical thinking

    c. increase number of students in class

    d. test students utilizing standardized tests

    e. require rote memorization of facts

6. The National Health Education Standards were intended to reform health education by emphasizing:

    a. essential knowledge and skills that teachers need to teach content

    b. essential knowledge and skills that students need to be healthy

    c. essential skills needed to be physically fit

    d. essential information on current health issues

    e. none of the above

7. There are several sets of "standards" mentioned in this article. Which one is NOT mentioned?

    a. National Standards for Quality Teaching

    b. The Standards for Teacher Educators

    c. National Health Education Standards

    d. National Health Instructors Standards

    e. Opportunity to Learn Standards for Health Education

8. Health educators have several responsibilities specific to teaching thinking. These responsibilities include:

    a. structuring curriculum, instruction, and assessment to enable students to be critical thinkers

    b. frequent testing of students on factual information

    c. checking students note-taking ability

    d. developing class lectures

    e. none of the above

9. Who made the following statement: "The right incentives and a supportive environment encourage educators to attempt to make changes in teaching"?

    a. Meyers

    b. Steinberg

    c. Haas and Keeley

    d. Smoke and Flame

    e. Keyser and Broadbear

10. Meyers suggested that a child's natural sense of wonder and inquisitiveness can be held down as early as these years in school:

    a. preschool

    b. kindergarten

    c. middle grades in elementary school

    d. junior high

    e. high school

# CHAPTER 13: HISTORICAL STEPS IN THE DEVELOPMENT OF THE MODERN SCHOOL HEALTH PROGRAM (VESELAK)

1. According to Veselak, what is NOT a phase of the modern school health program?

    a. healthful school living

    b. health education

    c. physical education

    d. school health services

    e. none of the above

2. In what year was the first formal lunch program installed in New York City schools?

    a. 1901

    b. 1906

    c. 1908

    d. 1910

    e. 1912

3. The National School Lunch Act served a catalyst for the development of the following:

   a.  kitchens and cafeteria facilities and services in public schools

   b.  free lunch program

   c.  requirement of hairnets on staff

   d.  fish on Fridays

   e.  free dinner program

4. The first state to pass a law making physical education a requirement was

   a.  New York

   b.  Minnesota

   c.  North Dakota

   d.  Massachusetts

   e.  Rhode Island

5. Between 1880 and 1890 almost every state in the United States passed a law requiring the teaching of the following:

   a.  personal hygiene

   b.  effects of alcohol and narcotics

   c.  physiology

   d.  physical education

   e.  evolution

6. What year did the National Conference on Graduate Study in Health Education, Physical Education and Recreation established desirable graduate training and qualifications for teachers working in the public schools?

   a.  1946

   b.  1948

   c.  1950

   d.  1952

   e.  1958

7. In 1872, Elmira, NY, employed a "sanitary superintendent" to help with medical inspections in the schools due to a high prevalence of what disease?

   a.  influenza

   b.  smallpox

   c.  head lice

   d.  anthrax

   e.  malaria

8.  The term "health education" was coined by this organization:

    a.  American Red Cross

    b.  Conference on the Care of Dependent Children

    c.  Massachusetts Institute of Technology

    d.  Women's Christian Temperance Union

    e.  Child Health Organization

9.  In what year was Safety Instruction included in health education programs?

    a.  1925

    b.  1928

    c.  1935

    d.  1938

    e.  1945

10. A report entitled *Health Instruction in the Secondary Schools: An Inquiry into its Organization and Administration*, that identified the number of schools that required health education classes and determined which schools provided health services, was commonly called:

    a.  United States Report on School Health

    b.  Healthy Schools

    c.  Kilander's Report

    d.  Kirkpatrick's Report

    e.  Robinson's Report

## CHAPTER 14: PHILOSOPHY AND PRINCIPLES OF THE SCHOOL HEALTH PROGRAM (OBERTEUFFER)

1.  According to Oberteuffer, we can describe "good" health as:

    a.  muscle and mind

    b.  a state of physical well-being

    c.  a status

    d.  an expression of function of the total person

    e.  a quality of life

2. The basic considerations suggested in the article are:

   a.  who are we dealing with

   b.  what cooperative effort is needed

   c.  does the program fit the social philosophy

   d.  all of the above

   e.  none of the above

3. School health should be a cooperative effort from all of the following EXCEPT:

   a.  doctors

   b.  nurses

   c.  school administrators

   d.  teachers

   e.  scientists

4. In an effort to meet the needs of a community, school health education must not overlook the following:

   a.  the capacity for self direction and the will of the individual

   b.  the resources available in the community

   c.  the name of the community

   d.  the professional preparation of the health educator

   e.  the name of the school mascot

5. Oberteuffer states that health education is:

   a.  essentially an operation, a means of producing something

   b.  sex education

   c.  physical education

   d.  freedom from disease

   e.  teaching health content

6. Health is a descriptive word used to describe:

   a.  characteristics of a person

   b.  the degree to which the aggregate powers of an individual are able to function

   c.  how a person feels

   d.  a class that everyone must take

   e.  a personal value

7. Dr. Thomas Shaffer described his conception of how to judge the fitness of athletes for competition by:

   a. how high they were able to jump

   b. how tall the person was

   c. by selection of athletic activity

   d. a person's overall readiness for athletics

   e. level of personal fitness

8. According to Oberteuffer, boards of health and boards of education must learn to work together because:

   a. they are both held responsible by the public for everything that happens in the school

   b. they fund school lunch programs

   c. people expect the two to work together

   d. they both perform the same job

   e. they are concerned about the welfare of children

9. School health programs require many people to operate successfully including staff in the following categories:

   a. medical, educational, administrative, psychiatric, and janitorial

   b. medical, educational, nursing, administrative, and psychiatric

   c. medical, educational, nursing, janitorial, and administrative

   d. medical, educational, janitorial, psychiatric, and administrative

   e. medical, educational, psychiatric, administrative, and nutritional

10. Oberteuffer emphasizes the need to preserve the following values within a free society EXCEPT:

    a. independence

    b. freedom from indigency

    c. freedom from persecution

    d. make choices

    e. pay our own way

## CHAPTER 15: BEHAVIORAL HEALTH AND HEALTH EDUCATION: AN EMERGING OPPORTUNITY (FERTMAN)

1. The roots of the term behavioral health can be traced directly to:

    a. comprehensive school health

    b. managed health care

    c. holistic health

    d. psychoneuroimmunology

    e. epidemiology

2. In what setting do health educators NOT work:

    a. clinical care

    b. public health

    c. volunteer agencies

    d. private sector in business and consulting

    e. health educators work in all of the above settings

3. The _____ model suggests that health educators move beyond their own settings to bring their broad set of health education skills and expertise to bear on shaping what is behavioral health:

    a. health belief model

    b. precede-proceed model

    c. health education socio-ecological model

    d. model for health education planning

    e. comprehensive health education model

4. Fertman argues that money should be taken from treatment services to fund prevention programs:

    a. true

    b. false

5. The focus on population, assessing and monitoring health behaviors, designing, implementing, and evaluating programs best describes:

    a. school health

    b. spiritual health

    c. alternative health

    d. consumer health

    e. public health

6. What term does the author say is missing from the report of the 2000 Joint Committee on Health Education and Promotion:

   a. public health

   b. school health

   c. community health

   d. behavioral health

   e. comprehensive health

7. According to Fertman, public health runs on:

   a. local funding

   b. federal and state funds

   c. grant funding

   d. private donations

   e. self-generated funding

8. The private sector experience of behavioral health is very different from the public sector experience of behavioral health:

   a. true

   b. false

9. Fertman states that the primary mode of insuring Americans in the 21st century is:

   a. Medicare

   b. Medicaid

   c. HMOs

   d. Managed care

   e. PPOs

10. To a large degree, behavioral health continues to focus on individuals with severe:

    a. mental health and substance abuse illnesses

    b. mental health and respiratory illnesses

    c. cardiovascular disease and substance abuse illnesses

    d. obesity and diabetes

    e. mental health and vascular illnesses

## CHAPTER 16: HEALTHY BEHAVIOR: THE IMPLICATIONS OF A HOLISTIC PARADIGM OF THINKING THROUGH BODYMIND RESEARCH (READ & STOLL)

1.  Cognitive control of physiological systems has been proven through:

    a.  cause and effect research

    b.  content analysis research

    c.  biofeedback research

    d.  systems influence research

    e.  policy research

2.  The _____ is said to be a powerful and complex switchboard of the body-mind gestaltic processes:

    a.  heart

    b.  brain

    c.  lungs

    d.  liver

    e.  kidney

3.  The treatment option that showed the most improvement on children's behavior was:

    a.  removing milk

    b.  psychotherapy

    c.  exercise

    d.  vitamins

    e.  removing sugar

4.  Read and Stoll state that the present allopathic monopoly over heath-care thinking was due to the acceptance of the _____ by the U.S. Congress.

    a.  Storey Report

    b.  Flexner Report

    c.  Crawford Report

    d.  McClarin Report

    e.  Domingo Report

5. The single most important ingredient for health behavioral change is:

   a. a desire to change

   b. access to health care

   c. a positive mental outlook

   d. a good attitude

   e. a regular exercise program

6. According to Read and Stoll, developing an "internal locus of control" is the first, and absolutely essential, step toward the effectiveness of any approach to health education.

   a. true

   b. false

7. Related to nervous system manifestations of allergy-causing substances, mood changes are most impacted by:

   a. mold

   b. bacteria

   c. pollens and dust

   d. virus

   e. food

8. The _____ was known by many ancient disciplines to be the "house of God" where everything seemed to center.

   a. 3rd lumbar vertebrae

   b. 2nd cranial nerve

   c. 4th ventricle of the brain

   d. 3rd molar

   e. 1st chakra

9. The mapping of the "addresses" of each gene on all forty-six human chromosomes best describes:

   a. complementary medicine

   b. conventional medicine

   c. digital divide project

   d. human genome project

   e. service learning project

10. _____ is based on a system that examines the ways in which psychological processes are intertwined with both the nervous and immune system.

    a. nuclear medicine

    b. stem cell research

    c. cognitive analysis

    d. psychoneuroimmunology

    e. epidemiology

# CHAPTER 17: PROBLEM-BASED LEARNING: CATALYST FOR BEHAVIORAL CHANGE (GARMAN, TESKE & CRIDER)

1. The hypothesis of this study was that active curricular incorporation and use of problem-based learning methodologies would result in increased "readiness" for positive behavioral change.

    a. true

    b. false

2. Participants for this investigation were from the state of _____.

    a. Alabama

    b. New Jersey

    c. Pennsylvania

    d. Florida

    e. Ohio

3. This investigation focused on students initially positioned in what stage of behavior change?

    a. preparation and action

    b. precontemplation and contemplation

    c. action and maintenance

    d. contemplation and preparation

    e. precontemplation and action

4. Which of following teaching formats was NOT used in this study?

    a. lecture recitation

    b. interactive distance learning

    c. role play, brainstorming, and buzz groups

    d. problem-based learning

    e. all of the above teaching formats were used

5. The efficacy of multiple instructional strategies in promoting lifestyle modification was assessed over the course of a (an) _____-week academic semester.

   a. 8

   b. 10

   c. 12

   d. 15

   e. 18

6. The majority of participants in this study were:

   a. male

   b. female

   c. transgendered

7. In response to the question of what "lifestyle habit" have you changed in the past 6 months, the most frequent response was:

   a. physical activity patterns

   b. alcohol consumption habits

   c. activity patterns

   d. nutritional concerns

   e. sexual activity

8. The survey course used in this study was titled:

   a. personal health management

   b. stress management

   c. health for daily living

   d. health issues of college students

   e. health and fitness management

9. Comparatively, lecture recitation places a greater emphasis for learning on the student, has the instructor function as a facilitator rather than a provider of knowledge, and requires the student to develop and refine critical thinking, creative problem solving analytical skills and other desirable learning characteristics.

   a. true

   b. false

10. The transtheoretical model is also known as the:

    a. change of life model

    b. alternative behavior model

    c. health action model

    d. stage of change model

    e. health constructs model

# CHAPTER 18: HEALTH PROMOTION AND EMPOWERMENT: REFLECTIONS ON PROFESSIONAL PRACTICE (LABONTE)

1. This study examines ideas generated over _____ years of professional training workshops:

    a. 2

    b. 4

    c. 6

    d. 8

    e. 10

2. What geographic location was NOT included in this investigation:

    a. Canada

    b. United States

    c. New Zealand

    d. Australia

    e. all of the geographic locations above were included

3. The behavioral or risk factor approach to health tends to take a "power-over" approach to health concerns:

    a. true

    b. false

4. The number of community health practitioners involved with this study was:

    a. 2,500

    b. 3,500

    c. 5,000

    d. 8,000

    e. 10,000

5. Which of the following is NOT true for the concept of "power with":
   a. respects others views
   b. looks to the reality of lived experiences
   c. relies upon the reality of things
   d. tries to find common ground
   e. all of the above are true regarding the concept of "power with"

6. Labonte talks about three broad clusterings of named health problems corresponding to:
   a. knowledge, attitudes, and practices
   b. diseases, behaviors, and social conditions
   c. cognitive, affective, and psychomotor domains
   d. nominal, ordinal, and interval issues
   e. gender, age, and ethnicity factors

7. The empowerment holosphere consists of how many spheres:
   a. two
   b. three
   c. four
   d. five
   e. six

8. According to Labonte, how long does it take before a group may form from disconnected individuals:
   a. one to two days
   b. one to two weeks
   c. one to two months
   d. one to two years
   e. one to two decades

9. The Holosphere Model presumes that professions and bureaucratic institutions are capable of transformation:
   a. true
   b. false

10. _____ describes the process of organizing people around problems or issues that are larger than group members' own immediate concerns:

    a. community organizations

    b. coalition advocacy

    c. political action

    d. personal care

    e. none of the above

# CHAPTER 19: HEALTH EDUCATION AS FREEING (GREENBERG)

1. According to Greenberg, the goal of health education should be:

    a. specific behavioral changes

    b. acquisition of knowledge

    c. free people to make own health-related decisions

    d. political advocacy

    e. none of the above

2. Which of the following "enslaving factors" should health education eliminate so as to free people to make their own related decisions?

    a. feelings of inferiority and hostility

    b. poor self-esteem

    c. emotional distress

    d. alienation

    e. all of the above

3. According to the philosophy of freeing health education, health educators must not be concerned with the particular behaviors of their clients.

    a. true

    b. false

4. Health behavioral choices of clients should be consistent with:

    a. their values and needs

    b. educational knowledge

    c. CDC health recommendations

    d. educator's area of specialty

    e. family upbringing

5. For a health educator, the most important health area for the client to emphasize and improve would be:

   a. physical health

   b. mental health

   c. social health

   d. spiritual health

   e. none of the above

6. In the case of the overweight businessman who is an amateur gourmet cook, according to this philosophy, the health educator would advise him to:

   a. lose weight

   b. eat smaller portion sizes

   c. use less oil and sugar in his recipes

   d. do nothing

   e. eat more fruits and vegetables

7. Powerlessness is defined as lack of rules, regulations, and standards that one can choose to live by.

   a. true

   b. false

8. Areas that the health educator can help the client improve and should work on include:

   a. values clarification activities

   b. health knowledge

   c. health skills

   d. internal locus of control

   e. all of the above

9. When one evaluates the effectiveness of health education, the health educator should measure all of the following EXCEPT:

   a. health-related behaviors

   b. self-esteem

   c. locus of control

   d. health knowledge

   e. skills tests

10. Greenberg recommends that further research continue to explore this health education philosophy including all EXCEPT:

   a. relationship between enslaving factors and health-related behaviors

   b. effective means to sell freeing health education to various constituents

   c. association of knowledge and health-related behaviors

   d. development of valid, reliable instruments to measure enslaving factors

   e. development and testing of instructional strategies aimed at diminishing enslaving factors

## CHAPTER 20: DEMOCRACY: THE FIRST PRINCIPLE OF HEALTH PROMOTING SCHOOLS (ANDERSON & RONSON)

1. Healthy Cities and Healthy Schools are movements around the world that emphasize all of the following EXCEPT:

   a. health improvement in all areas of health

   b. collaboration

   c. partnerships at all levels

   d. health care sector

   e. all of the above

2. Roots in "Healthy School" programs require

   a. vending machine regulations

   b. physical activity supervision

   c. democracy, active learning principles

   d. cafeteria worker training

   e. health education preparation

3. The greatest advance in health policy achieves as the result of scientific conceptions of health is:

   a. vaccinations

   b. clean air and water

   c. traffic death reduction

   d. universal health care in many countries

   e. all of the above

4. The underlying concept of health promotion is that in order to achieve good health, a person must have some measure of control over the decisions and conditions they encounter.

    a. true

    b. false

5. Principles listed as fundamental to the WHO Health Promoting Schools framework are all of the following EXCEPT:

    a. equity

    b. health services

    c. democracy

    d. teacher development

    e. community development

6. According to Fenstermacher, content only becomes knowledge when the learner:

    a. demonstrates content competency with certain score attainment

    b. acquires written skill coherence

    c. applies the information to real world problems

    d. plans for future academic engagement

    e. all of the above

7. Components of democracy can be inclusive of all of the following concepts EXCEPT:

    a. polling stations

    b. respect of alternative views and realities

    c. actively pursuing meaning from multiple texts

    d. a way of belonging

    e. contribution of the betterment of society

8. Giroux proposed that politics and pedagogy are inseparable because content or knowledge is not neutral.

    a. true

    b. false

9. Weare believes that four components exercised in the right proportion make up a health promoting school. Which of the following is NOT one of these components?

    a. participation that includes empowerment

    b. good relationships between pupils, staff, teachers

    c. people know what is expected of them and what they can expect of others

    d. students learn to think for themselves and work independently

    e. adherence to nationally set guidelines

10. In the example of a class examining the possible outcomes of a nation converting to a diet rich in fresh fruit and vegetables, under people considerations, one might look at:

    a. school district policy for vending machines.

    b. school policy for cafeteria menus

    c. food resources available via public health

    d. an understanding of sustainable development

    e. food and agriculture policies

# CHAPTER 21: HUMAN ECOLOGY AND HEALTH EDUCATION (HOYMAN)

1. The unitive view of man as a self-regulating, self-actualizing organism is a fundamental principle of:

    a. modern ecology

    b. human ecology

    c. biotic community

    d. biosphere

    e. none of the above

2. An ecological model of health and disease include all of the following EXCEPT:

    a. hereditary factors

    b. precontemplative factors

    c. environmental factors

    d. personal factors

    e. ecological factors

3. The ecological-epidemiologic approach to disease etiology and cures focuses on:

   a.  biologic containment

   b.  individual containment

   c.  prevention and control

   d.  pharmaceutical development

   e.  all of the above

4. Phenotype is determined by:

   a.  interaction of genotype and environment

   b.  genes a person inherits from his/her parents

   c.  congenital abnormalities

   d.  chromosomal disorders

   e.  none of the above

5. Components to improving Health Science curricula would be all of the following EXCEPT:

   a.  included in grades K–12

   b.  flexible scope and sequence

   c.  spiral learning progression

   d.  include evaluation as integral part of planning

   e.  all of the above

6. According to Hoyman, man is the dominant but endangered species on Earth.

   a.  true

   b.  false

7. Issues that impact both human ecology and health education are all EXCEPT:

   a.  wellness vs. optimum health

   b.  quantity vs. quality of life

   c.  prevention and control vs. eradication of disease

   d.  universal health care vs. market-driven health care

   e.  family planning vs. population control

8. A recommendation by Hoyman to improve teacher preparation is to provide to Juniors a required field course in community health education.

   a. true

   b. false

9. Health from an ecological perspective considers the whole multidimensional person in an dynamic ecological process.

   a. true

   b. false

10. Examples of functional health teaching that Hoyman discussed included all EXCEPT:

    a. population control

    b. sedentary lifestyle

    c. disease control

    d. cigarette smoking

    e. premarital sex

# CHAPTER 22: SPIRITUAL WELLNESS, HOLISTIC HEALTH, AND THE PRACTICE OF HEALTH EDUCATION (HAWKS)

1. According to Hawks, what often fails to harmonize with the multidimensional, dynamic, and functional nature of health?

   a. medical practices

   b. current practice of health education

   c. insurance reimbursements

   d. teacher preparation

   e. all of the above

2. To improve the likelihood of successful outcomes to the attainment of health education objectives, Hawks suggests all of the following EXCEPT:

   a. reviewing definitions and goals of the profession

   b. consider philosophical inconsistencies

   c. a unified code of ethics for the profession

   d. outline a foundational role for spiritual health in health education

   e. all of the above

3. Although health educators espouse the belief that health education is multidimensional, the primary outcome that is measured is:

   a. physical well-being

   b. spiritual wellness

   c. self-esteem

   d. locus of control

   e. levels of stress

4. According to Hawks, the health education profession as inherited a preoccupation with which dimension of health?

   a. physical

   b. emotional

   c. environmental

   d. social

   e. spiritual

5. Most individuals are motivated to change health behaviors when they see a vital connection to the behavior and life longevity.

   a. true

   b. false

6. Which goal does Hawks contend is unreachable in health education?

   a. increasing health knowledge

   b. behavior change

   c. decision-making skills

   d. political advocacy

   e. social empowerment

7. Health education practice is limited as the result of:

   a. inability to measure physical health

   b. ever-changing definition of health

   c. vast public health system

   d. limited health care options

   e. inconsistency of practice and philosophy

8.  To make each dimension of health as a legitimate outcome goal for health education, Hawks suggests all of the following EXCEPT:

    a.  clearly defined

    b.  operationalized

    c.  compartmentalized

    d.  development of valid, reliable instruments to measure

    e.  all of the above

9.  An acceptable definition of spiritual health is a commitment to a worldview that provides personal clarity to understanding the purpose of life and one's place in it.

    a.  true

    b.  false

10. Which of the following is a definition for emotional health?

    a.  ability to experience and express human feelings

    b.  quality of relationships

    c.  satisfaction in one's social roles

    d.  sense of belonging

    e.  feelings of love and acceptance

# CHAPTER 23: NEW HEALTH PROMOTION MOVEMENT: A CRITICAL EXAMINATION (ROBERTSON & MINKLER)

1.  Prominent features to the new health promotion movement include all of the following EXCEPT:

    a.  community participation in identifying health problems

    b.  going beyond individual emphasis of health problems

    c.  equating being ill with being guilty of unhealthy lifestyles

    d.  include social and economic determinants of health

    e.  understanding empowerment as key health promotion strategy

2. Which of the following factors should health education professions focus on when working on health promotion as defined by this new movement:

   a. micro-level change

   b. individual life-style changes

   c. professional ownership

   d. public ownership

   e. all of the above

3. When one sees health as a means, the goal of health promotion should be social justice.

   a. true

   b. false

4. Organizations that serve as mediating structures when trying to improve health include all EXCEPT:

   a. medical clinics

   b. neighborhood organizations

   c. churches

   d. voluntary organizations

   e. schools

5. The separation between individuals and their health may be problematic due to:

   a. the cost of maintaining physical health

   b. the access to affordable health care

   c. individual's influence on their social health

   d. importance of spiritual health

   e. minimizes everyday reality of a person's life

6. To increase community competence the health education professional must be willing to do all of the following EXCEPT:

   a. provide access to information

   b. use medical experts to propose health solutions

   c. support indigenous community leadership

   d. assist the community in overcoming bureaucratic obstacles

   e. increase community's ability to problem solve

7. Empowerment is the notion that one has the ability to control the factors that determine health in a community.

   a. true

   b. false

8. According to McKnight, which of the following features are NOT characteristic of community?

   a. emphasis on capacity of its members

   b. an informality

   c. recognized deficiency among its members

   d. a reliance on common history

   e. incorporation of celebration, tragedy, and fallibility

9. Within the context of the new health promotion movement, when a health education professional frames a health problem within the context of the individual level, it cannot be considered empowering.

   a. true

   b. false

10. Which of the following attributes would NOT describe community participation?

    a. social process

    b. defined geographic area

    c. pursuit of identifying needs

    d. establishment of mechanisms to meet needs

    e. free or cheaper forms of service delivery

## CHAPTER 24: POTENTIAL UNTAPPED: HEALTH EDUCATION AND HEALTH PROMOTION AS A MEANS TO PEACE (LEVITON)

1. Leviton defined the term "horrendous death" as:

   a. resulting from terrorism

   b. resulting from war

   c. people-caused preventable deaths

   d. all of the above

   e. none of the above

2. Peace was defined as:

   a. an absence of war

   b. living in social harmony

   c. enhanced health and well-being of people

   d. enhanced health and well-being of the planet

   e. all of the above

3. Horrendous death is a threat to the quality of individual and global health. Leviton identifies two types of horrendous death differentiated by all of the following characteristics EXCEPT:

   a. intention to kill

   b. racism

   c. accidental death

   d. misuse of tobacco

   e. global travel

4. Thanatology is defined by Kastenbaum as the study of life ending in death and is characterized by all of the following themes EXCEPT:

   a. causation

   b. denial

   c. grief

   d. expectations for the future

   e. motivator for action

5. Increased awareness of horrendous death might positively impact health educators' view of health and their perceived role as a professional.

   a. true

   b. false

6. Lifegenic factors increase the probability of living long and well and include:

   a. meaningful education

   b. meaningful employment

   c. financial security

   d. purpose and meaning in life

   e. all of the above

7. To date, the approach of the U.S. government in developing policies concerning horrendous death can be characterized by all of the following descriptors EXCEPT:

   a. fragmented

   b. driven by a need for retribution

   c. focused on homicide

   d. focused on crisis management

   e. focused on terrorism or war

8. According to Leviton, Quality of Global Health (QGH) is defined as having a maximum of lifegenic factors and a minimum of or absence of horrendous death occurrences.

   a. true

   b. false

9. This article identifies several root causes for acts of horrendous death including:

   a. poverty

   b. hunger

   c. illiteracy

   d. totalitarianism

   e. all of the above

10. Health Education and Health Promotion have assets that can be applied effectively to prevent horrendous death and promote peace including all of the following EXCEPT:

    a. grounded in the scientific method

    b. concern for the health and well-being of people

    c. prevention-oriented

    d. finance-driven

    e. education-based

# CHAPTER 25: PUTTING POLITICS BACK IN PUBLIC HEALTH EDUCATION (COULTER, ALLBRECHT, GULITZ, FIGG, & MAHAN)

1.  The model proposed by Coulter, Allbrecht, Gulitz, Figg, and Mahan would ensure that students have sound academic and practical preparation for legislative advocacy should include all of the following components EXCEPT:

    a.  communication skills

    b.  issues preparation

    c.  research-based training

    d.  political environment exposure

    e.  application of newly acquired skills / knowledge (mock hearing)

2.  Issues preparation includes what learning objective?

    a.  select issues with an individual health impact

    b.  articulate values underlying political positions

    c.  defend policy using value-laden beliefs

    d.  work with business partners

    e.  all of the above

3.  Identifying topics of significant public health concerns means to select issues from a community-based perspective.

    a.  true

    b.  false

4.  Legislators concerned with passing laws with a parochial interest, are more concerned with issues that impact:

    a.  national concerns

    b.  regional interests

    c.  churches

    d.  other concerned legislators

    e.  all of the above

5.  An example of an area of significant public health concern may be:

    a.  mental health legislation

    b.  universal health care legislation

    c.  health insurance policy

    d.  maternal and child health policy

    e.  all of the above

6. Elements of the Toulmin Argumentation Model that are helpful to students with persuasive strategies include all of the following EXCEPT:

   a. identifying the constituent groups

   b. offering persuasive and disarming counter arguments

   c. inoculate the audience by anticipating possible objections

   d. forming possible rebuttals to the claim

   e. none of the above

7. When interpreting data for its relevance to practice, statistical significance is equal to clinical (or practical) significance.

   a. true

   b. false

8. Which of the following is NOT a test for determining the quality and quantity of evidence:

   a. is the source objective and competent?

   b. is the information correct?

   c. are as many sources as possible used?

   d. does the information appeal to the masses?

   e. is the information verifiable?

9. The students found the personnel of the mock panel rude.

   a. true

   b. false

10. Outcomes of this teaching activity included:

    a. students not making an adjustment from a paper presentation to addressing a legislative panel

    b. students' understanding of panel interaction

    c. students' lack of preparation for panel presentation

    d. none of the above

    e. all of the above

# CHAPTER 26: HEALTH CARE REFORM: INSIGHTS FOR HEALTH EDUCATORS (O'ROURKE)

1. Health educators are not affected by the health care reform debate because of their roles as:

   a. experts in medical care

   b. health professionals

   c. citizens

   d. tax payers

   e. consumers of service

2. Success of framing a policy debate includes all of the following EXCEPT:

   a. the focus of the debate

   b. the possible outcomes

   c. paradigm shift

   d. the eventual outcome

   e. all of the above

3. Medical care is synonymous with health care.

   a. true

   b. false

4. Increasing medical care expenditures, to improve health, is usually seen in all areas EXCEPT:

   a. infrastructure

   b. size of medical care

   c. quality of the workforce

   d. paying more for services

   e. utilization review

5. In the 1979 Surgeon General's Report, U.S. mortality is due to:

   a. 40% unhealthy behavior, 30% environmental factors, 20% human biology, 10% health care

   b. 30% unhealthy behavior, 30% environmental factors, 20% human biology, 20% health care

   c. 10% unhealthy behavior, 20% environmental factors, 20% human biology, 50% health care

   d. 50% unhealthy behavior, 20% environmental factors, 20% human biology, 10% health care

   e. none of the above

6. To control medical costs, one could do all of the following EXCEPT:

   a. controlling costs

   b. reducing administrative waste

   c. expand insurance coverage

   d. utilization review

   e. none of the above

7. Countries that spend more on medical care report better health indicators for their population.

   a. true

   b. false

8. Which of the following is NOT a focus for medical care?

   a. quality of life

   b. begins with the sick

   c. seeks to keep the sick alive

   d. make the sick well

   e. minimize disabilities

9. There is a positive relationship between medical care and health.

   a. true

   b. false

10. According to Sigerist, which of the following would NOT be a way to promote health?

    a. provide a decent standard of living

    b. provide universal access to medical care

    c. provide good labor conditions

    d. provide education

    e. provide a means of rest and relaxation

# CHAPTER 27: THE ROLE OF HEALTH EDUCATION ASSOCIATIONS IN ADVOCACY (AULD & DIXON-TERRY)

1. The organization and operation of a 501(c)(3) organization can include all of the following purposes EXCEPT:

    a. promotion of social welfare

    b. charitable or religious purposes

    c. education or safety purposes

    d. prevention of cruelty to children or animals

    e. private foundation

2. Tax–exempt designations that are common among health groups include:

    a. 501(c)(3)

    b. 501(c)(4)

    c. 501(c)(6)

    d. a and c

    e. all of the above

3. 501(c)(6) are not limited in their endorsement of political candidates.

    a. true

    b. false

4. The definition of a lobbying contact is:

    a. a person paid by another to make lobbying contacts

    b. an oral or written communication with members of Congress regarding federal legislation

    c. any lobbying contacts with person covered under the Lobbying Disclosure Act

    d. lobby activities

    e. none of the above

5. Which of the following staffing issues would affect the amount of political activity for an organization?

   a. amounts of funds committed to advocacy

   b. having a satellite office in Washington, DC

   c. employing lobbyist(s) to maintain ongoing contacts with policymakers

   d. developing a communication plan with Congress

   e. all of the above

6. Which of the following is NOT listed as a purpose of the Coalition of National Health Education Organizations (CNHEO):

   a. facilitate national level coordination among member organizations

   b. elect a lead organization for Health Education

   c. provide a forum to identify and discuss health education issues

   d. take action on issues affecting members' interest

   e. serve as a resource for external agencies

7. "Health Education in the 21st Century" identifies advocacy as one of the four critical areas for improving graduate education in the next millennium.

   a. true

   b. false

8. Which of the following is NOT an example of political issue that CNHEO has addressed on behalf of the health education profession?

   a. reproductive health legislation

   b. tobacco legislation

   c. Healthy People 2010

   d. identifying health educators as part of the SOC used by DLC

   e. none of the above

9. The Health Education Advocacy Summits provide health education organizations the opportunity to come together to develop common advocacy agenda and to collectively advocate for these issues on Capitol Hill.

   a. true

   b. false

10. According to Auld and Dixon-Terry, which of the following is NOT one of the challenges ahead for health organizations in the twenty-first century?

    a. sustained presence on Capitol Hill

    b. broaden annual political objectives to be more inclusive

    c. expand ways of effectively mobilizing memberships

    d. advocate for funds to expand research base of health education discipline

    e. make a long-term commitment to advocacy

# CHAPTER 28: THE ROLE OF HEALTH EDUCATION ADVOCACY IN REMOVING DISPARITIES IN HEALTH CARE (ALLEGRANTE, MORISKY, & SHARIF)

1. In Healthy People 2010, all the following areas called for a reduction in health disparities EXCEPT:

    a. infant mortality

    b. cardiovascular disease

    c. tuberculosis

    d. diabetes

    e. HIV/ AIDS

2. Health disparities have become increasingly more evident for all of the following groups EXCEPT:

    a. women

    b. people with low income

    c. people with disabilities

    d. elderly

    e. white-collar workers

3. Disparities between minorities and the white population have increased in the last decade on virtually every measure of health.

    a. true

    b. false

4. African-Americans find better access and treatment in which of the following health care services:

    a. emergency room services

    b. organ transplantation

    c. total joint replacement

    d. treatment of chest pain

    e. none of the above

5. Socioeconomic factors that influence health status include:

    a. education

    b. income

    c. occupation

    d. all of the above

    e. none of the above

6. All of the following have a strong predictive factor in disease prevention EXCEPT:

    a. satisfying jobs

    b. governmental jobs

    c. decent housing

    d. good schools

    e. regular leisure activities

7. Perceived systematic discrimination may play an important role in low health status among people of color.

    a. true

    b. false

8. The least powerful constituencies in health care are:

    a. health education professionals

    b. physicians

    c. hospitals

    d. insurance companies

    e. pharmaceutical industries

9. The purpose of media advocacy is to inform legislative members of Congress on pertinent health education issues.

    a. true

    b. false

10. Which of the following is NOT listed as an advocacy effort concerning HIV/AIDS?

    a. inform the public about the risk

    b. foster public support for prevention programs in schools

    c. pharmaceutical development for treatment options

    d. develop consortium approaches to delivery of HIV services

    e. develop community-based HIV prevention programs

# CHAPTER 29: LESSONS FROM DEVELOPING COUNTRIES: HEALTH EDUCATION IN THE GLOBAL VILLAGE (PINZON-PEREZ)

1. The primary goal of this article is to:

    a. emphasize need for cross-cultural interaction between countries

    b. encourage understanding of impact of Internet on the global village

    c. share lessons learned from international health education experience

    d. describe health care systems around the world

    e. discuss global and multicultural health issues

2. Immigration issues have become a major concern for health care systems in industrialized nations.

    a. true

    b. false

3. Pinzon-Perez indicates that the number of foreign-born residents has reached the highest level in U.S. history. How many immigrants are in the United States?

    a. 11 million

    b. 24 million

    c. 28 million

    d. 31 million

    e. 44 million

4. Pinzon-Perez suggests that Maslow's hierarchy of human needs should be applied to help health educators better understand the priorities of others in the global village. Which need is NOT part of the theory?

    a. physiological and safety

    b. belongingness and love

    c. esteem

    d. physical fitness

    e. self-actualization

5. Kofi Annan is quoted as saying "today's real borders are not between nations, but between _____."

    a. powerful and powerless

    b. free and fettered

    c. privileged and humiliated

    d. all of the above

    e. none of the above

6. Pinzon-Perez uses the term "relative poverty." Which statement best reflects her meaning?

    a. Poverty is a major concern, especially for immigrants.

    b. Better economic conditions lessen the effects of poverty.

    c. Improved living conditions lessen the effects of poverty.

    d. Better educational opportunities lessen the effects of poverty.

    e. Even with a "sense of improvement," immigrants may not experience equity.

7. Environmental health is a core global issue and includes all of the following concerns EXCEPT:

    a. global pollution

    b. industrial contamination

    c. lack of drinkable water

    d. sewage disposal

    e. global warming

8. Cross, Bazron, Dennis, and Isaacs created a cultural proficiency model encompassing the following steps. Which category is NOT a step on the ladder?

   a.  cultural destructiveness

   b.  cultural incapacity

   c.  cultural blindness

   d.  cultural deafness

   e.  cultural competence

9. In this commentary, Pinzon-Perez calls for health educators to achieve a state of advanced cultural competence characterized by attitudes that value differences and actions that demonstrate respect for diverse populations.

   a.  true

   b.  false

10. Pinzon-Perez calls for health educators to fight discrimination in a number of ways. Which methods does she support?

   a.  educating children

   b.  promoting cultural competence

   c.  advocating for social justice

   d.  teaching respect for others

   e.  all of the aboveAppendix E: Ches Questions

# REFERENCES

Allegrante, J. P., Morisky, D. E., & Sharif, B. A. (1999). The role of health education advocacy in removing disparities in Health Education. *The Health Education Monograph, 17*(2), 1–9.

American Association of Health Education. (2005). Philosophy of health education: A position statement of the American Association of Health Education (AAHE). Retrieved from http://www.aahperd.org/aahe/pdf_files/pos_pap/Philosophy.pdf.

American Association of Health Education. (2008). Health literacy: A position statement of the American Association of Health Education (AAHE). Retrieved from http://www.aahperd.org/aahe/pdf_files/pos_pap/HealthLiteracy.pdf.

Anderson, A., & Ronson, B. (2005). Democracy—The first principle of health promoting schools. *International Electronic Journal of Health Education, 8*, 24–35.

Auld, E., & Dixon-Terry, E. (1999). The role of health education associations in advocacy. *Health Education Monograph, 17*(2), 10–14.

Bensley, L. B. (1993). This I believe: A philosophy of health education. *Eta Sigma Gamma Monograph Series, 11*(1), 1–7.

Beyrer, M. K., & Nolte, A. E. (Eds.). (1993). Reflections: The philosophies of health educators of the 1990s. *Eta Sigma Gamma Monograph Series, 11*(2), 1–118.

Black, J. M. (2006). Approaches and resources for examining the history of health education. *Health Education Monograph Series, 23*(1), 1–6.

Blomquist, K. B. (1986). Modeling and health behavior: Strategies for prevention in the schools. *Health Education, 17*(3), 8–11.

Brennan, A. J., & Galli, N. (1985). Health educators: Role modeling and smoking behavior. *Journal of Drug Education, 15*(4), 343–352.

Carroll, C. R. (1993). Some guiding principles on health and health education: A philosophical statement. *Eta Sigma Gamma Monograph Series, 11*(2), 17–25.

Clark, N. M. (1994). Health educators and the future: Lead, follow or get out of the way. *Journal of Health Education, 25*(3), 136–141.

Coalition of National Health Education Organizations. (1999). *Code of ethics for the health education profession.* Retrieved from http://www.cnheo.org/code2.pdf.

Coulter, M. L., Allbrecht, T., Guliotz, E., Figg, M., & Mahan, C. (1999). Putting politics back in public health education. *Journal of Health Education, 30*(6), 372–374.

Creswell, W. H., & Newman, I. M. (1989). *School health practice* (9th ed.). St Louis, MO: Times Mirror/Mosby College.

Fertman, C. I. (2002). Behavioral health and health education: An emerging opportunity. *American Journal of Health Education, 33*(2), 115–117.

Garman, J. F., Teske, C. J., & Crider, D. A. (2001). Problem-based learning: Catalyst for behavioral change. *International Electronic Journal of Health Education, 4*(1), 74–80.

Green, L. W., Kreuter. M. W., Deeds, S. G., & Partridge, K. B. (1980). *Health education planning: A diagnostic approach.* Palo Alto, CA: Mayfield.

Greenberg, J. S. (1978). Health education as freeing. *Health Education, 9*(2), 20–21.

Hawks, S. (2004). Spiritual wellness, holistic health, and the practice of health education. *American Journal of Health Education, 35*(1), 11–16.

Hoyman, H. S. (1971). Human ecology and health education. *Journal of School Health, 41*(10), 538–547.

Joint Committee on National Health Education Standards. (1995). *National health education standards: Achieving health literacy.* Atlanta, GA: American Cancer Society.

Keyser, B. B., & Broadbear, J. T. (1999). The paradigm shift toward teaching for thinking: Perspectives, barriers, solutions and accountability. *International Electronic Journal of Health Education, 2*(3), 111–117.

King, K. (1982). Selected behavioral strategies for the health educator. *Health Education, 13*(3), 35–37.

Kolbe, L. J. (1982). What can we expect from school health education? *Journal of School Health, 52*(3), 145–150.

Labonte, R. (1994). Health promotion and empowerment: Reflections on professional practice. *Health Education Quarterly, 21*(2), 253–268.

Landwer, G. E. (1981). Where do you want to go? *Journal of School Health, 51*(8), 529–531.

Leviton, D. (2002). Potential untapped: Health education and health promotion as a means to peace. *International Electronic Journal of Health Education, 1*, 12–26.

Nolte, A. (1976). The relevance of Abraham Maslow's work to health education. *Health Education, 7*(3), 25–27.

Oberteuffer, D. (2001). Philosophy and principles of the school health program. *Journal of School Health, 71*(8), 373–375.

O'Rourke, T. (2002). Health care reform: Insights for health educators. *American Journal of Health Education, 33*(5), 297–300.

*Oxford dictionary of current English* (4th ed.). (2006). New York: Oxford University Press.

Paul, R. W. (1984). Critical thinking: Fundamental to education for a free society. *Educational Leadership, 42*(1), 4–14.

Pigg, R. M. (1993). Three essential questions in defining a personal philosophy. *Eta Sigma Gamma Monograph Series, 11*(2), 94–101.

Pinzon-Perez, H. (2003). Lessons from developing countries: Health education in the global village. *American Journal of Health Education, 34*(2), 101–103.

Rash, J. K. (1985). Philosophical bases for health education. *Health Education, 16*(2), 48–49.

Read, D., & Stoll, W. (1998). Healthy behavior: Implications of a holistic paradigm of thinking through body-mind research. *International Electronic Journal of Health Education, 1*, 2–18.

Robertson, A., & Minkler, M. (1994). New health promotion movement: A critical examination. *Health Education Quarterly, 21*(3), 295–312.

Russell, R. D. (1975). *Health education.* Washington, DC: National Education Association.

Russell, R. D. (1983). Is behavior change a legitimate objective for the health educator? *Health Education, 14*(2), 16–19.

Smith, B. J. (2006). Connecting a personal philosophy of health to the practice of health education. *Health Education Monograph Series, 23*(1), 11–13.

Tappe, M. K., & Galer-Unti, R. A. (2001). Health educator's role in promoting health literacy and advocacy for the 21st century. *Journal of School Health, 71*(10), 477–482.

Thomas, S. B. (1984). The holistic philosophy and perspective of selected health educators. *Health Education, 15*(1), 16–20.

Timmreck, T. C., Cole, G. E., James, G., & Butterworth, D. D. (1988). Health education and health promotion: A look at the jungle of supportive fields, philosophies and theoretical foundations. *Health Education, 18*(6), 23–28.

Ubbes, V. A., Black, J. M., & Ausherman, J. A. (1999). Teaching for understanding in health education: The role of critical and creative thinking skills within constructivism theory. *Journal of Health Education, 30*(2), 67–73, 135.

Veselak, K. (2001). Historical steps in the development of the modern school health program, *Journal of School Health*, *71*(8), 369–372.

Welle, H. M., Russell, R. D., & Kittleson, M. J. (1995). Philosophical trends in health education: Implications for the 21st century. *Journal of Health Education*, *26*(6), 326–332.

Willgoose, C. E. (1985, October). *Health education as a basic*. Reston, VA: Association for the Advancement of Health Education, 1–8.

# INDEX